Atlas of
Early Lung
Cancer

ATLAS OF EARLY LUNG CANCER

National Cancer Institute
National Institutes of Health
U.S. Department of Health
and Human Services

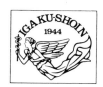

IGAKU-SHOIN
New York • Tokyo

Published and distributed by

IGAKU-SHOIN Ltd.,
5-24-3 Hongo, Bunkyo-ku, Tokyo

IGAKU-SHOIN Medical Publishers, Inc.,
1140 Avenue of the Americas,
New York, N.Y. 10036

This work was supported in part by
National Institutes of Health contracts:
NO 1-CN-45037, NO 1-CN-45007, and
NO 1-CB-53886.

Library of Congress Cataloging in Publication Data
Main entry under title:

Atlas of early lung cancer.

   Includes index.
   Contents: Introduction / Nathaniel I. Berlin —
Anatomy and histology / Myron R. Melamed, Muhammad
B. Zaman, Nael Martini — Staging of lung cancer /
Nael Martini . . . et al. — [etc.]
   1. Lungs—Cancer—Atlases. I. National Cancer
Institute (U.S.) [DNLM: 1. Lung neoplasms—Atlases.
WF 17 A862]
RC280.L8A84 1983   616.99'424075   82-23278
ISBN: 0-89640-078-6

Printed and bound in Japan
10 9 8 7 6 5 4 3 2 1

Contributors

National Cancer Institute

Nathaniel I. Berlin, M.D., Ph.D.
Former Director, Division of Cancer
Biology and Diagnosis[*1]

Johns Hopkins University School of Medicine

Wilmot C. Ball, Jr., M.D.
Associate Professor of Medicine

Darryl Carter, M.D.
Former Associate Professor
of Pathology[*2]

Yener S. Erozan, M.D.
Associate Professor of Pathology

John K. Frost, M.D.
Professor of Pathology
Director, Division of Cytopathology

Prabodh K. Gupta, M.D.
Associate Professor of Pathology

Bernard R. Marsh, M.D.
Associate Professor of Laryngology
and Otology
Director, Broyles Bronchoscopic
Clinic

Frederick P. Stitik, M.D.
Clinical Associate Professor
of Radiology[*3]

Mayo Clinic and Mayo Foundation

David T. Carr, M.D.
Former Consultant, Division of
Thoracic Diseases and Internal
Medicine, and Former Consultant
Division of Medical Oncology[*4]

Robert S. Fontana, M.D.
Consultant, Division of Thoracic
Diseases and Internal Medicine

W. Eugene Miller, M.D.
Consultant, Department of Diagnostic
Radiology

John R. Muhm, M.D.
Consultant, Department of Diagnostic
Radiology

David R. Sanderson, M.D.
Chairman, Division of Thoracic
Diseases and Internal Medicine

Lewis B. Woolner, M.D.
Senior Consultant, Department of
Surgical Pathology

Memorial Sloan–Kettering Cancer Center

Nael Martini, M.D.
Chief of Thoracic Surgery

Myron R. Melamed, M.D.
Chairman, Department of Pathology

Muhammad Zaman, M.D.
Assistant Attending Pathologist,
Cytology Service

[*1] Currently Director, Northwestern
University Cancer Center

[*2] Currently Professor of Pathology, Yale
University School of Medicine

[*3] And Professor of Radiology, Eastern
Virginia School of Medicine

[*4] Currently Head, Section of Pulmonary
Medicine, M.D. Anderson Hospital and
Tumor Institute of the University of Texas,
Houston

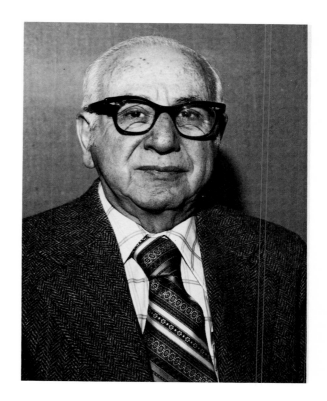

In memory of a great man:
**William Pomerance, M.D.
(1906-1978)**

*The great man does not think
beforehand of his words, that they
may be sincere, nor of his actions,
that they may be resolute — he
simply speaks and does what
is right.*

Mencius

Preface

"Now this is not the end. It is not even the beginning of the end. But it is, perhaps, the end of the beginning."

These words, spoken by Winston Churchill at the height of World War II, could be applied today to the nation's war against cancer. They aptly reflect the current status of the ongoing studies of the Cooperative Early Lung Cancer Group of the National Cancer Institute and account for the format of this publication. There is no final summary or concluding section. Such is not possible at this time, when information is incomplete and methodology is undergoing continuous refinement. Numerous comments and opinions are expressed throughout the text, and these have been made as explicit as possible. The contributors assume full responsibility for any controversial statements.

This is an atlas, and emphasis has appropriately been placed on graphic demonstration. There are few references, because the material presented is largely new. Many treatises have been written on the subject of lung cancer, and the National Cancer Institute has already published a **Manual of Procedures** detailing the techniques utilized by the Cooperative Early Lung Cancer Group in its investigations.

The atlas has been organized into a series of concise, integrated sections. Certain illustrations appear in more than one section, to eliminate the need to refer to other pages.

The introduction describes the formation of the Cooperative Group and the design of its research programs. The sections on anatomy and staging define the structures from which lung cancers arise and the basis for assessing size, extent, and histologic appearance. The two established methods of detecting early lung cancer are presented. The cytopathology section illustrates the spectrum of cellular abnormalities observed in the sputum of patients who have established cancers, evolving cancers, and benign conditions that may mimic cancer. The sections on bronchoscopy and pathology depict the features of radiographically inapparent ("occult") bronchogenic carcinoma detected cytologically. The radiology section portrays the various radiographic manifestations of early lung cancer together with associated pathologic findings. Finally, there are a number of case presentations selected to demonstrate important clinical aspects and problems.

Work on this volume was initiated by Dr. Nathaniel Berlin, when he was Director of the Division of Cancer Biology and Diagnosis of the National Cancer Institute. It was completed under the guidance of his successor, Dr. Alan Rabson, and Dr. William Pomerance, late Chief of the Division's Diagnosis Branch.

This has been a collaborative endeavor. It would not have been accomplished without the help of present and former colleagues, both medical and paramedical, at the National Cancer Institute and at the Johns Hopkins Medical Institutions, the Mayo Clinic, and the Memorial Sloan-Kettering Cancer Center. Space does not permit individual citation, but to borrow from Churchill again, "From the highest to the humblest...all are of equal honor; all have had their part to play."

Final editing was conducted at Mayo. Special acknowledgment should be made of the contributions of Dr. Werner Heidel of the Section of Publications, Mr. Robert C. Benassi of the Section of Medical Graphics, Mr. James S. Martin of the Section of Photography, and their associates at that institution.

The Contributors

Contents

ATLAS OF EARLY LUNG CANCER

INTRODUCTION

Nathaniel I. Berlin, M.D., Ph.D.

The number of people who die from lung cancer continues to increase. Cigarette smoking has been identified as the major, but not the sole, cause of lung cancer. Total cigarette sales are still rising, although there has been some decline in cigarette smoking by middle-aged and older men and a significant decline in smoking by physicians. Less than 10% of patients with lung cancer are "cured" of their disease, that is, are alive 5 years after confirmation of the diagnosis. Since prevention of lung cancer is possible, but has thus far been a disappointment, and since cure by surgery, radiation, or drugs is currently infrequent, there remains at present only the possibility that "early" diagnosis might reduce mortality.

To test this hypothesis a "Cooperative Early Lung Cancer Group" was established. The origin of this group can be traced back to the middle 1960's, when the Diagnosis Research Branch of the National Cancer Institute (NCI) was transferred to the office of the Clinical Director, and I first came to know Dr. John Frost of the Department of Pathology of the Johns Hopkins University. At that time, the NCI was supporting a multi-institutional study of circulating tumor cells. As that investigation was drawing to a close, Dr. Frost suggested that the skills of cytopathology might be applied to the diagnosis of lung cancer, in a manner similar to their utilization for diagnosis of cancer of the uterine cervix.

Coincidentally, Dr. Lawrence Tuttle, then at the National Institute for Environmental Health Sciences, called to my attention a remarkable motion picture produced by Dr. Shigeto Ikeda, a Japanese physician interested in lung cancer. Dr. Ikeda's film presented a detailed account of the development and use of a flexible fiberoptic bronchoscope.

Dr. Ikeda was subsequently invited to the United States, at which time he discussed with physicians of the NCI and the Johns Hopkins University staff the technical aspects and clinical applications of his fiberoptic bronchoscope. He also arranged for the Johns Hopkins staff to obtain one of these instruments.

Dr. Frost began to assemble a team that developed a multidisciplinary approach to the diagnosis of lung cancer. The group included Dr. Wilmot Ball, a chest physician, Dr. Bernard Marsh, an otolaryngologist and bronchoscopist, Dr. Frederick Stitik, a diagnostic radiologist, Dr. R. Robinson Baker, a thoracic surgeon, Dr. Yener Erozan, a cytopathologist, and Dr. Morton Levin, an eminent epidemiologist, who was responsible for the earliest studies relating cigarette smoking to lung cancer.

Dr. Frost and his colleagues developed both short- and long-range plans. The short-range plan was directed toward improving methodology. The long-range plan called for application of the new methodology to a randomized controlled clinical program for detecting and localizing "early" lung cancer. These plans were submitted to the NCI as an unsolicited contract proposal. The Frost protocol was reviewed by a site visit team and by the Diagnosis Research Committee. It was funded in 1969 and is now known as the "Johns Hopkins Lung Project."

In 1970, the Mayo Clinic, with Dr. Robert Fontana as principal investigator, submitted a proposal for a long-term, controlled evaluation of lung cancer screening. This program, designated the "Mayo Lung Project," was funded the following year. The Mayo program utilized much of the methodologic base developed at Johns Hopkins.

In 1973, the Memorial-Sloan Kettering Cancer Center, with Dr. Myron Melamed as principal investigator, became the third member of the group. The Memorial protocol, entitled the "National Lung Program," was similar to the Johns Hopkins long-term clinical program for lung cancer detection. Preliminary plans were developed for a fourth institution to join the group, but this did not come about. A statistical coordination center was developed at the University of Cincinnati, under the direction of Dr. C. Ralph Buncher, to provide the essential data management and analysis support for this project.

The reasons for having first two and later three institutions in the group were to provide an increased number of persons to be screened, to test comparability of data and reproducibility of observations, and, as a consequence, to obtain earlier results and increased statistical reliability of the results. This has been achieved in part. Each institution has now screened approximately 10,000 male cigarette smokers more than 45 years old.

The screening program at Mayo differs slightly from those at Johns Hopkins and Memorial. However, at all three institutions the subjects have been randomized into two groups—a close surveillance study group and a comparison or "control" group, which is examined less frequently. Lung cancers detected on the first screening have been designated "prevalence" cancers, whereas those detected on subsequent screenings have been termed "incidence" cancers.

At Mayo, all candidates received a chest x-ray and a sputum cytology examination when first seen. Those persons who have been randomized into the "close surveillance" study group are rescreened radiologically and cytologically every 4 months. The comparison or "control" group has been advised to have an annual chest x-ray examination and sputum test.

At Johns Hopkins and at Memorial, the "close surveillance" study group receives a chest x-ray annually and a sputum cytology examination every 4 months. The comparison or "control" group receives a yearly chest x-ray only.

The populations at the three institutions also differ slightly. At Mayo, those who are being screened are male Mayo Clinic outpatients without a history or suspicion of respiratory tract cancer. At Johns Hopkins and Memorial, those undergoing screening have been recruited from the population at large by a variety of techniques.

When Mayo became the second institution in the cooperative group, frequent joint meetings were begun for the purpose of exchanging information. Joint meetings have continued. Today, the "Cooperative Early Lung Cancer Group" is organized into an Executive Committee as well as committees on statistics, radiology, pathology, bronchoscopy, surgery, patient management, and mortality. A **Manual of Procedures** has been developed which describes the methodology in detail. This **Atlas** is designed as companion to the **Manual of Procedures**.

Historically, it has long been known that cytologic examination of specimens of sputum could detect some lung cancers, sometimes years before the tumor became obvious radiographically. The rigid, or open-tube, bronchoscope and its telescopes did not permit a sufficiently extensive examination of the bronchi, especially those in the upper lobes, to identify the cancer.

It was not until Drs. Ikeda and Marsh, using Ikeda's fiberoptic bronchoscope, demonstrated the ability to localize radiographically "occult" tumors among patients who had cancer cells in their sputum that screening for lung cancer acquired a new dimension. Previous attempts to reduce the mortality from lung cancer by screening, either by x-rays or by x-rays and cytology, only pointed out the need for more study.

The "Cooperative Early Lung Cancer Group" investigations have now reached the point where it is possible to describe the characteristics of "early" lung cancer as seen in a screening program. The value of cytologic examination of the sputum, radiologic examination of the lungs, and fiberoptic bronchoscopy is being carefully assessed. A sufficient number of cancers have been diagnosed, both at the first and at subsequent screenings, to provide the basis for describing the full range of abnormal cells in the sputum, the radiologic spectrum of "early" lung cancer, and the "early" bronchoscopic appearance. A sufficient number of cancers have been surgically resected and the pathologic specimens examined in detail to allow definition of the histopathologic characteristics of "early" lung cancer.

This **Atlas** describes the multiple manifestations of "early" lung cancer and provides representative examples and case histories. The precise value of cytologic and radiologic screening for lung cancer has not yet been determined with reference to reduction of mortality from lung cancer. However, it has been demonstrated that if diligently searched for in a "high-risk" population (men more than 45 years old who are smoking one pack of cigarettes or more per day), small lung cancers can be found. Moreover, if this "high-risk" group is rescreened at regular intervals, lung cancer will be found at a predictable rate.

That the work has advanced as rapidly as it has is due to the collaborative efforts of the "Johns Hopkins Lung Project," the "Mayo Lung Project," and the "National Lung Program." The three members of the "Cooperative Early Lung Cancer Group" have been working together effectively—sharing data, techniques, and experience. These three institutions have brought together in this **Atlas** what is now known about "early" lung cancer.

Section 1

ANATOMY AND HISTOLOGY

Myron R. Melamed, M.D.

Muhammad B. Zaman, M.D.

Nael Martini, M.D.

There are certain aspects of the anatomy and histology of the lung which are particularly important in the diagnosis and management of early lung cancer. These include the segmental anatomy of the bronchi and lungs, the nature of the epithelia that line the air passages, and the distribution of the lymphatics and lymph nodes that drain the lungs. This review is intended to emphasize those features and to serve as a point of reference for comparison with the descriptions of cytology and pathology of early lung cancer that follow.

1

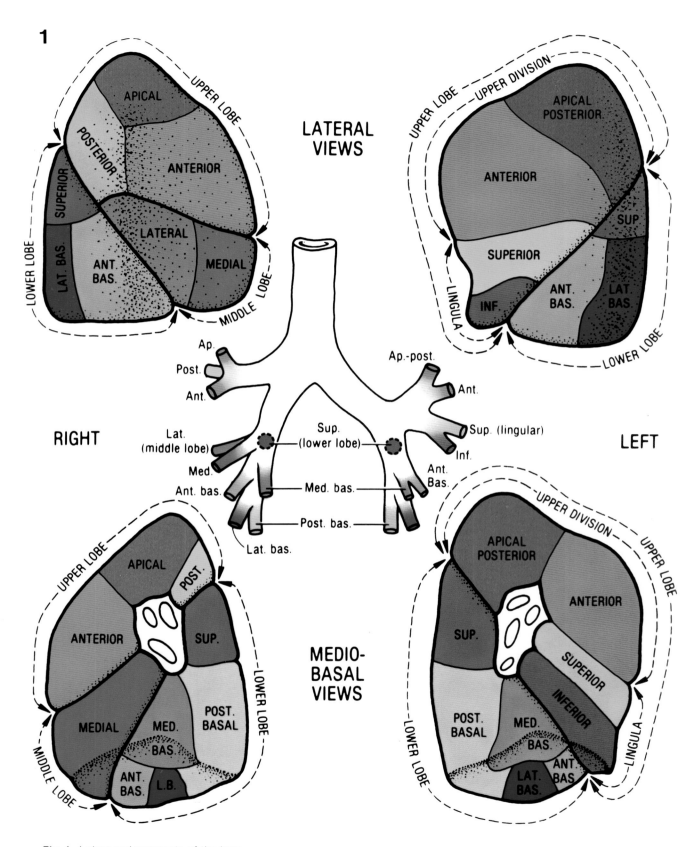

Fig. 1. Lobes and segments of the lung.

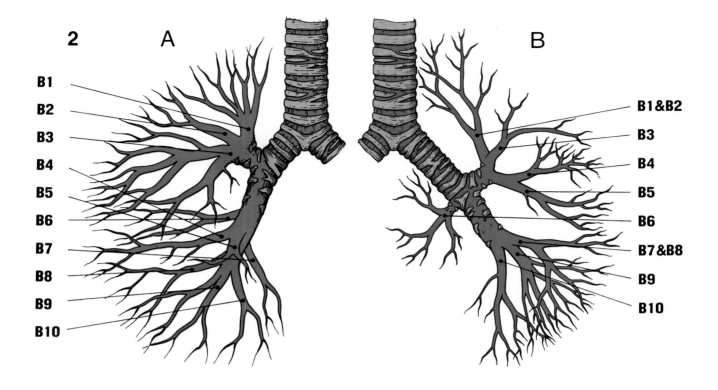

2   **A**   **B**

B1
B2
B3
B4
B5
B6
B7
B8
B9
B10

B1 & B2
B3
B4
B5
B6
B7 & B8
B9
B10

Fig. 2. Lobar and segmental bronchi of right (**A**) and left (**B**) lungs. The name corresponding to the number of each segmental bronchus is as follows:

Right Lung

Upper lobe	B1 - Apical
	B2 - Posterior
	B3 - Anterior
Middle lobe	B4 - Lateral
	B5 - Medial
Lower lobe	B6 - Superior
	B7 - Medial basal
	B8 - Anterior basal
	B9 - Lateral basal
	B10 - Posterior basal

Left Lung

Upper lobe	B1 & 2 - Apical-posterior
	B3 - Anterior
Lingula	B4 - Superior
	B5 - Inferior
Lower lobe	B6 - Superior
	B7 & 8 - Anteromedial basal
	B9 - Lateral basal
	B10 - Posterior basal

Bronchopulmonary Anatomy

The lungs are paired organs that lie within the thorax and that function by exchanging dissolved gases in the blood with respired air. The exchange of gases takes place in alveolar spaces within the lung parenchyma, and these spaces communicate, via the branching tracheobronchial tree, with the upper airway passages. Each of the bronchial branches with its corresponding segment of pulmonary parenchyma constitutes an independent unit.

The trachea extends from the larynx in the neck into the chest, where it bifurcates into right and left main-stem bronchi at the level of the fourth thoracic intervertebral disk. The two main-stem (first generation) bronchi continue to the hilar regions of the right and left lungs and divide there into lobar (second generation) bronchi.

The right lung is partially separated by fissures into upper, middle, and lower lobes, and the left lung is divided into an upper and a lower lobe. Each lobe is supplied by a single lobar bronchus.

The lobes are subdivided into anatomic segments, each of which is supplied by its own segmental (third generation) bronchus.

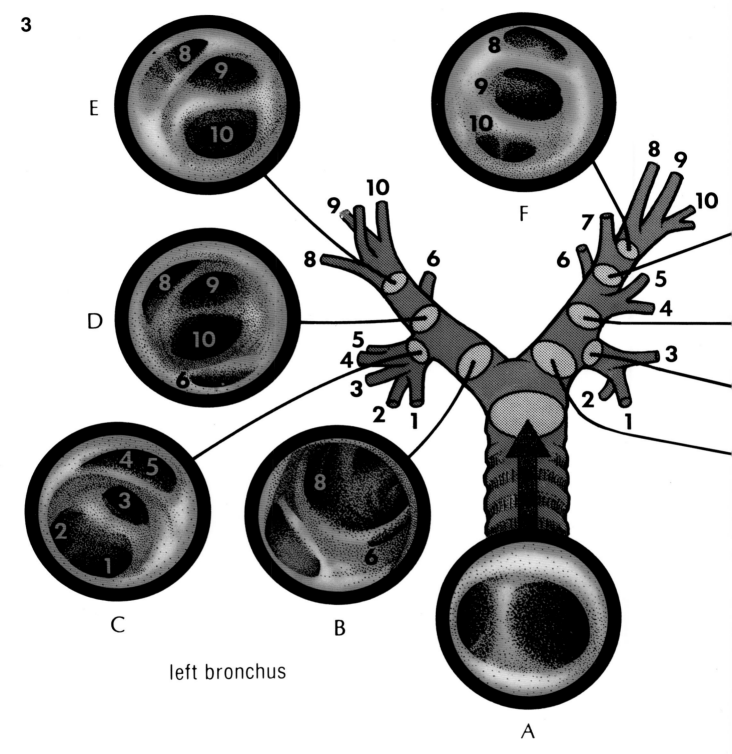

3

left bronchus

Fig. 3. Schematic representation of the orifices of the various segmental bronchi shown in Figure 2 as they would be observed bronchoscopically. The large arrow indicates both the direction of insertion of the bronchoscope and the direction of the bronchoscopic view. The position of the bronchoscope is indicated by the ovals placed in the bronchial tree for each view. A = tracheal bifurcation; B = main-stem bronchus; C = upper-lobe bronchus; D = intermediate bronchus (**right**), lower-lobe bronchus (**left**); E = bronchi to basilar segments, lower lobes; F = bronchi to anterior (8), lateral (9), and posterior (10) basilar segments, right lower lobe.

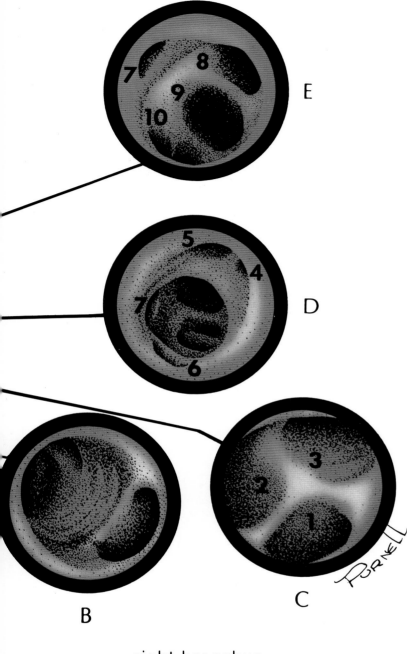

right bronchus

There are 10 bronchopulmonary segments on the right and 8 on the left.

The lobes and segments of the lungs are shown diagrammatically in Figure 1. The corresponding lobar and segmental bronchi are illustrated schematically in Figure 2 **A** and **B** for the right and left lungs, respectively. Each pulmonary segment is identified by a name according to its position within the lobe, and the bronchial branch to each segment (the segmental bronchus) is given the same name or, more recently, is numbered according to an international nomenclature. For the sake of symmetry in numbering right and left sides, the apical-posterior bronchus of the left upper lobe is numbered LB1 & 2, and the anteromedial basal segment of the left lower lobe is numbered LB7 & 8. This is the nomenclature that we have adopted, and it is utilized throughout this atlas.

With the advent of fiberoptic bronchoscopy, it has become possible to visualize fourth-, fifth-, and sometimes sixth-generation bronchial branches. Endoscopic anatomy is now of considerable practical importance, and techniques have been devised to teach this anatomy by using glass or plastic models. Figure 3 is a schematic representation of the segmental bronchial orifices as visualized during a bronchoscopic examination.

The segmental bronchi divide into progressively smaller branches within each segment of the lung. The very small peripheral branches, which measure 1 mm or less in diameter, are called bronchioles. They terminate in respiratory bronchioles and ducts that communicate with the alveoli.

The lungs are normally expanded with air, and they completely fill the thoracic cavity on each side. They are attached only by structures at the hilus, including the pulmonary and bronchial blood vessels, lymphatics, nerves, and supporting connective tissue. The outer surface of the lung, like the inner surface of the thoracic cavity, is covered by a thin, smooth pleural membrane whose lining consists of a single layer of mesothelial cells. Opposing pleural surfaces on the lung (visceral) and chest wall (parietal) are moist; this serves to lessen friction during respiration and helps to keep the lungs fully expanded by the surface tension between visceral and parietal pleura. Fibrous adhesions between lung and chest wall are common, and they may develop after any inflammatory process involving lung or pleura.

The pulmonary and bronchial vessels divide and follow the segmental distribution of the bronchi after entering the hilus of the lung.

Histology

The trachea is a semirigid tube that is kept open by a series of about 20 C-shaped rings. The open end of each ring is directed posteriorly. The rings continue along both main-stem bronchi and into their lobar branches. Rigid support is less necessary for the intrapulmonic bronchi; thus, the cartilaginous plates within walls of the segmental bronchi are incomplete, and they

become reduced progressively and are irregularly distributed in succeeding bronchial branches. At the same time, the muscularis, which is incomplete in the trachea and the main-stem bronchi, becomes progressively more prominent, and it completely encircles small bronchi and their branches. Bronchioles less than 1 mm in diameter have no cartilage at all.

Mucous and serous glands are numerous in the mucosa all along the respiratory tract, from the nose and mouth to the bronchioles. In the tracheobronchial tree, the glands lie both outside and within the muscularis, with ducts extending to the bronchial lumen. Distally, as the bronchioles lose their cartilage, the glands also are lost.

The mouth, oropharynx, and hypopharynx are lined by stratified squamous epithelium, and exfoliated squamous cells from these surfaces are normally present in sputum (Fig. 4). For the most part, this is nonkeratinizing epithelium, but at sites of trauma, such as on the hard palate and gingiva, the epithelium does keratinize. Chronic irritation from smoking or ill-fitting dentures can also cause keratinization of buccal mucosa or palate, where the thickened epithelium may develop a white appearance (leukoplakia).

Trachea and Bronchi.—The respiratory mucosa that lines the trachea and bronchi is normally composed of at least four and probably five principal cell types: namely, basal or reserve cells, intermediate cells, goblet cells, ciliated columnar cells, and nonciliated columnar cells (Fig. 5).

4

Fig. 4. Histologic section of stratified squamous epithelium in the pharynx. Most of the mucosa is nonkeratinizing, but some keratinization does occur over bony prominences or on the edge of the tongue; chronic irritation will cause an increase in keratinization. Cells desquamated from these surfaces are normally present in cough specimens of sputum.

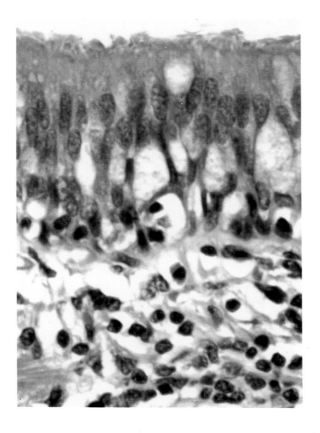

Fig. 5. Normal respiratory mucosa lining trachea and bronchial branches. Lying immediately on the basement membrane is a single, interrupted layer of small, rounded, basal or reserve cells with very dark nuclei and scanty cytoplasm. Above these are a layer of cell nuclei that are larger and more vesicular, representing intermediate cells that are derived from the basal cell layer and are partially differentiated. Overlying them are the fully differentiated, ciliated columnar cells with occasional interspersed mucus-containing goblet cells. The luminal surface of the ciliated columnar cells has a dark-staining terminal bar (basal bodies by electron microscopy, see Figure 7) to which the cilia attach. The bronchial epithelium is tightly coherent and exfoliates only after vigorous cough or with trauma such as endoscopy. The few small round cells within clear spaces in the basal layers of epithelium are lymphocytes (see also Figure 6). Note the incomplete smooth muscle layer in the bronchial wall underlying the epithelium.

Basal cells are ovoid or polygonal small cells that measure about 10 to 12 μm in diameter. They rest directly on the basement membrane, wedged between the attenuated basal cytoplasm of other cell types. Basal cells have irregularly round or ovoid nuclei, often with a nucleolus, and they are undifferentiated—that is, cytoplasm is scanty and specialized cytoplasmic organelles are few (Fig. 6). Like basal epithelial cells of other mucous membranes, they proliferate and differentiate to form the other cell types.

Intermediate cells, which are similar to the basal cells and are derived from them, may be found just above the basal cell layer. They are slightly larger and have somewhat more abundant cytoplasm. These cells are also capable of differentiating into and replacing ciliated columnar or mucus-secreting cells (Fig. 6).

Ciliated columnar cells normally account for about 85% of the tall columnar epithelial cells. They are attached to the basement membrane and extend the full thickness of the epithelium. The nuclei are oval, only slightly larger than nuclei of basal cells, and usually located near the middle of the cells or toward the basal end. The cytoplasm is very often tapered at the basal end of the cell to accommodate the interspersed basal epithelial cells. On its free surface there is a thick terminal bar to which the cilia attach. In good preparations, the terminal bar can be seen as a row of granules, probably corresponding to the basal bodies of the cilia at their attachment in the cytoplasmic border and to intervening short microvilli (Fig. 7). There are variable numbers of lysosomes in the cytoplasm of ciliated cells, and these may sometimes be visible by light microscopy as darkly staining cytoplasmic granules.

6

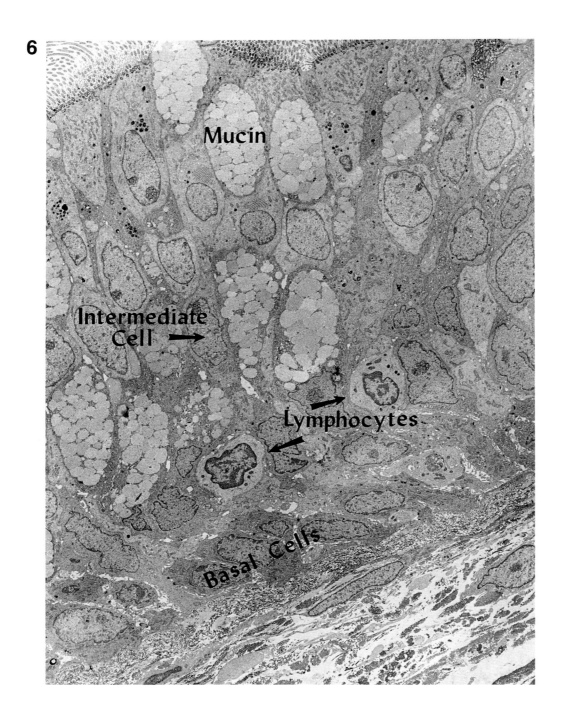

Mucin

Intermediate
Cell ➔

Lymphocytes

Basal Cells

Fig. 6. Electron micrograph of somewhat hyperplastic
bronchial mucosa, showing a layer of polygonal basal
cells lying on the basement membrane, slightly larger
intermediate cells in a more superficial position, and
ciliated columnar and mucus-filled goblet cells lining
the lumen. There are two lymphocytes within the basal
cell layer. (x2,240.)

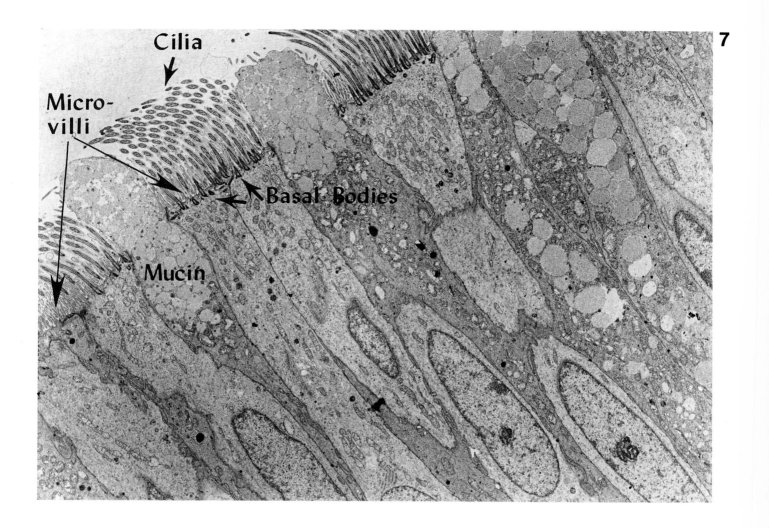

7

Fig. 7. Electron micrograph of the luminal surface of the bronchus. The cilia can be seen attaching to a linear array of basal bodies within the cytoplasm just beneath the free surface of the columnar cells. Microvilli are interspersed among the cilia and are not related to the basal bodies. Together, the basal bodies and the microvilli appear by light microscopy as a terminal bar. Cytoplasmic droplets of mucin in the goblet cells accumulate on the luminal side of the nucleus and are extruded into the bronchus, as shown here. (x4,320.)

8

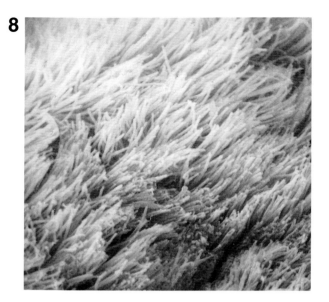

Fig. 8. Scanning electron micrograph of the normal bronchial mucosal surface, showing "shag rug" appearance of cilia. (x2,500.)

9

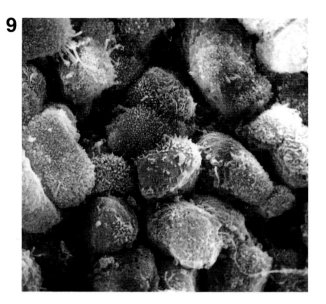

Fig. 9. Scanning electron micrograph of the bronchial surface of a squamous cell carcinoma. The cells are rounded and loosely arranged, and they have lost their cilia. Microvilli can be seen but are variable in size and distribution. It is easy to see why these loosely coherent cells are desquamated by the force of a cough. (x2,200.)

Scanning electron micrographs provide a striking view of the cilia covering the mucosal surface of a normal bronchus (Fig. 8). This differs dramatically from the bronchial surface of carcinoma, in which the cells have lost their cilia and are loosely and irregularly arranged (Fig. 9).

Nonciliated columnar cells are fewer than cells of the other types. They have surface microvilli rather than cilia, with a brushlike free border as seen by light microscopy. It is not known whether these cells have a specialized function or whether they represent a transitional stage in the formation of ciliated cells. Mature ciliated columnar cells have microvilli as well as cilia (Fig. 7).

Mucous or goblet cells normally make up about 15% of the columnar epithelial cells. They are tapered at the base to accommodate the interspersed basal epithelial cells and distended above by pale-staining mucus—hence the shape that gave them the name "goblet." They have round nuclei, which are usually located toward the base of the cell below the mucus droplet. In electron micrographs, the cytoplasmic mucus is composed of multiple droplets that coalesce as they near the free surface of the cell (Fig. 7). A well-developed stack of folded membranes and vesicles—the Golgi apparatus—is present just above the nucleus and is believed to be the site of formation and concentration of the mucus secretory product.

Bronchioles.—The smaller bronchial branches, or bronchioles, lose the goblet cells in their epithelium as they lose the cartilaginous plates and glands in their wall. Nonciliated cuboidal cells gradually replace the ciliated columnar cells (Fig. 10). In very small bronchioles, there are bulging, nonciliated cells with apical cytoplasmic granules that stain with toluidine blue or the periodic acid-Schiff reaction (Fig. 11 and 12). These are called Clara cells and are of unknown function, although it has been suggested that they may play a role in producing surfactant.

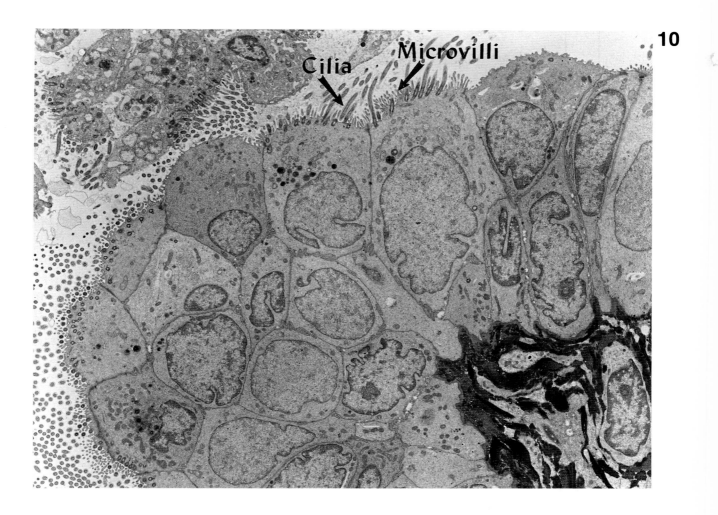

10

Cilia   Microvilli

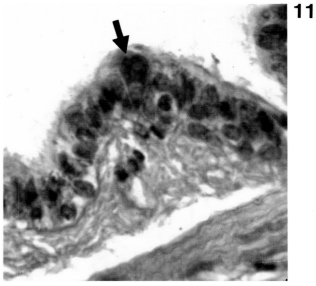

11

Fig. 10. Electron micrograph of epithelium from a bronchiole. Nonciliated cuboidal cells are replacing the ciliated columnar epithelium. The epithelium here is slightly hyperplastic. (x3,840.)

Fig. 11. A small bronchiole with a single Clara cell (**arrow**) stained by the periodic acid-Schiff reaction to show red-staining secretory granules in the apical cytoplasm.

12

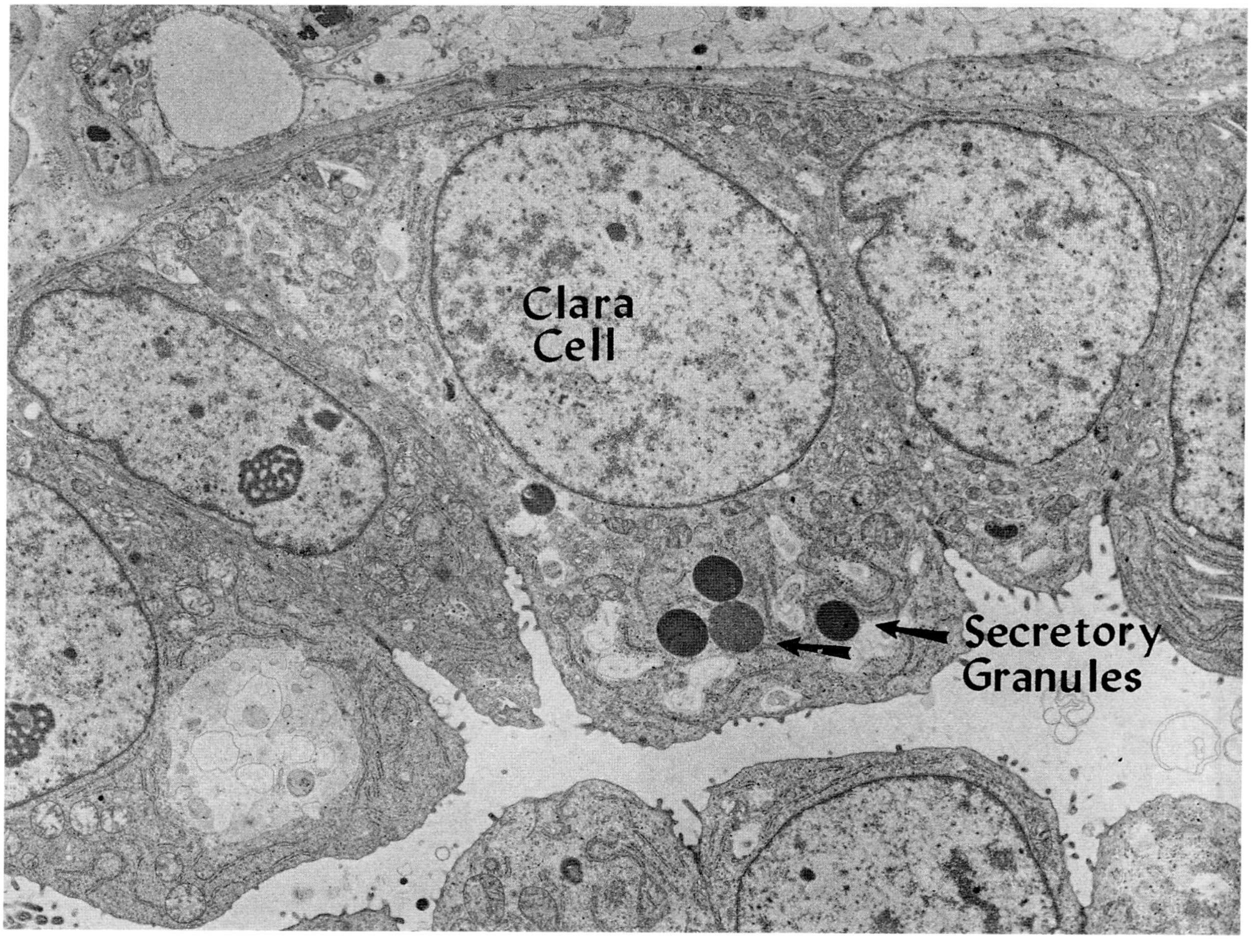

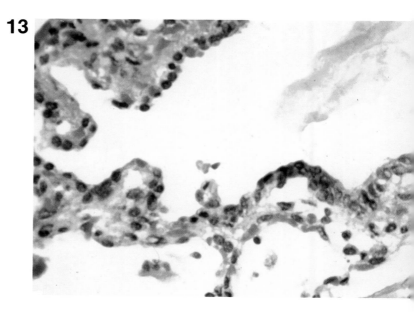

Clara
Cell

Secretory
Granules

Fig. 12. A terminal bronchiolar adenocarcinoma showing one of the tumor cells differentiated into a Clara cell and containing cytoplasmic secretory granules. (x5,940.)

13

Fig. 13. A terminal bronchiole in continuity with a respiratory bronchiole and alveolar duct. Note the progression from low-cuboidal, nonciliated epithelium, to very flattened epithelium in the alveolar duct. (x140.)

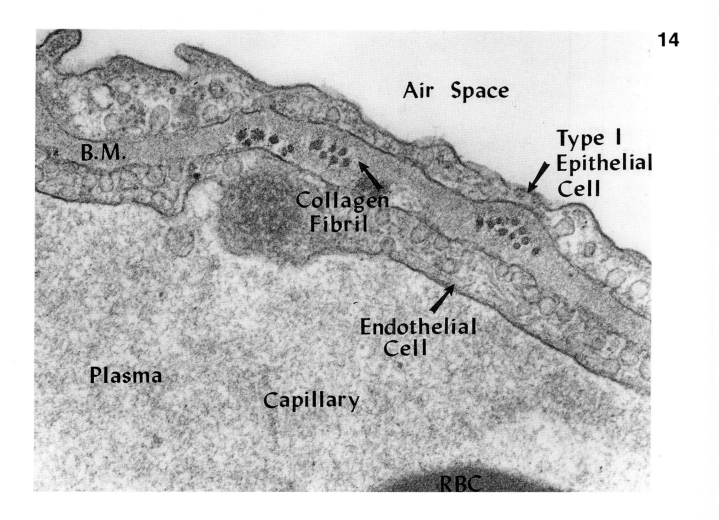

Fig. 14. Alveolar wall and capillary showing a flattened, membranous (type I) pneumocyte lining the alveolar surface on one side and an endothelial cell lining a capillary on the opposite side; between is a slightly thickened basement membrane (**B.M.**) with collagen fibrils. (x64,000.)

Terminal bronchioles continue into one or several respiratory bronchioles, which each divide into two or more alveolar ducts that then open into alveolar sacs and alveoli (Fig. 13). The respiratory bronchioles measure 0.5 mm or less in diameter and are lined by nonciliated cuboidal epithelium with some residual ciliated epithelium.

The alveoli are lined by thinned-out epithelial cells called type I, or membranous, pneumocytes, which resemble endothelial cells (Fig. 14). A few, more prominent cells, called type II, or granular, pneumocytes, also line the alveolar surface, and these are thought to help form surfactant. They have numerous cytoplasmic inclusions that are responsible for the granular appearance (Fig. 15 and 16).

15

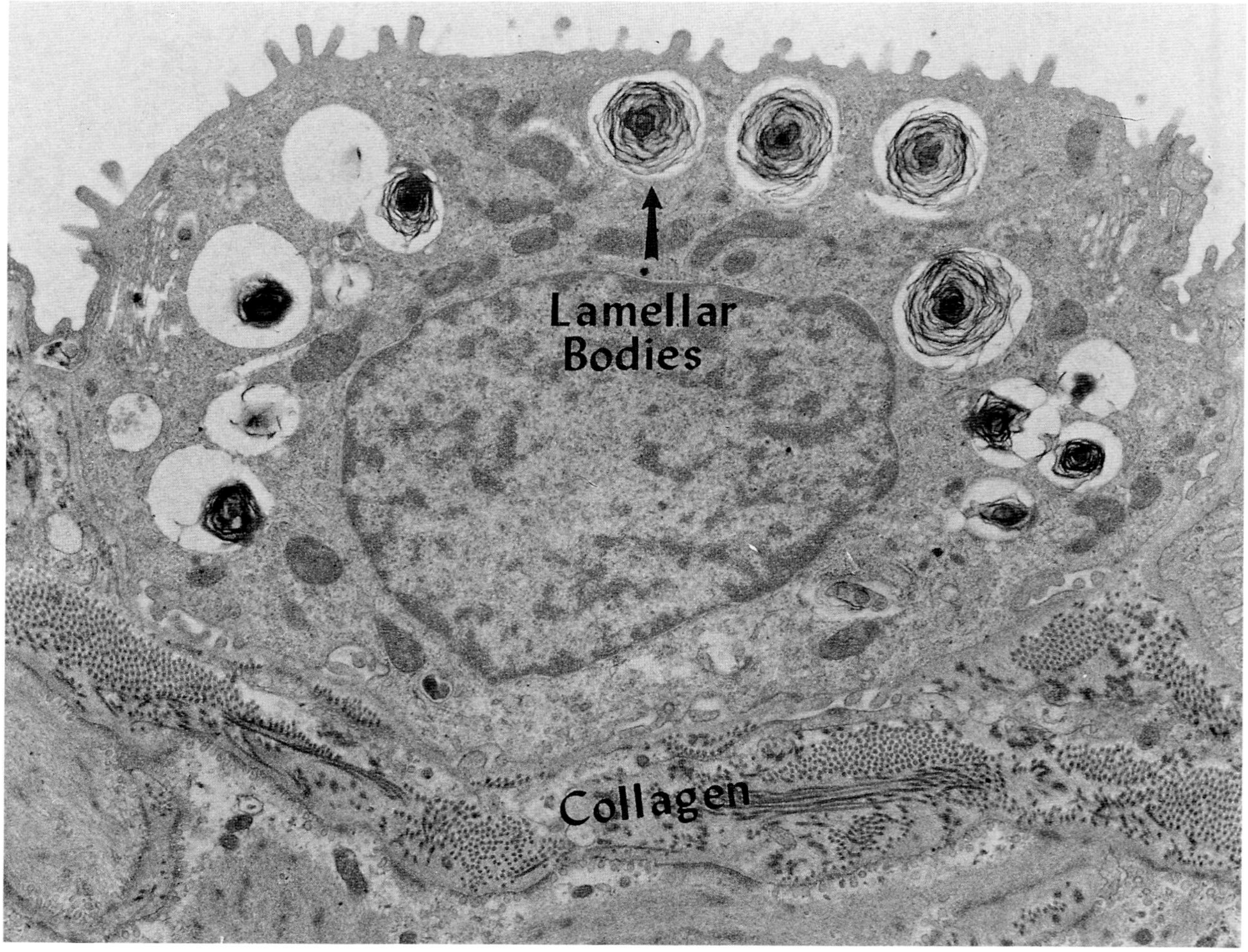

Fig. 15. Type II (granular) pneumocyte. Note the concentrically laminated lamellar bodies in the cytoplasm which characterize these cells. (x13,600.)

16

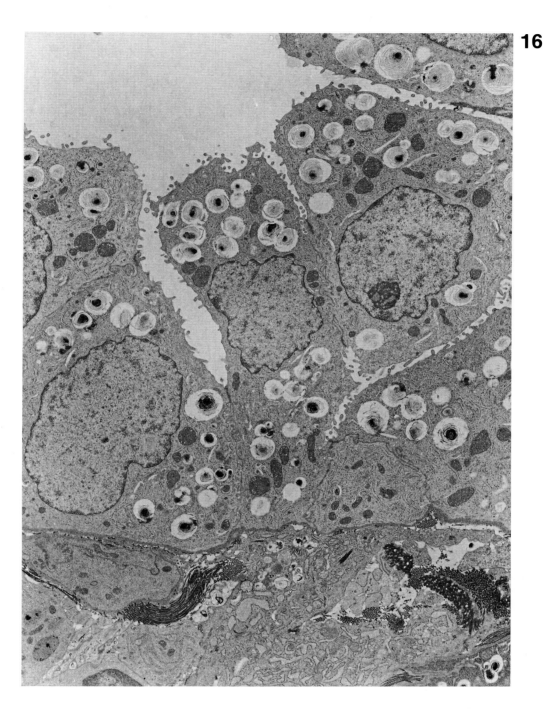

Fig. 16. Type II pneumocytes often become hyperplastic and proliferate in response to irritation or inflammation. In this case, the entire alveolus is lined by type II pneumocytes. They may desquamate into the alveolar lumen; together with histiocytes, they probably constitute some of the large monocytic cells seen in typical deep-cough specimens of sputum (see Figure 17). (x5,760.)

Fig. 17. Alveolar air spaces in the lung, showing many "dust" cells—that is, dust-filled histiocytes (**arrow**)—and a few unpigmented monocytic cells that probably are type II pneumocytes. (x280.)

Fig. 18. Bronchus showing slight basal cell hyperplasia and early squamous metaplasia. (x280.)

17

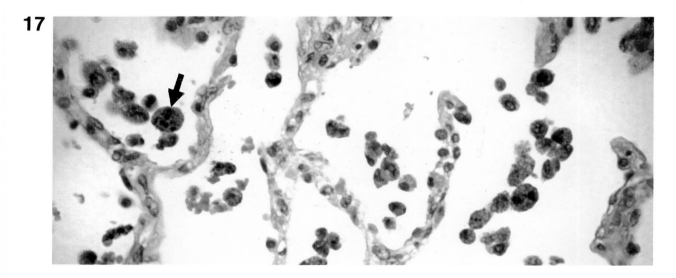

18

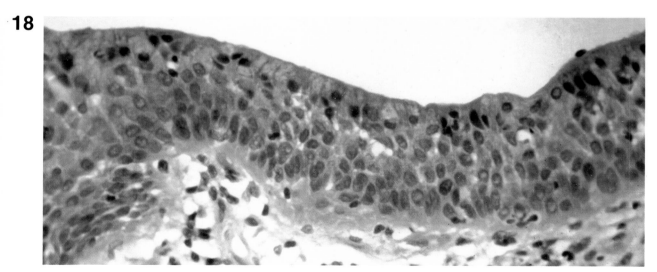

Within the alveolar space are varying numbers of phagocytic histiocytes or "dust" cells, which act as scavengers in removing particulate matter from the respired air. These cells lie free in the alveolus. They are present in large numbers in a satisfactory deep-cough sputum specimen (Fig. 17).

Nonspecific Irritative Changes.—There are a number of reactions of the bronchial epithelium to irritation or inflammation. Most common is basal cell hyperplasia and squamous metaplasia (Fig. 18) and goblet cell hyperplasia (Fig. 19). When these processes are extensive, they can influence the cytologic makeup of the sputum.

19

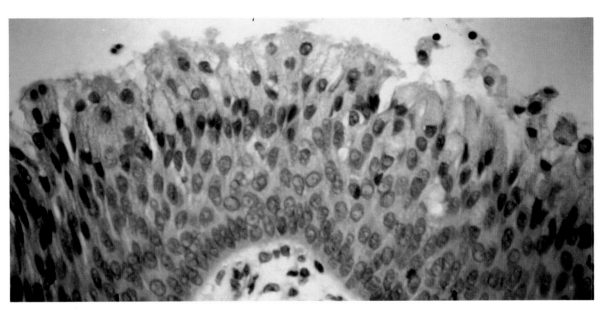

Fig. 19. Bronchus with pronounced hyperplasia and goblet cell metaplasia. (x280.)

Lymphatics

The pulmonary lymphatics originate as a plexus of endothelial-walled capillary channels surrounding and accompanying peripheral pulmonary blood vessels and bronchioles. These give rise to larger collecting trunks with thin muscular walls which course along the pulmonary vessels and bronchi proximally until they become tributaries of intrapulmonic and hilar lymph nodes.

The pulmonary lobes and segments do not constitute independent or distinct lymphatic units. Vessels coursing between adjacent lobes drain lymphatics from pulmonary tissue in both lobes. Nor is there anatomic uniformity from individual to individual. In general, however, lymphatics of the lower lobes drain into nodes at the level of the tracheal bifurcation (subcarinal lymph nodes), and lymphatics of the upper lobes drain into nodes along the lateral tracheal chain (paratracheal lymph nodes).

To permit more precise evaluation of the extent of tumor and the distribution of nodal metastases at the time of thoracotomy for lung cancer, systematic dissection of hilar and mediastinal lymph nodes should be performed as part of the operative procedure, particularly when complete resection of the primary tumor has been feasible. The lymph nodes are identified by their anatomic location, and the extent of nodal involvement is indicated for each site. The diagram in Figure 20 (which was devised in collaboration with the Tokyo National Cancer Center Hospital) is used to identify the various lymph nodes and has been adopted by the American Joint Committee for Lung Cancer Staging.

It should be emphasized that lymph nodes are quite variable in size and in distribution and that lymphoid tissue may be present throughout the respiratory tract. In addition to the large tonsillar masses in the pharynx, lymphoid tissue, either nodular or diffuse, is present in the tracheobronchial mucosa and within the pulmonary parenchyma, usually in subpleural sites. Thus, the presence of lymphocytes in specimens of sputum, particularly after vigorous cough or following bronchoscopy, does not necessarily signify disease.

Patients with early lung cancer and either absence of or limited nodal involvement are expected to have the best chance of prolonged survival after resection. It is hoped that a meticulous assessment of the lymph nodes at thoracotomy will provide better information about the sequence of node involvement with increasing tumor size at each location. Ultimately, this should be of help in selecting the optimum management for each patient.

Fig. 20. Diagrammatic representation of lymph node locations and nomenclature used for their identification.

Unless otherwise stated, all light microscopic sections were stained with hematoxylin and eosin. Transmission electron micrographs were kindly provided by Dr. Robert Erlandson and scanning electron micrographs by Dr. Patricia Saigo.

SITES OF LYMPH NODES

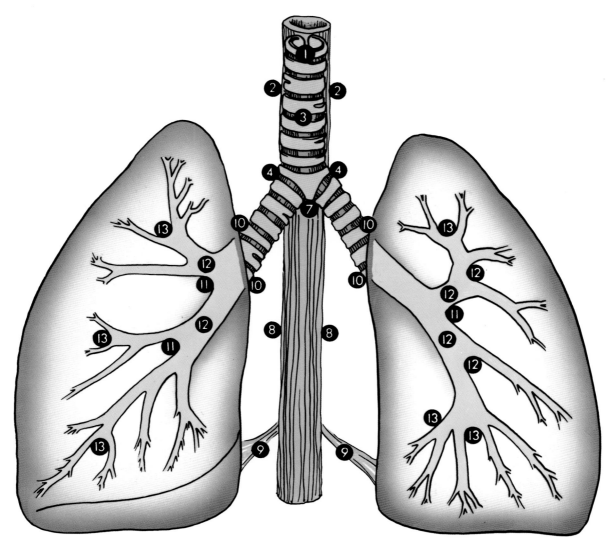

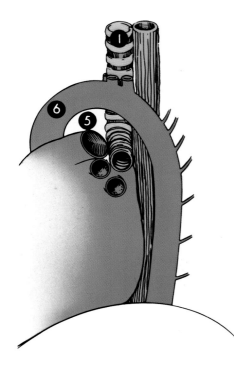

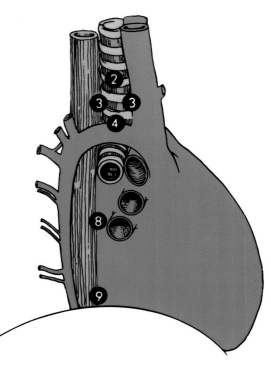

1. Highest mediastinal
2. Upper paratracheal
3. Pre or retrotracheal
4. Lower paratracheal
   or tracheobronchial
5. Subaortic
6. Aortic [phrenic]
7. Subcarinal
8. Paraesophageal
9. Pulmonary ligament
10. Hilar
11. Interlobar
12. Lobar
13. Segmental

Section 2

STAGING OF LUNG CANCER

Nael Martini, M.D.

Myron R. Melamed, M.D.

Lewis B. Woolner, M.D.

David T. Carr, M.D.

The lack of a uniform and reliable method of describing the extent of the disease has been one of the major obstacles in selecting proper treatment and evaluating reports of end results of treatment of lung cancer.

The staging system proposed and developed in 1973 by the American Joint Committee for Cancer Staging and End-Results Reporting is a simple and easily applied method for estimating and recording the anatomic extent of the tumor and its metastases. It was derived from the analysis of data from more that 2,000 patients with proven lung cancer. This staging system uses the TNM designations, in which T = primary tumor, N = regional lymph nodes, and M = distant metastases.

It has been approved by the TNM Committee of the International Union Against Cancer, the organization initially responsible for the development of the TNM system of all cancer staging.

To the letter T is appended a suffix to describe increasing size of the tumor and involvement by direct extension (TX, T1, T2, T3). Suffixes for the letter N describe the absence or increasing degrees of regional nodal involvement, and suffixes for the letter M describe the absence or presence of distant metastases. The definitions of the various TNM categories and their stage groups are shown in Tables 1 and 2. Diagrams depicting examples of the various tumor presentations are illustrated in Figure 1. These tables and figures conform with the 1977 revision of the system by the Task Force on Lung Cancer of the American Joint Committee.

All patients are assigned a clinical-diagnostic stage before treatment. The data necessary for the clinical-diagnostic stage are obtained from the medical history, physical examination, bronchoscopy, esophagoscopy, mediastinoscopy or mediastinotomy, routine and special x-ray studies, thoracentesis, and biopsy of accessible sites of distant metastases short of a formal thoracotomy. (Not all procedures are carried out on all patients.) Additional data needed for a surgical-evaluative staging are obtained at exploratory thoracotomy. For resected tumors, a postsurgical-treatment (pathologic) staging may be recorded. More recently, a re-treatment staging has been recommended with each new development in the course of the follow-up and before the initiation of further treatment. Autopsy staging may also be performed. All patients, therefore, are staged before treatment is instituted, and other stagings are recorded as appropriate. Histologic or cytologic proof of cancer is required. Because of the specific problem of radiologically occult cancer of the lung, a TX NO MO category was included.

A worksheet has been prepared by the American Joint Committee to help in the classification of lung cancer. Copies of the worksheet are available from the American Joint Committee, 55 East Erie Street, Chicago, IL 60611.

Table 1. Definitions of T, N, and M Categories for Carcinoma of the Lung

Each case must be assigned the highest category of T, N, and M which describes full extent of disease in that case.

T   PRIMARY TUMORS

T0 No evidence of primary tumor

TX Tumor proven by the presence of malignant cells in bronchopulmonary secretions but not visualized radiologically or bronchoscopically, or any tumor that cannot be assessed

TIS Carcinoma in situ

T1 A tumor that is 3.0 cm or less in greatest diameter, surrounded by lung or visceral pleura and without evidence of invasion proximal to a lobar bronchus at bronchoscopy

T2 A tumor more than 3.0 cm in greatest diameter, or a tumor of any size which invades visceral pleura or which has associated atelectasis or obstructive pneumonitis that extends to the hilar region. At bronchoscopy, the proximal extent of demonstrable tumor must be within a lobar bronchus or at least 2.0 cm distal to the carina. Any associated atelectasis or obstructive pneumonitis must involve less than an entire lung, and there must be no pleural effusion.

T3 A tumor of any size with direct extension into an adjacent structure such as the parietal pleura, the chest wall, the diaphragm, or the mediastinum and its contents or demonstrable bronchoscopically to involve a main bronchus less than 2.0 cm distal to the carina, or any tumor associated with atelectasis or obstructive pneumonitis of an entire lung or pleural effusion.

N   REGIONAL LYMPH NODES

N0 No demonstrable metastasis to regional lymph nodes

N1 Metastasis to lymph nodes in the peribronchial or ipsilateral hilar region (or both) (including direct extension)

N2 Metastasis to lymph nodes in the mediastinum

M   DISTANT METASTASIS

M0 No distant metastasis

M1 Distant metastasis such as in scalene, supraclavicular, cervical, or contralateral hilar lymph nodes, brain, bones, liver, or contralateral lung

Table 2. Staging Grouping in Carcinoma of the Lung

Occult Carcinoma

> **TX   N0   M0**

An occult carcinoma with bronchopulmonary secretions containing malignant cells but without other evidence of the primary tumor or evidence of metastasis to the regional nodes or distant metastasis (If subsequently proved to be bronchogenic carcinoma becomes stage I, II or III)

Stage I

> **TIS   N0   M0**
> **T1   N0   M0**
> **T1   N1   M0**
> **T2   N0   M0**

Carcinoma in situ
A tumor that can be classified T1 without any metastasis or with metastasis to the lymph nodes in the peribronchial and/or ipsilateral hilar region only, or tumor that can be classified T2 without any metastasis to nodes or distant metastasis

Stage II

> **T2   N1   M0**

A tumor classified as T2 with metastases to the lymph nodes in the peribronchial and/or ipsilateral hilar region only

Stage III

> **T3 with any N or M**
> **N2 with any T or M**
> **M1 with any T or N**

Any tumor more extensive than T2 or any tumor with metastasis to the lymph nodes in the mediastinum or with distant metastasis

T1

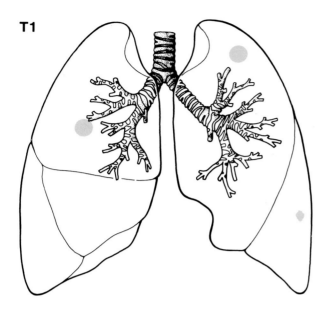

T1

A solitary tumor that is 3.0 cm or less in greatest diameter, surrounded by lung or visceral pleura and without evidence of invasion proximal to a lobar bronchus at bronchoscopy. Three examples of T1 lesions are shown.

T2

The primary tumor is more than 3.0 cm in greatest diameter as depicted in 2a or a tumor of any size which invades visceral pleura, as depicted in 2b, or which has associated atelectasis or obstructive pneumonitis that extends to the hilar region, as depicted in 2c. At bronchoscopy, the proximal extent of demonstrable tumor must be at least 2.0 cm distal to the carina. Any associated atelectasis or obstructive pneumonitis must involve less than an entire lung, and there must be no pleural effusion.

T2

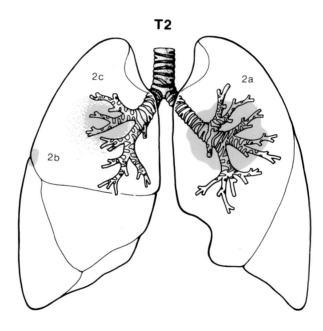

T3

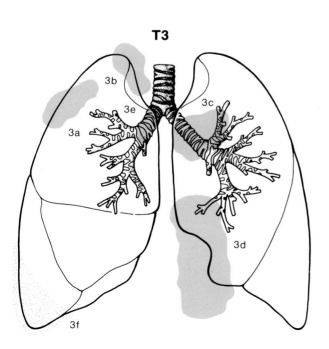

T3

A primary tumor of any size with direct extension into an adjacent structure such as parietal pleura, chest wall (3a), or mediastinum and its contents (3b), with direct invasion of the aorta, main pulmonary artery or veins, or recurrent or phrenic nerves (3c), or with invasion of the pericardium or diaphragm (3d). T3 lesions include tumors demonstrable bronchoscopically to be less than 2.0 cm distal to the carina (3e) and any tumor associated with a pleural effusion (3f) or with atelectasis obstructive pneumonitis of an entire lung.

Histopathologic Classification

The purpose of these paragraphs is to provide background for the terminology used to identify the various types of bronchogenic carcinomas discussed in the chapters that follow. Histopathology occupies section 6.0 of the latest revision of the American Joint Committee's (AJC) system of staging of cancer of the lung.*

Subdivision 6.1 states:

There are four major cell types of lung cancer:
1. Squamous cell (epidermoid) carcinoma
2. Adenocarcinoma including alveolar cell or terminal bronchiolar carcinoma
3. Undifferentiated large cell carcinoma
4. Undifferentiated small cell (oat cell) carcinoma

The AJC classification is immediately preceded by the caveat:

Staging grouping is significant for all cell types listed in 6.0 HISTOPATHOLOGY except undifferentiated small cell (oat cell) carcinoma in which there is no significant relation between stage and survival rates. Nevertheless, the anatomic extent of small cell cancers may be recorded by the TNM system for future reference.

The AJC classification of lung tumors is the newest and simplest. The committee in charge of its formulation is composed of contributors to this atlas and Dr. Clifton F. Mountain. Dr. Raventos died and was replaced by Fred Stitik who is a contributor to atlas.

World Health Organization (WHO) Classification

By tradition, the World Health Organization's (WHO) international classification of lung tumors also merits consideration. ·· The WHO classification is somewhat more detailed than the AJC classification, but regarding the four major cell types of lung cancer, the differences are slight.

The WHO classification of the four major cell types is presented here, together with representative photographs of the histologic features of the more common varieties.

Terminology from both the AJC and the WHO classifications is used interchangeably throughout this atlas.

*American Joint Committee for Cancer Staging and End-Results Reporting: Staging of cancer of the lung. *In* Manual for Staging of Cancer, 1977. American Joint Committee, 55 East Erie Street, Chicago, IL 60611, 1977, pp 59-65.

··Kreyberg L, Liebow AA, Uehlinger EA: Histologic Typing of Lung Tumours. World Health Organization, Geneva, 1967.

I. Epidermoid (Squamous) Carcinoma

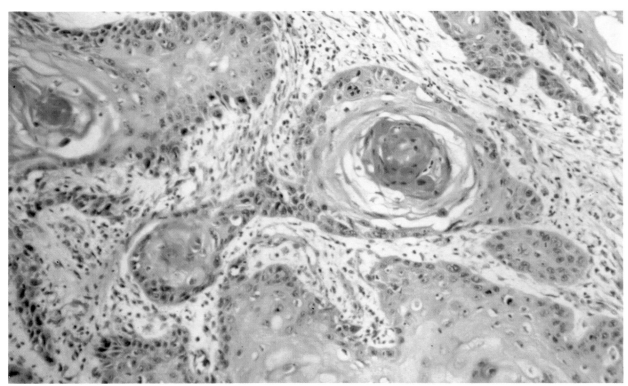

1. Well differentiated

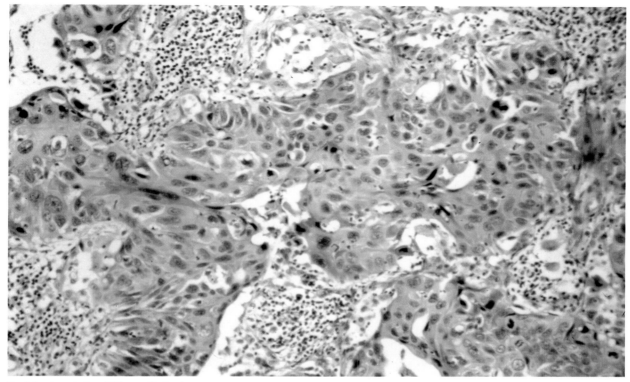

2. Moderately differentiated

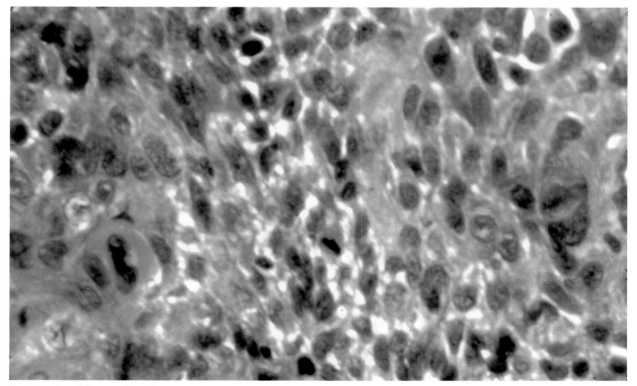

3. Poorly differentiated

II. Small Cell Anaplastic Carcinomas

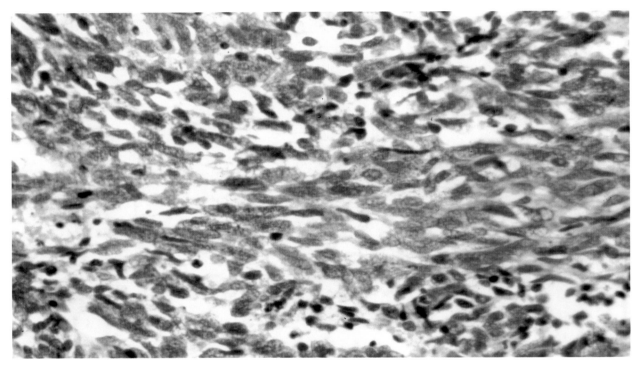

1. Fusiform cell type

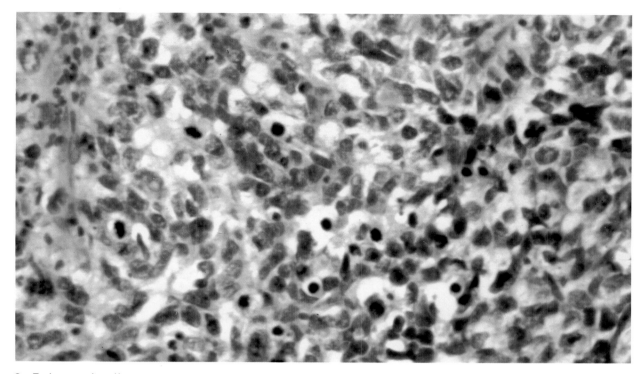

2. Polygonal cell type

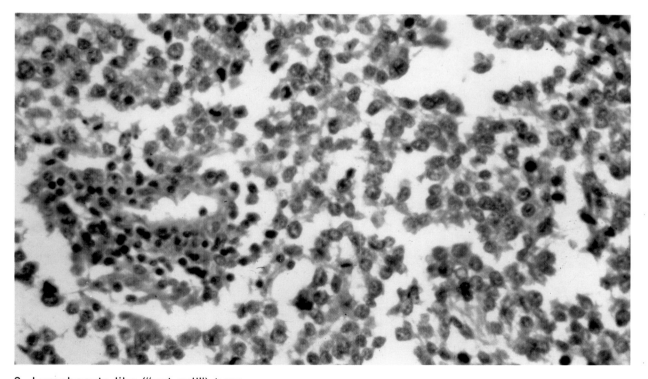

3. Lymphocyte-like ("oat-cell") type

III. Adenocarcinomas

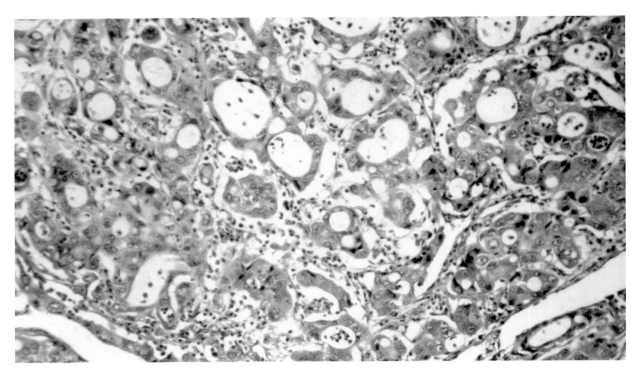

1. Bronchogenic, acinar type

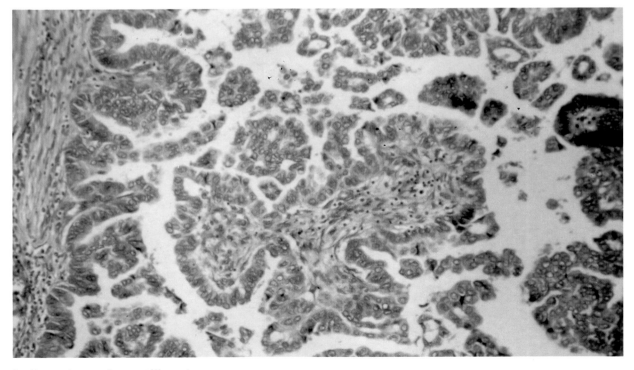

2. Bronchogenic, papillary type

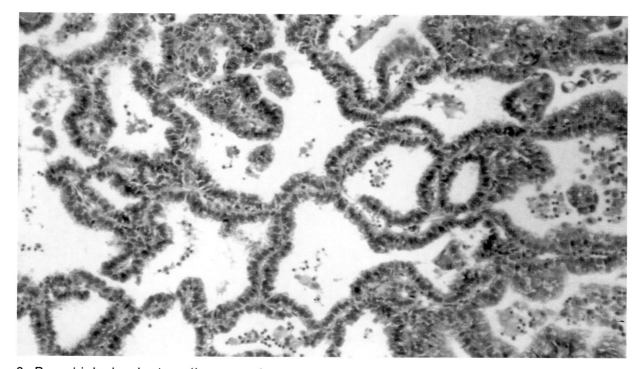

3. Bronchioloalveolar type (low power)

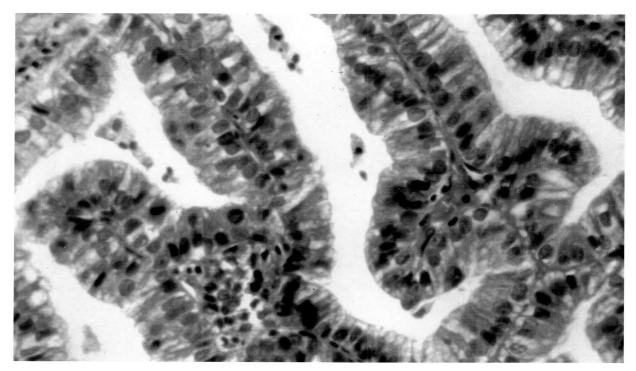

4. Bronchioloalveolar type (high power)

IV. Large Cell Carcinomas

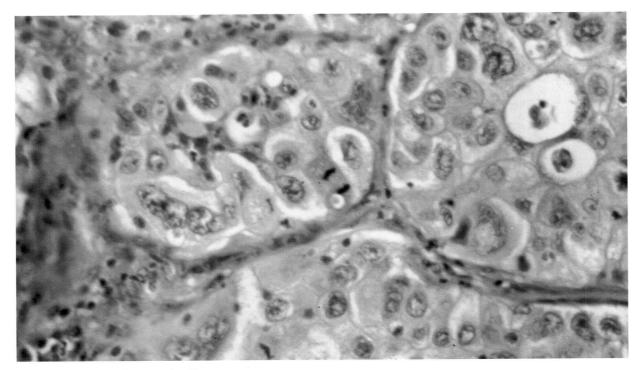

1. Solid tumor with mucin-like content

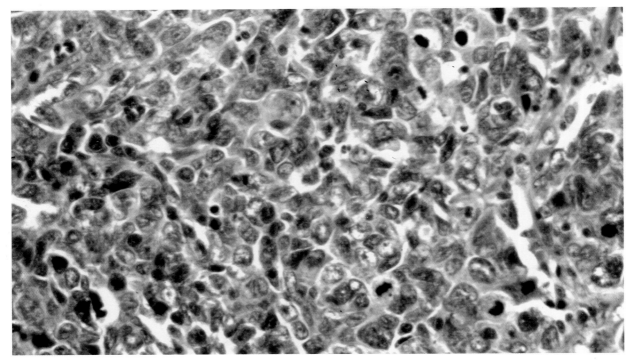

2. Solid tumor without mucin-like content

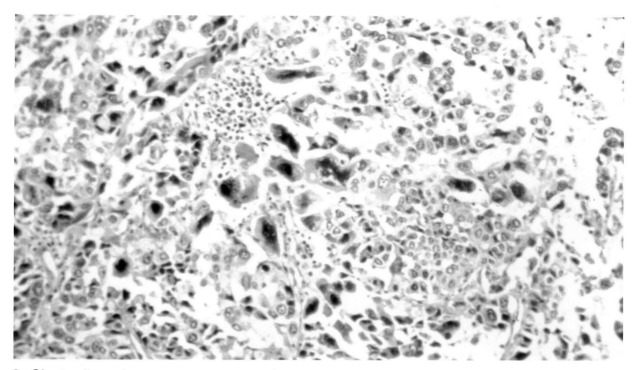

3. Giant cell carcinoma

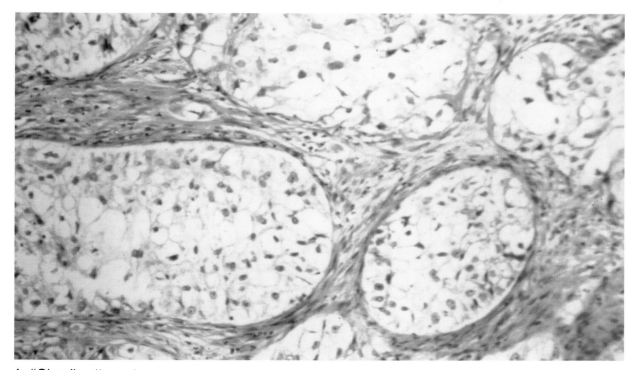

4. "Clear" cell carcinoma

Section 3

CYTOPATHOLOGY

John K. Frost, M.D.

Yener S. Erozan, M.D.

Prabodh K. Gupta, M.D.

Darryl Carter, M.D.

Introduction

Screening a population for lung cancer by sputum cytology testing will permit earlier detection, especially of squamous cell carcinomas and serious squamous cellular atypias, than is possible in routine clinical practice. This section describes the spectrum of cytologic abnormalities which has been encountered during the screening programs of the NCI Cooperative Early Lung Cancer Group. Appropriate emphasis has been given to squamous cell abnormalities. Cytologic findings have been correlated with histopathologic observations wherever possible.

There are four parts to the section. Part I describes benign cellular changes that may simulate cancer. Part II summarizes the cytopathology of the four major cell types of bronchogenic carcinoma: squamous cell (epidermoid), adenocarcinoma, large cell undifferentiated, and small cell.

Part III, on early squamous cell carcinoma, and Part IV, on developing squamous epithelial atypias, are the most important yet are conceptually the most difficult parts of the section. They deal with less well-defined entities that have been, and continue to be, the object of intensive study by the Cooperative Group. These two parts illustrate problems that may be expected in any lung cancer screening program involving pulmonary cytology.

Considerable cytologic data have already been compiled by the Cooperative Group, permitting certain conclusions to be offered now. Preliminary observations of ongoing studies are also described in order to present the current state of the art in pulmonary cytology.

A standard final magnification of 1,250 times and the Papanicolaou staining technique have been used in all illustrations, unless otherwise specified.

Part I: Nonmalignant Changes

There are many variations of normal cells in sputum and bronchial secretions which may mimic cancer and render differential diagnosis difficult. The more common variations have been well documented in the literature. In this part, some of the most significant and confusing of the benign structural alternations will be presented. They include changes resulting from chronic inflammation and irritation, hypersensitivity, irradiation, drug therapy or chemotherapy, and viral diseases. Although lung tissues react to their environment in only a few basic ways, combinations of changes can produce a wide range of morphologic abnormalities that may be mistaken for cancer.

Normally functioning cells display rounding and regularity of the nucleus, with predictable configurations of nuclear chromatin, chromatinic rim, parachromatin, and nucleoli (Fig. 1**A** through **C**).

Increased cellular activity, including stimulation, repair, and replication, is characterized by increased undulation of the nuclear membrane (Fig. 2**G** and 3**A**), chromatin granularity (Fig. 2**E**, 2**G**, 3**A**, 3**E**, and 4**F** and **G**), parachromatin clearing (Fig. 2**G**, 3**E**, and 4**F**), prominent nucleoli (Fig. 2**G**, 3**E**, 4**G**, and 4**K**), mitosis, multinucleation (Fig. 4**B**), and cytoplasmic immaturity (Fig. 2**E**, 2**G**, 3**A**, 4**C**, and 4**H** and **I**).

Decreased cellular activity secondary to injury, aging, degeneration, or death produces blurring of the nuclear chromatin, clumping, alteration of chromasia (Fig. 3**D** and 4**A** through **C**), cytoplasmic acidophilia, fragmentation, and loss of cell borders (Fig. 3**D**, 4**A**, 4**G**, and 4**K**).

Mixtures of these three levels of cellular activity may cause structural abnormalities closely resembling cancer. However, true malignant disease exhibits additional morphologic characteristics (Part II) that are specifically associated with cancer.

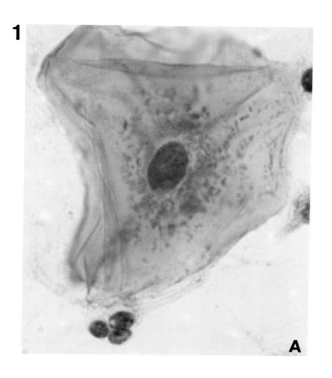

Fig. 1. **A**, Intermediate squamous epithelial cell from sputum. Nucleus is central and measures about 12 μm, or size of well-preserved neutrophil (below). Cytoplasm is wafer thin. This type of cell originates from mouth and pharynx and denotes saliva rather than "deep" endobronchial sputum. **B**, Columnar epithelial cells, mucus-secreting (goblet) and ciliated. Nuclei are eccentric, with abundant cytoplasm near lumen and tail formation near basement membrane. Normal goblet cells have multiple, lacy cytoplasmic vacuoles. With irritation and hypersensitivity, secretion increases and becomes tenacious, and signet-ring cells result (see Fig. 2**D**). Diagnostic cilia are numerous and of uniform length, periodicity, and thinness. Rootlets of cilia, viewed in profile, form a terminal plate. Cilia with such characteristics are not found on exfoliated cancer cells. Frequent from sinuses and nasopharynx, these cells do not denote "deep" endobronchial sputum. **C**, Carbon-bearing histiocyte, with cytoplasm containing carbon particles that nearly obscure two nuclei. Although these cells may be shed transiently from sinuses after inhalation of carbon, they are shed for years from lungs and constitute best indication of true "deep" sputum.

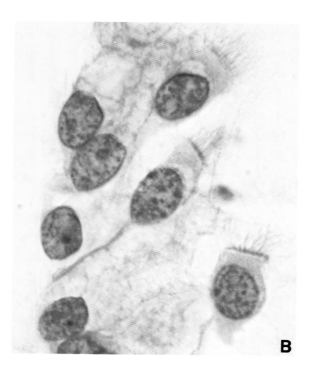

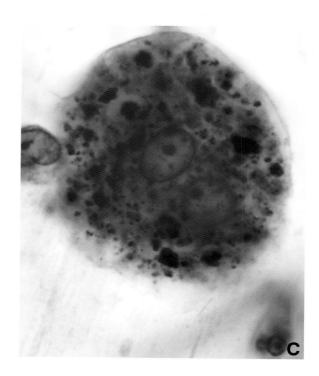

2

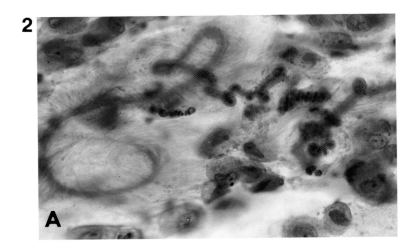

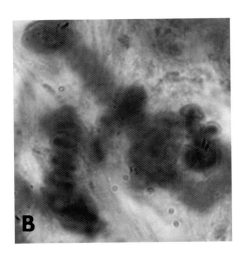

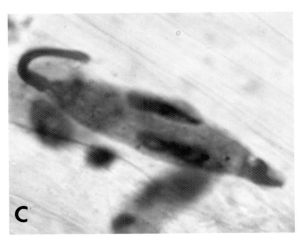

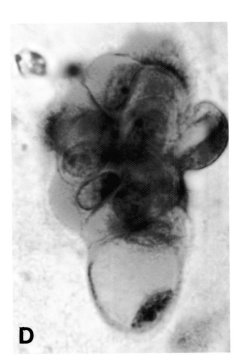

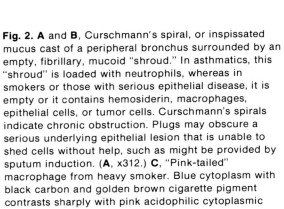

Fig. 2. A and **B**, Curschmann's spiral, or inspissated mucus cast of a peripheral bronchus surrounded by an empty, fibrillary, mucoid "shroud." In asthmatics, this "shroud" is loaded with neutrophils, whereas in smokers or those with serious epithelial disease, it is empty or it contains hemosiderin, macrophages, epithelial cells, or tumor cells. Curschmann's spirals indicate chronic obstruction. Plugs may obscure a serious underlying epithelial lesion that is unable to shed cells without help, such as might be provided by sputum induction. (**A**, x312.) **C**, "Pink-tailed" macrophage from heavy smoker. Blue cytoplasm with black carbon and golden brown cigarette pigment contrasts sharply with pink acidophilic cytoplasmic processes extending from both poles.

Immunofluorescence has identified alpha₁-antitrypsin in these pink tails. **D**, Hypersecretory, reactive, ciliated columnar-tissue fragment (Creola body). There are large hyperchromatic nuclei with nucleoli. Hyperdistended secretory vacuole is in cell at bottom. Cursory examination suggests adenocarcinoma; however, diagnostic cilia (see Fig. 1**B**) in right upper corner indicate a benign condition. This is a common finding in sputum from an allergic individual or in bronchial secretion associated with inflammation. **E**, Active reserve cells, frequent in bronchoscopic brush samples and occasionally found in sputum. Scanty cytoplasm and hyperchromatic nuclei suggest small cell carcinoma; however, round nuclei are irregular only from molding by adjacent nuclei, and chromatinic pattern is uniform without variation from cell to cell. **F**, Atypical reactive cells from sputum. Foamy cytoplasm with enlarged vacuoles suggests atypical secretory cells. Minimal degeneration evidenced by slight chromatin blurring may account for some hyperchromasia. Picture is suggestive of malignancy but actually represents organizing pneumonia. **G**, Extremely atypical reactive cells from sputum. Hyperchromasia with marked parachromatin clearing, uniform dispersion of granular chromatin, prominent nucleoli, and undulated nuclear membrane indicate increased activity. Slight chromatin blurring and nuclear membrane wrinkling indicate degeneration. Pseudopearl formations, possible secretion (top), and suggestive keratinizing cytoplasmic (ecto-endoplasm) tendencies (bottom) suggest metaplastic epithelium, but they could be extremely active macrophages. These changes represent organizing pneumonia, but they could easily be misdiagnosed as adenocarcinoma if degeneration is overlooked and strict criteria for malignancy are not observed.

2

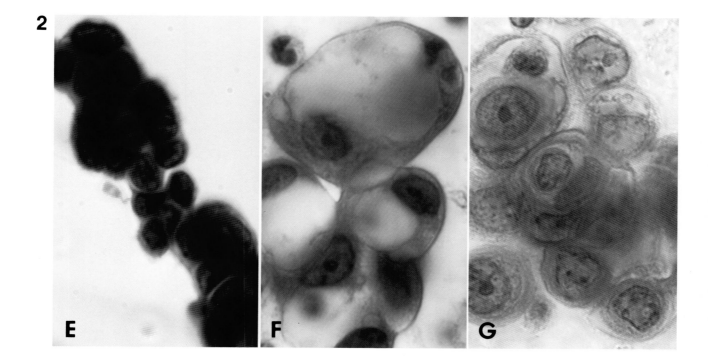

E   **F**   **G**

Fig. 3. Irradiation and cytotoxic drugs affect rapidly multiplying cells of bronchoalveolar epithelium. **A** through **C**, Irradiation. Bronchial epithelial cells, reacting to irradiation, exhibit macrocytosis, nuclear enlargement (karyomegaly), hyperchromasia, and nuclear membrane undulation. There are also degenerative changes, notably blurring and hyperchromasia. All are columnar cells, with suggestive ecto-endoplasmic squamous features in **B**. Although neoplasm must be considered in differential diagnosis, their features are not diagnostic of malignancy. **D** and

E, Chemotherapy. Columnar cells in **D**, even though hyperchromatic and bizarre, are extremely poorly preserved, with an ''air-dried'' artifact producing severe cytoplasmic acidophilia and blurring of nuclear details. Extremely reactive columnar cells in **E** were obtained by bronchoscopic lavage. Large central cell is hyperchromatic, with moderately coarse, uniformly distributed chromatin and rounded nucleoli. Upper cell has chromatin blurring, clearing, and wrinkling due to degeneration. At another level of focus, cilia were identified on these cells.

3

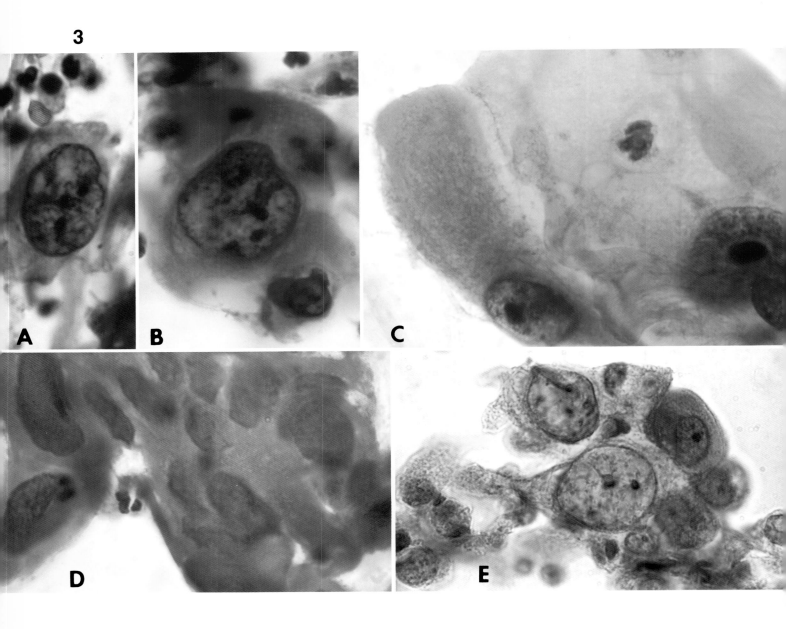

Fig. 4. Viral infection. **A**, Columnar cells in tissue fragment. There is karyomegaly, with some hyperchromasia and chromatin granularity, but blurring of degeneration negates their significance. **B**, Herpes simplex infection. Extreme multinucleation is evident. Degenerative chromatin granules are concentrated near nuclear membrane; this leaves a prominent gelatinous nuclear centrum. Cytoplasm is scant but is well defined and pigmented. **C**, Herpes simplex infection. Intranuclear inclusions show irregularities associated with fine threads of degenerated chromatin which traverse halo from inclusion to nuclear membrane. **D** through **F** and **H** through **J**, Bronchoscopic specimens. Cells have high nucleo-cytoplasmic ratio and eccentric, large, hyperchromatic nuclei with chromatin clumping and irregularities of nuclear membrane. Chromatin blurring suggests degeneration, however, and these cells are not diagnostic of cancer. Rather, they are reactive and degenerative columnar cells. **G** and **K**, Bronchoscopic specimens. Cells show high nucleo-cytoplasmic ratio with hyperchromasia, prominent nucleoli, and a uniformly thick, round chromatinic rim.

4

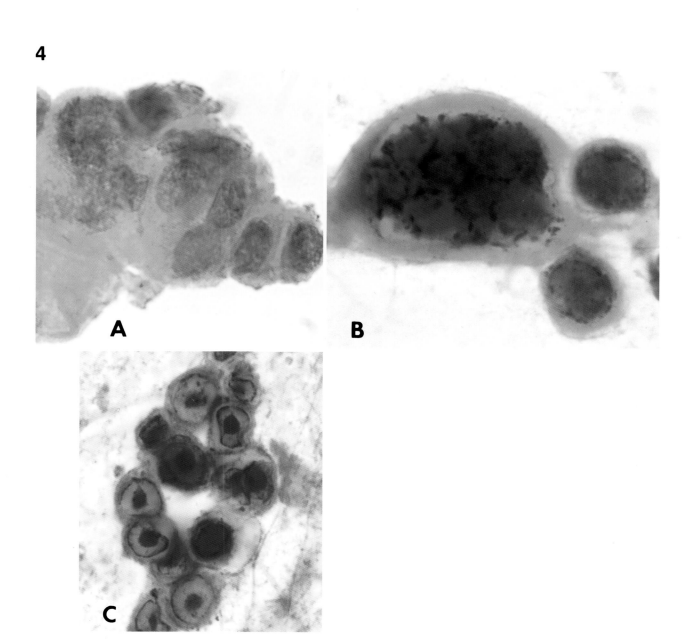

There is squamous differentiation in lower cell. Background is bloody, yet characteristic features of malignancy are lacking. These are reparative and degenerative changes accompanying a viral infection.

4

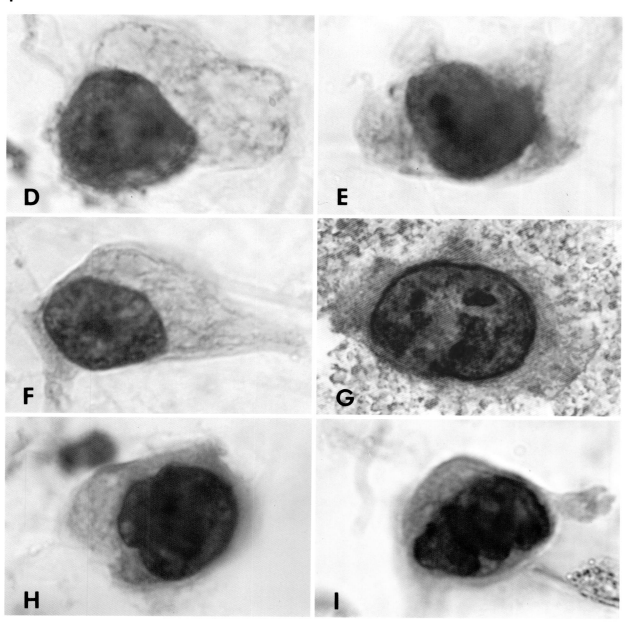

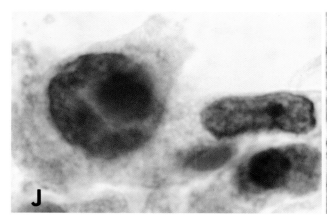

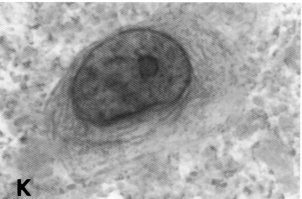

4

Part II: Typical Pulmonary Carcinoma

Early in the course of bronchogenic carcinoma, particularly squamous cell carcinoma, malignant cells may be shed into the bronchial lumen. Because the tumor is part of the surface epithelium, its cells have access to the lumen.

Early shedding of tumor cells may present an excellent opportunity for characterization of a developing cancer and for definitive diagnosis at a curable stage. Accurate cytologic diagnosis demands an adequate sample of cells that are representative of the tumor and that have been properly preserved and satisfactorily processed. This is accomplished by a combination of sputum induction by means of aerosol inhalations plus three morning "pooled" collections of spontaneously expectorated sputum.

Small **squamous cell carcinomas** (WHO I) have been detected in a cytologically positive, radiographically negative ("occult") stage, localized, resected, and then followed. This has substantially increased the basic knowledge of these early tumors. They may be encountered in various stages of their

development: typical invasive squamous cell carcinoma (Part II); early invasive, microinvasive, and in situ carcinomas (Part III); and developing carcinomas and epithelial atypias (Part IV).

Less is known regarding developmental stages of **adenocarcinoma** (WHO III). The smallest adenocarcinomas encountered by the Cooperative Early Lung Cancer Group appear to have originated principally in the peripheral air passages. Early in its development, a peripheral adenocarcinoma may block the small airway from which it arises. Later on, it may reestablish communication with an open bronchus and shed cells into the lumen.

Large cell undifferentiated carcinoma (WHO IV) shows insufficient differentiation of either cells or tissue pattern to allow further identification as squamous cell carcinoma or adenocarcinoma. At times it may present evidence of either or both, in tissue and in cellular specimens.

Small cell carcinoma (WHO II) shows no differentiation on light microscopy, even though it may be biologically or immunologically active.

Fig. 5. Squamous cell carcinoma. **A** through **D**, Cell spreads. Large tumor cells with bizarre hyperchromatic nuclei exhibit good criteria of malignancy, including significant irregularities of nuclear membrane (**C**), irregular clumping of chromatin, parachromatin clearing, and prominent nucleoli (**D**). Acidophilic keratinizing cytoplasm (**A-C**), ecto-endoplasmic keratinizing pattern (**C**), basophilic keratinizing granule (**D**), and pearl formation (**C**) are hallmarks of squamous cell differentiation. Necrotic cellular debris and prominent nucleoli suggest advanced cancer with invasion. **E** and **F**, Tissue section shows poorly differentiated squamous cell carcinoma with large bizarre nuclei, prominent nucleoli, and pearl formation (**F**). (Hematoxylin and eosin; **E**, x125.)

5

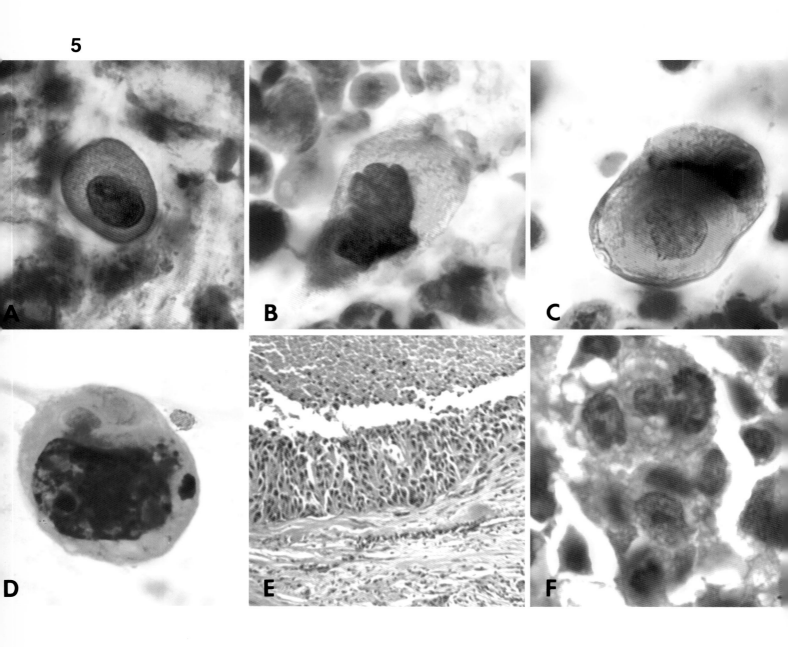

Fig. 6 and 7. Squamous cell carcinoma. Fig. 6A through C. Cell spreads. Malignant squamous cells show nuclear pleomorphism and hyperchromasia. A represents small tissue fragment with prominent, rounded nucleoli. B is a binucleated cell. All have keratinizing cytoplasm. E and F, Tissue section from necrotic, cavitating squamous cell carcinoma. (Hematoxylin and eosin; E, x56.)

Fig. 6D and 7A. Cell spreads. Prominent nucleoli and irregular parachromatin clearing (Fig. 6D) suggest invasion. Multinucleation (Fig. 6D) can be seen in both invasive and in situ squamous cell carcinoma.

6

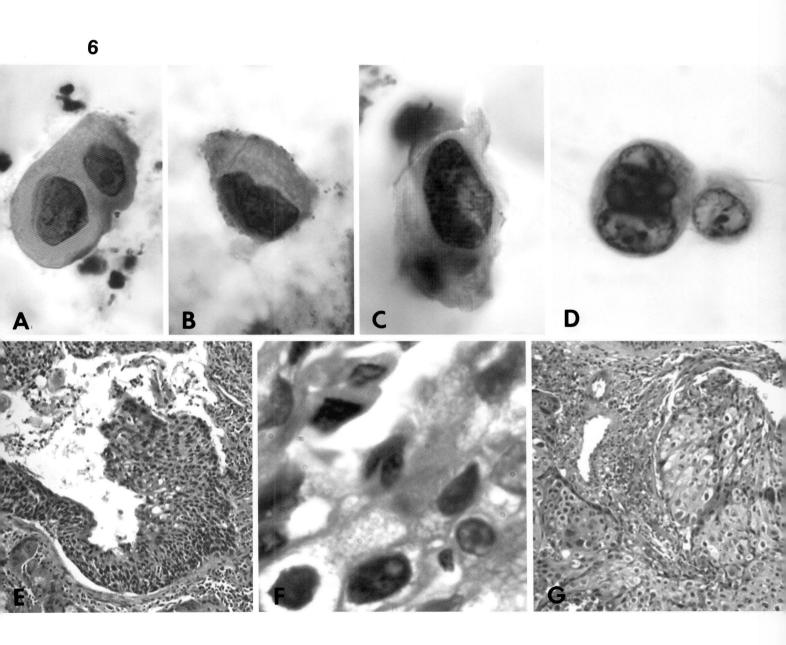

Fig. 6G and **7E**. Tissue section. Invasive squamous cell carcinoma is present. Pearl formation in tissue (Fig. 7**E**) matches that of cell spread (Fig. 7**A**). (Hematoxylin and eosin; Fig. 6**G**, x312.)

Fig. 7. B through **D**, Cell spreads. Degenerated cancer cells show poor squamous differentiation and pearl formation (**D**). **F** and **G**, Tissue sections. This peripheral lesion is poorly differentiated squamous cell carcinoma with abortive pearl formation. (Hematoxylin and eosin; **F**, x312.)

7

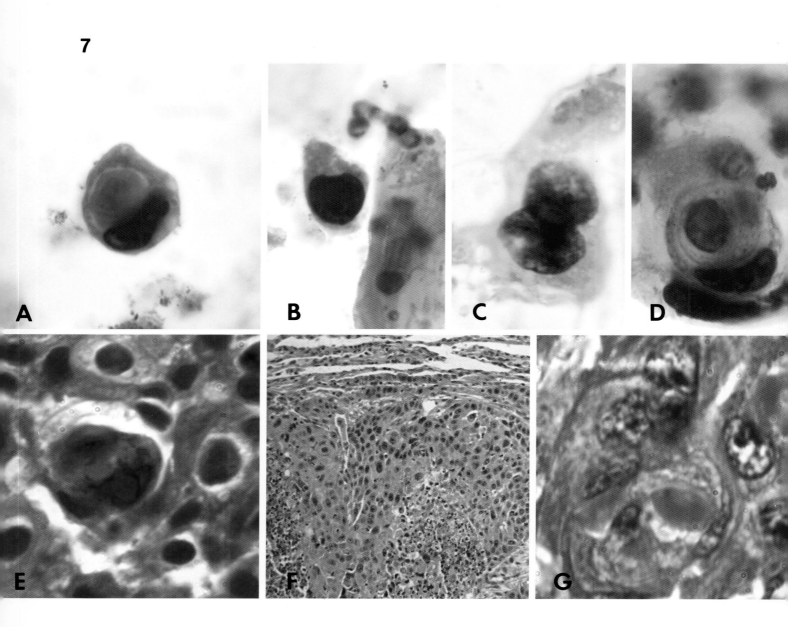

Fig. 8. A and **D**, Mucus-producing papillary adenocarcinoma. **A**, Cell spread. Papillary frond has epithelial luminal border along right margin. Nuclei are round or ovoid with modest chromatin-parachromatin irregularities and prominent nucleoli. Nuclei are eccentric from multiple cytoplasmic vacuoles. There is one large hyperdistended secretory-type vacuole at lower right. **D**, Tissue section. Note mucous and papillary pattern with epithelial luminal borders. (Hematoxylin and eosin; x312.) **B** and **C, E** and **F**, Poorly differentiated adenocarcinoma. **B** and **C**, Cell spreads. Phagocytosis in resolving pneumonitis (see Fig. 2**F**, **G**) would need to be considered if this were not clearly a cancer. There are good criteria of malignancy, including irregular chromatin-parachromatin pattern, irregularities of nuclear membrane, and high nucleo-cytoplasmic ratio. Reminiscent of large cell carcinoma (see Fig. 10), lesion has some features of functional differentiation, such as multiple cytoplasmic vacuoles, a few intracytoplasmic granules, and eccentric nuclei. **E** and **F**, Tissue sections. Identical malignant criteria are present, with large, irregular nucleoli. Good epithelial luminal border (**E**) and periodic acid-Schiff (PAS)-positive cytoplasmic vacuoles indicate adenocarcinoma. (Hematoxylin and eosin.)

8

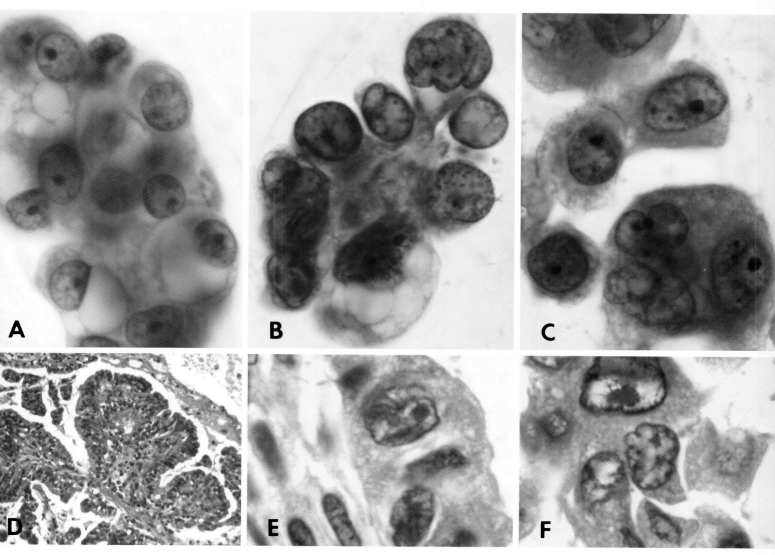

Fig. 9. Small peripheral adenocarcinoma, bronchiolo-alveolar type. **A** through **D**, Cell spreads. There are single cells and tissue fragments in sputum. Nuclei are pleomorphic and moderately hyperchromatic, with irregularities in distribution of chromatin. Some nuclei are eccentric and have prominent nucleoli (**D**) and foamy cytoplasm. Tissue fragments suggest papillary adenocarcinoma (**A**, **B**). Yet although fragments are only loosely held together (**A**, **D**), they remain attached by sticking (**C**, **D**), and these features are more characteristic of bronchiolo-alveolar type of cancer (**A**, x500.) **E** and **F**, Tissue sections. Tumor is growing along surfaces of alveolar walls, with little desmoplastic reaction (**E**). One cell type that is found in this tumor (**F**) is tall and columnar and produces abundant, sticky mucus. (Hematoxylin and eosin; **E**, x125.)

9

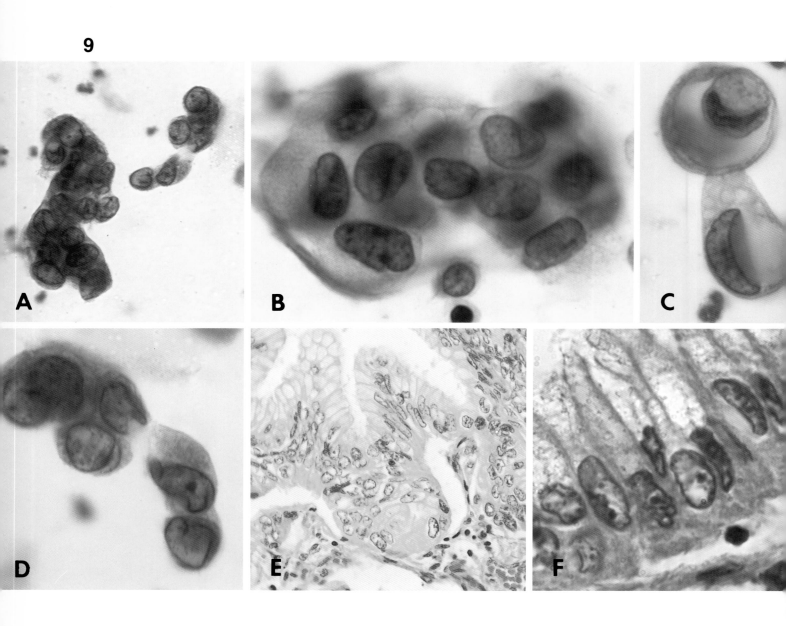

Fig. 10. Large cell carcinoma. **A** through **D**, Cell spreads. Extremely large nuclei, prominent irregular chromatin and nucleoli (**C**), abnormal distribution of highly cleared parachromatin (**B-D**), irregular chromatinic rim, and pleomorphism indicate malignancy. There is scanty, lacy cytoplasm with indistinct cellular borders. Careful search failed to reveal squamous, columnar, or sarcomatous functional differentiation, and this leaves diagnosis as large cell carcinoma by exclusion. **E** and **F**, Tissue sections. There is abundant clear cytoplasm without differentiation. Nucleoli are prominent and often irregular (**F**, compare with **C**). (Hematoxylin and eosin; **E**, x312.)

10

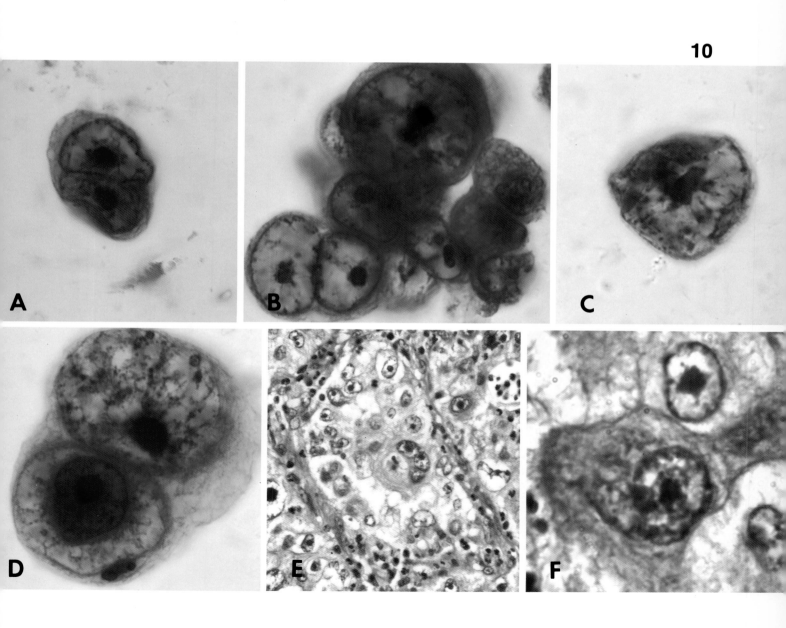

Fig. 11. Small cell carcinoma. **A** through **D,** Cell spreads from three patients at same magnification (x1,250) Cellular size varies from smallest-celled tumor (**D**) to largest (**C**), but there is relative uniformity within each tumor. All cells are small (compare with neutrophil and macrophage, **C**). Cytoplasm is extremely scanty but intact (**B, C**). Basically rounded nuclei are irregular because of extreme molding by neighboring cells of tissue fragment (**B-D**) and of unpredictable irregularities of chromatinic rim (**A-C**). Hyperchromatic, coarse chromatin and cleared parachromatin are irregularly distributed (**A, B**), with definite but inconspicuous nucleoli (**C, D**). This arrangement of loose tissue fragments is characteristic of small cell carcinoma, as are cells in columns (**C, D**) or pearl-like formations (**B**). In carefully interpreted cell spreads, small cell carcinoma can be recognized as being distinct from squamous cell, large cell, and adenocarcinoma. However, it may also be found with them in tumors of mixed differentiation. It is important, but at times difficult, to differentiate between small cell carcinoma and bare nuclei (note intact cytoplasm on a few cells in each figure, especially **C**), or lymphocytes or reserve cells (see Fig. 2**E**). **E** and **F,** Tissue sections from patient of **C**. Cytologic features are similar. (Hematoxylin and eosin; **E,** x312.)

11

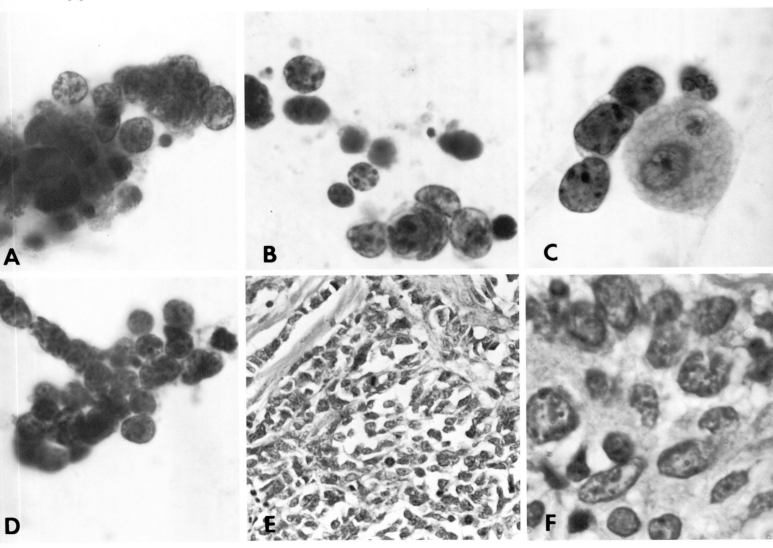

Part III: Early Squamous Cell Carcinoma

Early squamous cell carcinoma exhibits morphologic abnormalities that differ from more advanced, invasive squamous cell cancer. Although it is better not to attempt definitive biologic characterization of each morphologic change in early squamous cell cancer at this time, certain key features can be illustrated. These features define **early invasive carcinoma** (Fig. 12 through 14); **microinvasive carcinoma** (Fig. 15 through 18); **in situ carcinoma with gland involvement** (Fig. 19 and 20); and **in situ carcinoma on the mucosal surface** (Fig. 21 through 23).

Early squamous cell cancers shed a higher proportion of atypical metaplastic cells than do the advanced, invasive tumors. However, early cancers also contain cells with distinct malignant characteristics. Their nuclear membranes tend to be severely undulated, as in the atypias, but there are also a few unpredictable, sharp irregularities that are more often observed in advanced, invasive cancers. Nuclear chromatinic rims are thicker than normal, as in atypias, but begin to exhibit extreme variations in thickness typical of advanced cancer. Chromatin tends to be coarsely granular, as with atypias, but there are a few large, irregular clumps that are more common in the advanced cancers.

Early squamous cell cancers have a high proportion of round, symmetric cells. These cells are also frequent in atypias, but with cancer there is an increase of bizarre, elongated shapes. Spindle cells with sharply pointed fusiform nuclei, so common with advanced, invasive tumors, are unusual in early epidermoid tumors, although an occasional elongated or cigar-shaped nucleus may be encountered.

Early squamous cell cancers tend toward higher nucleo-cytoplasmic ratios and smaller overall cell size than are found in advanced, invasive squamous cell carcinomas. Many of the smaller cells become highly keratinized.

Nucleoli tend to be absent or inconspicuous in in situ carcinoma and in the squamous atypias. They appear in small numbers with microinvasive squamous cell cancer, and they become more prominent and numerous in early invasive cancer. They become still larger, more irregular, and more frequent in the advanced, invasive carcinomas.

Occasional large, bizarre, typically malignant cells are present in these early cancers. However, their numbers are less than in the invasive cancers. In early squamous cell cancer, there is a higher ratio of malignant tissue fragments to individual cancer cells than occurs in either precancerous atypias or advanced invasive tumors. Often the tissue fragments have a "pseudosyncytial" appearance, with indistinct cellular borders. The necrotic background that is so common with advanced cancers is virtually absent in early tumors.

Case 1 (Fig. 12, 13, and 14)

Early invasive squamous cell carcinoma, 3 mm in diameter, within extensive area of in situ carcinoma, treated by right lower lobectomy (Fig. 12 and 13). Patient continued to smoke and continued to shed metaplastic squamous cells with increasing degrees of atypia (slight to moderate to marked) for 3 years. He eventually shed cancer cells from a second primary squamous cell lung cancer (Fig. 14). The chest x-ray was negative except for changes secondary to previous thoracotomy and pulmonary resection.

Fig. 12. A through **D**, Cell spreads indicative of in situ carcinoma. **A**, Small, round tumor cell with pleomorphic nucleus and no nucleolus. **B**, Tumor cells and a columnar cell (10 o'clock). Some nuclei are degenerated and smudgy. However, diagnosis of cancer should not be made on this basis alone, for similar changes may occur in viral infection (see Fig. 4) or in degenerated squamous metaplasia. **C**, Tumor cells with nuclear irregularities, thickening of chromatinic rim, and no nucleoli. One cell is binucleated and has a very high nucleo-cytoplasmic ratio. **D**, Multinucleated tumor cell without nucleoli. Degenerative changes of upper nucleus should make one cautious about interpretation. **E** and **F**, Tissue sections. In situ squamous cell carcinoma of right lower lobe with extensive involvement of surface epithelium and deep extension down into submucosal glands (**E**, right); 3-mm focus of early invasive cancer is not shown. (Hematoxylin and eosin; **E**, x40, **F**, x500.)

12

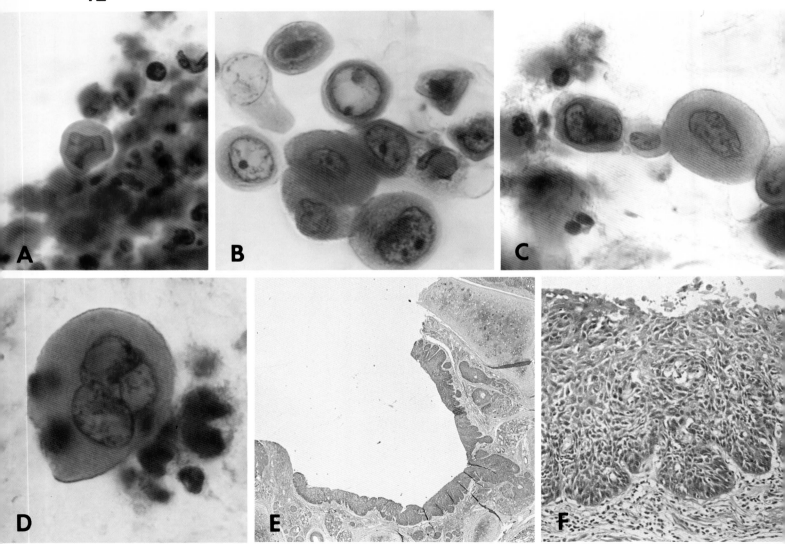

Fig. 13. **A** through **H**, Cell spreads. Small, round, and uniformly sized cells with granular chromatin, undulated thickened chromatinic rim, and high nucleo-cytoplasmic ratio. In addition to these features of in situ squamous cell carcinoma, prominent rounded nucleoli and evidence of keratinization (**D**, **F**, **H**) suggest invasive disease. Cytoplasmic vacuolation (**G**, center and above) is due to degeneration.

13

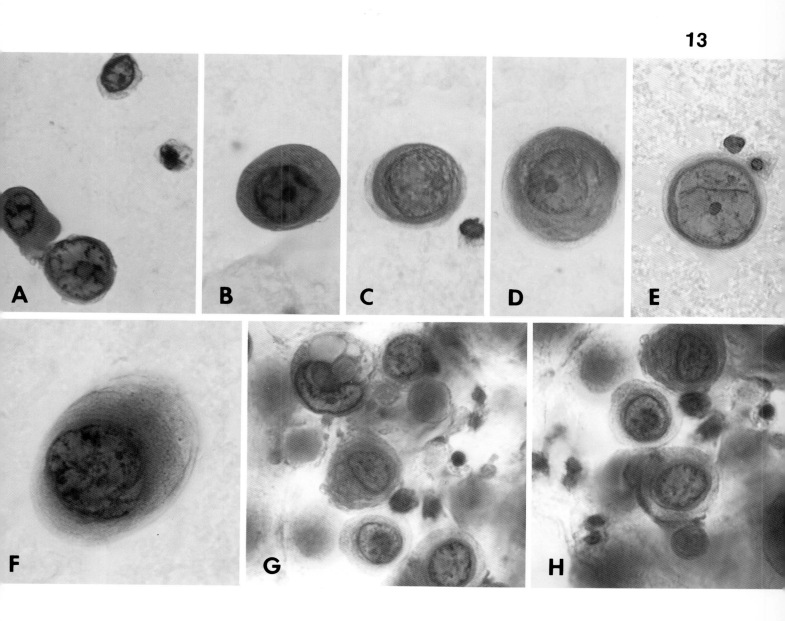

Fig. 14. A through **D**, Cell spreads. More advanced
invasive squamous carcinoma cells are seen, with
elongation, bizarre keratinization, and irregularly
pointed triangular nuclei (**A**, **C**, **D**). Note necrotic
background characteristic of invasive cancer. (**B**, **C**,
x500.) **E** and **F**, Tissue sections. New primary cancer
has developed in left upper lobe. Section shows area of
in situ carcinoma associated with invasive squamous
cell carcinoma. (Hematoxylin and eosin; **E**, x125.)

14

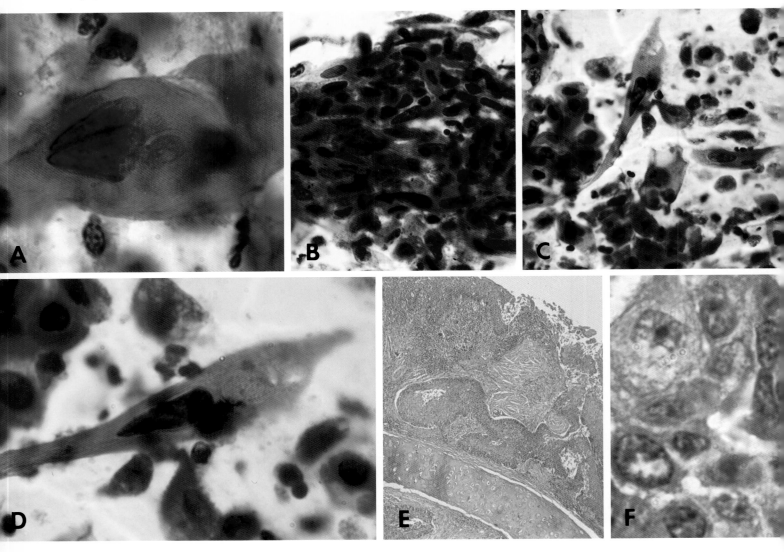

Case 2 (Fig. 15 through 18)

Microinvasive squamous cell carcinoma with extensive in situ carcinoma. Chest x-ray was negative.

Fig. 15. A through **C**, **E** and **F**, Cell spreads. Small cells have high nucleo-cytoplasmic ratios. Nuclei are hyperchromatic and some have irregular borders (**B**, **E**). These small, round cancer cells are a prominent feature of early squamous cell carcinomas. **D** and **G**, Cell spreads. Larger cancer cells are present with more irregular chromatin distribution and nuclear pleomorphism (**D**).

15

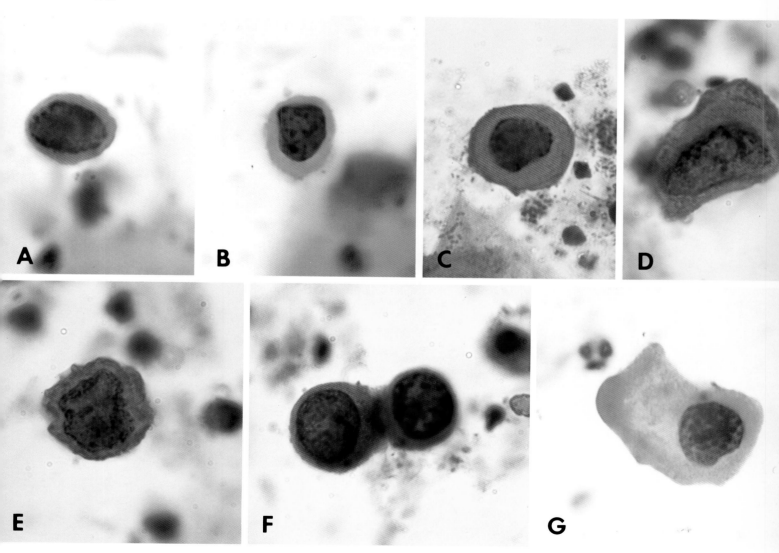

Fig. 16. A through **G**, Cell spreads. Many features of in situ carcinoma are present, especially in **A**. In addition, there are thickness and irregularity of chromatinic rim (**B, C, E**), nuclear pleomorphism (**C, D, F**), irregular chromatin aggregation and parachromatin clearing (**B, D, E, G**), and nucleoli (**A, C, E**) that suggest invasive squamous cell cancer.

16

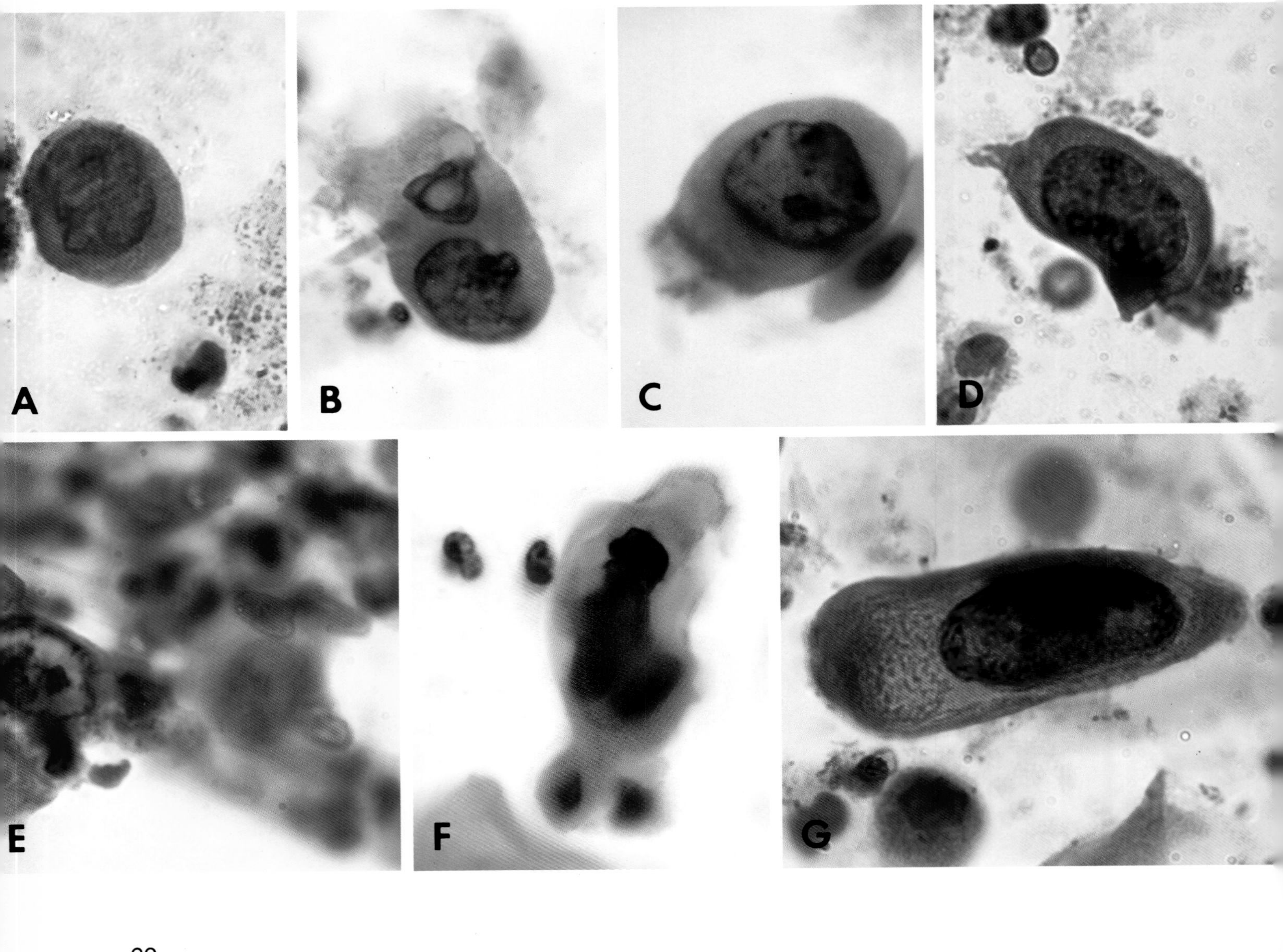

Fig. 17. A through **E**, Cell spreads. These are more typical of invasive squamous cell cancer, with irregular chromatin-parachromatin distribution, parachromatin clearing, chromatin clumping (**A**), hyperchromasia, irregular nuclear membrane (**A, D, E**), irregular thickness of chromatinic rim (**A**), and nucleoli (**A, B**). There is atypical functional differentiation with tailing of cytoplasm (**D, E**) and abortive pearl (**E**) formation. Note tissue fragments (**B-E**). Although a few cells of this type occur with in situ and microinvasive squamous cell carcinomas, they are more common in advanced invasive tumors.

17

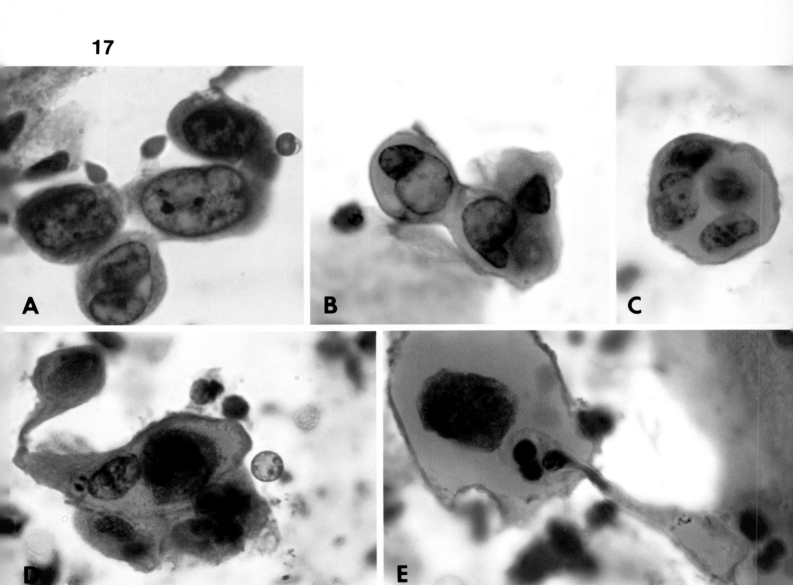

Fig. 18. A and **B**, Cell spreads. These are tissue fragments of keratinized squamous cancer. Atypical functional differentiation, such as pearl formation (**B**), is not necessarily an indication of malignancy, but when observed in a cancer cell it suggests invasion. Irregular chromatin distribution and extreme differences in size among nuclei in a tissue fragment are likewise suggestive. **C** through **E**, Tissue sections. Segmental bronchus of left upper lobe contains extensive in situ squamous cell carcinoma with deep glandular involvement and an area of microinvasion (**C**). Higher power of microinvasive area (**D**, **E**) shows marked pleomorphism, hyperchromasia, and nuclear criteria of squamous cell cancer. There is a large keratinized cell near basement membrane (**D**) as well as on surface (**E**). (Hematoxylin and eosin; **C**, x312.)

18

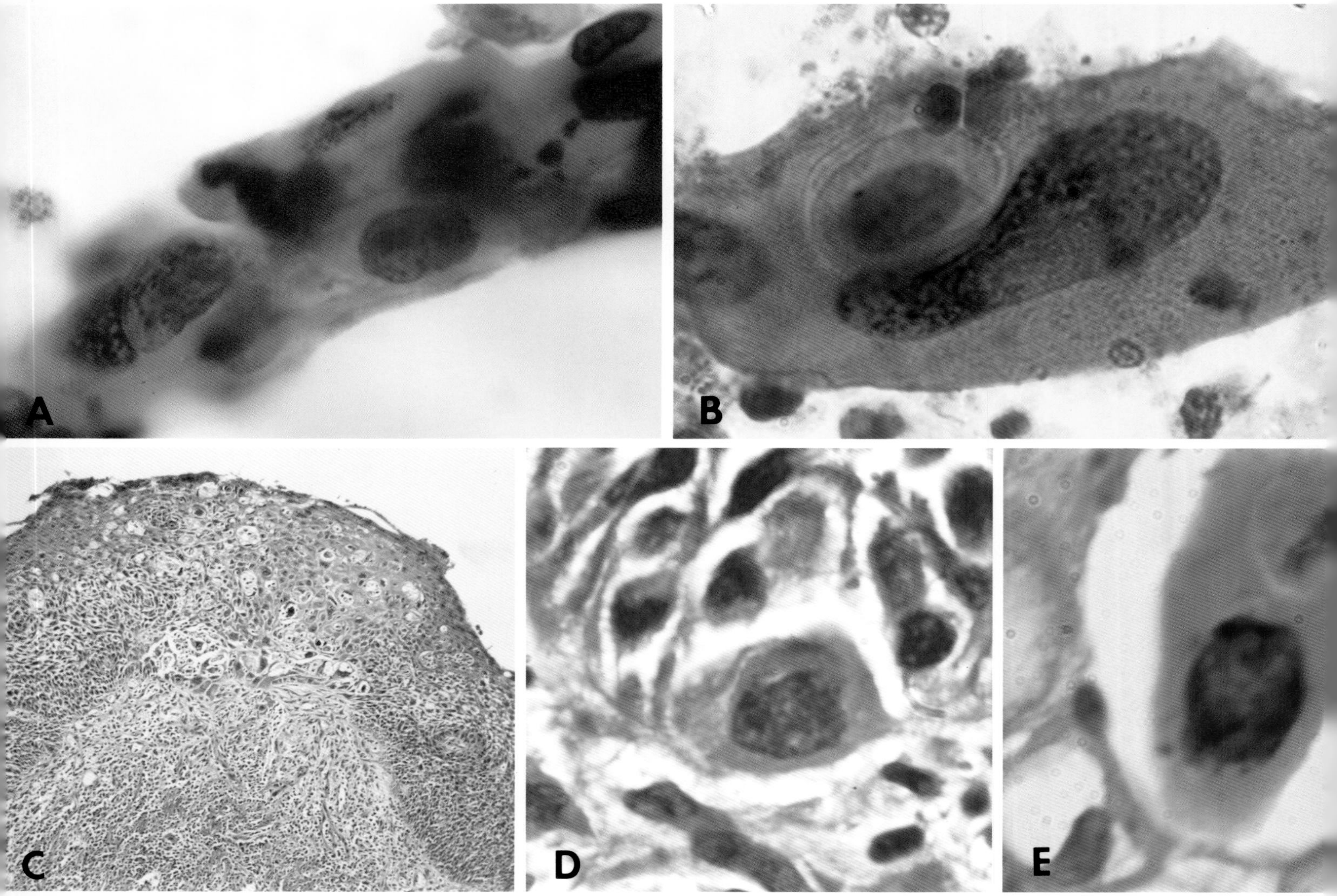

Case 3 (Fig. 19 and 20)

In situ squamous cell carcinoma with deep-gland involvement. Chest x-ray was negative.

Fig. 19. A through **F**, Cell spreads. Small, round cells show high nucleo-cytoplasmic ratio. Nuclei are hyperchromatic, rounded, and undulated but somewhat pyknotic. Chromatin is coarsely granular and uniformly distributed. Cytoplasm of some cells is acidophilic, and this suggests keratinization (**A**, **C-E**), but degenerative changes in the cytoplasm (small vacuoles) and in nuclei (dark, smudgy chromatin) may be a contributing factor.

19

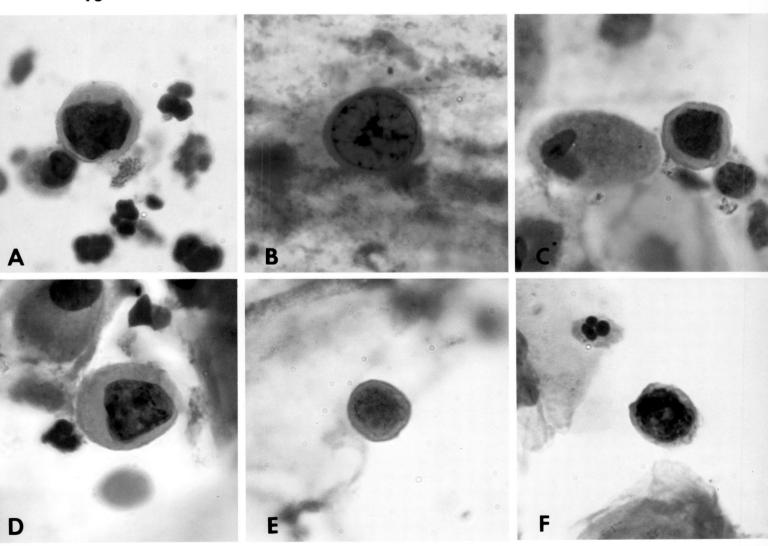

Fig. 20. A and **B**, Cell spreads. These show multinucleation with nuclear variation (**A**) and a tissue fragment (**B**) with abortive pearl formation. Cytoplasmic borders are ill defined. **C** and **D**, Tissue sections. In situ carcinoma on surface and in mucous glands of bronchial wall. At base of a gland (**D**) are pearl formation and some abortive keratinization. Intact basement membrane is at lower left. (Hematoxylin and eosin; **C**, x56.)

20

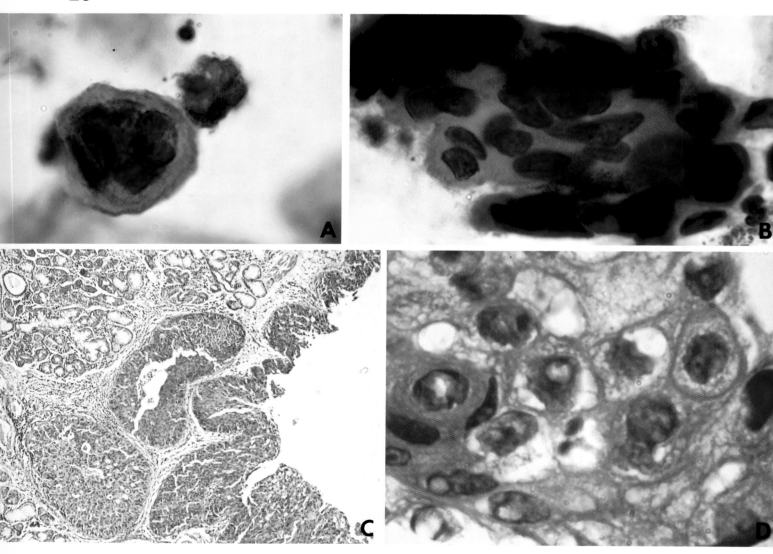

Case 4 (Fig. 21)

Surface in situ squamous cell carcinoma with moderate gland involvement. Chest x-ray was negative.

Fig. 21. A and **B**, Cell spreads. Squamous cell cancer fragments are seen. Cellular borders are moderately distinct, and there is abortive pearl formation (**A**). **C** and **D**, Tissue sections. In situ squamous cell carcinoma is present, mostly on surface, with moderate gland involvement. Cells on surface (**D**) are also pyknotic, with tailing and keratinization. (Hematoxylin and eosin; **C**, x56.)

21

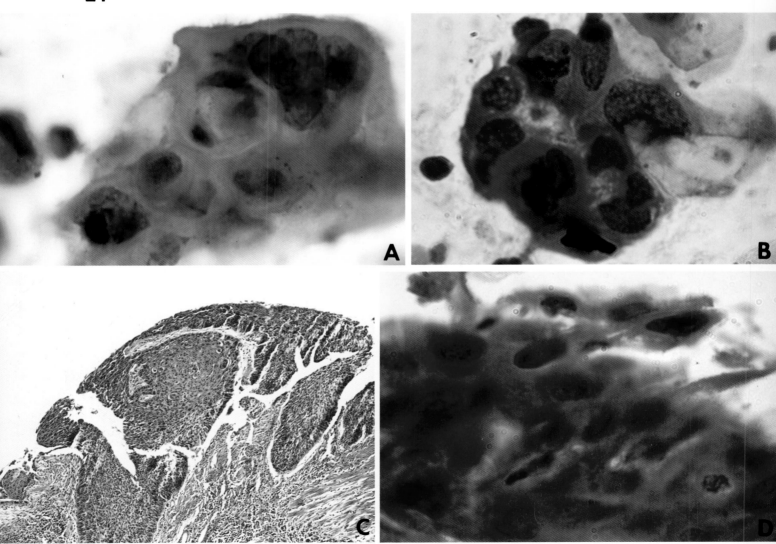

Case 5 (Fig. 22 and 23)

Squamous cell carcinoma in situ on surface
with minimal gland involvement. Chest x-ray
was negative.

Fig. 22. A through **K**, Cell spreads. Small (**A-E**) and
larger (**F-K**) cells are characteristic of in situ squamous
cell carcinoma, with basically rounded nuclei, granular
chromatin, and undulation of chromatinic rim.
Hyperchromasia is due mainly to varying degrees of
karyopyknosis. There is some cytoplasmic tailing (**E**, **K**),
acidophilia (**A**, **B**, **E-I**), and ecto-endoplasmic
dyskeratosis (**J**).

22

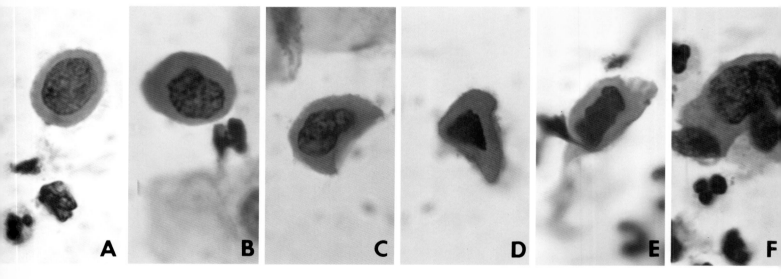

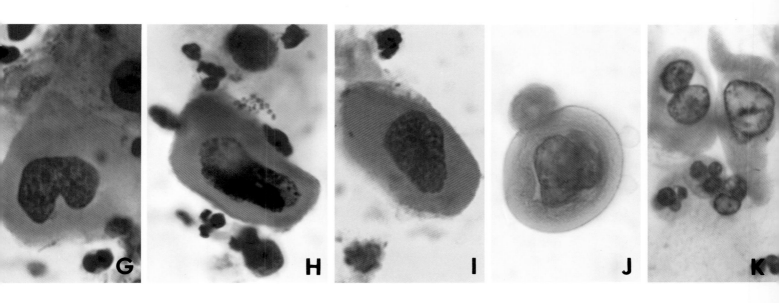

Fig. 23. A through **D**, Cell spreads. Essentially rounded nuclei with undulation are seen. There are cellular features suggesting an impending prophase (**C**), with coarse chromatin granularity, parachromatin clearing, uniform distribution, and disappearance of chromatinic rim in many areas about nuclear membrane. There is multinucleation (**D**) but with degeneration and nuclear wrinkling. Note abortive cytoplasmic tail formation (**A**, **D**) and small tissue fragment (**C**). **E** and **F**, Tissue sections. In situ squamous cell carcinoma appears mainly on surface, with only minimal superficial gland involvement. At lumen (**F**), numerous cells show varying degrees of keratinization. (Hematoxylin and eosin; **E**, x56.)

23

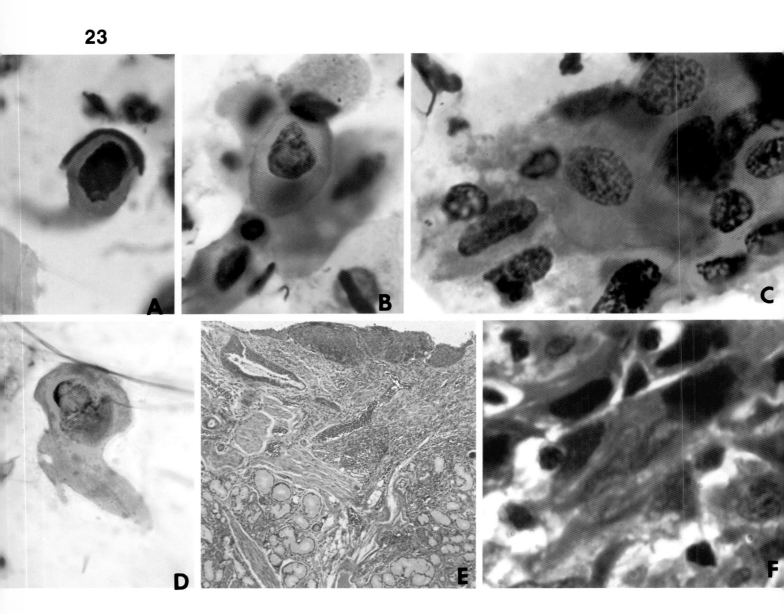

Part IV: Developing Squamous Cell Carcinoma and Squamous Epithelial Atypias

For a better understanding of the cytologic findings that represent less than unequivocal cancer, three degrees of cellular **atypia** are recognized. They have been designated **marked** (grave, suspicious), **moderate**, and **slight** (mild).

Columnar cellular atypias occur in various epithelial injuries and repair (see Fig. 2 through 4). They may also be observed in the early stages of squamous metaplasia, in which both columnar and squamous features can occur together (see Fig. 2 through 4, 24, 27, 28, and 30), and in well-differentiated adenocarcinomas. Atypical columnar cells tend to have eccentric nuclei or prominent nucleoli.

In most instances, however, the term "atypia" is applied specifically to **squamous** cells and indicates that an epithelial abnormality of at least the specified degree of severity is present. A more serious degree of atypia or even frank cancer may be present but not detectable because of poor preservation of the specimen or too few significant cells. Thus, observations of increasing degrees of atypia in successive specimens (Fig. 24 through 26) may simply reflect improved sampling of sputum or bronchial secretion rather than actual progression of disease.

Alterations in the nucleus provide the most reliable evidence of changing degrees of cellular atypia. With increasing atypia, the nucleus itself tends to remain basically round, but the nuclear membrane becomes more severely undulated, and the chromatinic rim thickens uniformly. The chromatin becomes more hyperchromatic and coarsely granular, and the parachromatin clears. Nucleoli are usually absent, and their presence would suggest either misidentification of a columnar cell or invasive cancer. The nucleo-cytoplasmic ratio tends to increase with increasing degrees of atypia, but abundant squamous cytoplasm may still be present.

Atypical functional differentiation may occur, particularly in the more severe atypias. Such abnormalities as tail formation, pearl formation, ecto-endoplasm, and keratinizing granules may be seen. Atypical squamous cells are usually found singly, but small tissue fragments do occur in the more severe degrees.

Squamous **metaplasia** is best identified cytologically when the cytoplasm of the cell is functionally differentiated into a thin squame (see Fig. 25C), which is typically smaller than a normal squamous cell (see Fig. 1A). When immature or only moderately mature, the metaplastic cell does not exhibit squamous thinning and approaches the proportions of a parabasal cell (see Fig. 25A).

Case 6 (Fig. 24 through 26)

Slight atypia progressing to cancer in 19 months. Initial cytologic screening showed slight atypia (Fig. 24A-D). Frequent examinations over the next 19 months revealed increasing degrees of atypia.(Fig. 24E, F; 25). Twenty months after initial screening, cancer was diagnosed cytologically (Fig. 26), and in situ squamous cell carcinoma of right upper lobe was identified. Chest x-rays were persistently negative.

Fig. 24. A through **D**, Initial sputum specimen. Diagnostic of at least slight squamous atypia, this sample had few significant cells, all of which are shown. Single cells with hyperchromatic nuclei suggest columnar atypia by eccentric position of nucleus (**A-C**) and by nucleoli (**A**, **B**). However, cytoplasmic ecto- endoplasm (**B**) suggests squamous differentiation. Extremely small cells (**D**) are often shed in minor inflammatory atypias. Features suggesting a more severe lesion include nuclear irregularities not facing cytocentrum (**C**), irregular chromatin (**B**, **C**), and nucleus "hugging" cell membrane (**A**).

24

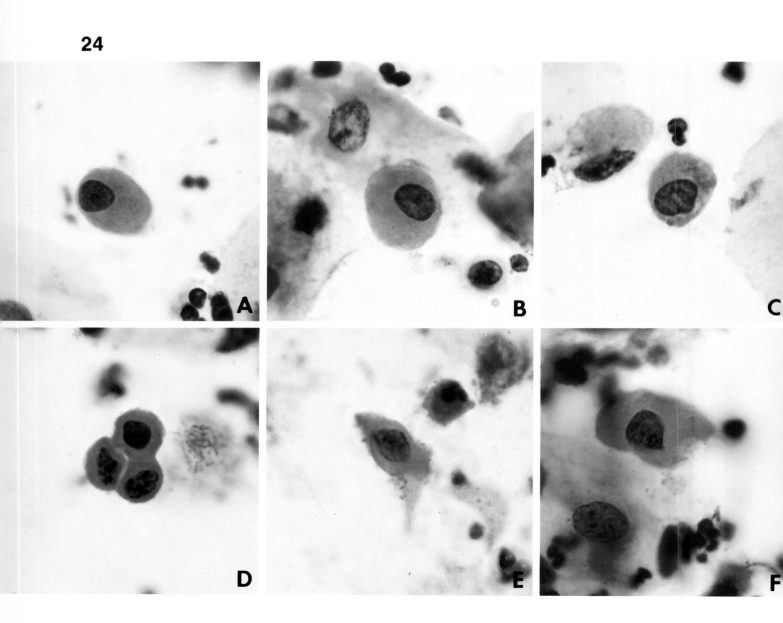

Fig. 24E and **F** and **25A** through **F**. Sputum during subsequent 19 months. Moderate atypia was diagnosed (Fig. 24**E**, **F**; 25**A-C**) and, eventually, marked atypia (Fig. 25**D-F**). Nuclear membrane is irregular (Fig. 24**F**; 25**B**, **E**) and sharply spiculated (Fig. 25**E**). There are modest chromatin clumping (Fig. 24**E**, **F**; 25**B**, **D**, **F**) and abnormal parachromatin clearing (Fig. 24**F**; 25**A**, **B**, **D**, **F**), but karyopyknosis and degeneration have blurred discriminating criteria. Note abnormal cytoplasmic tailing (Fig. 24**E**) and two tissue fragments (Fig. 25**B**, **F**), with keratinizing granule and abortive pearl formation (Fig. 25**F**). Background is mildly inflammatory.

25

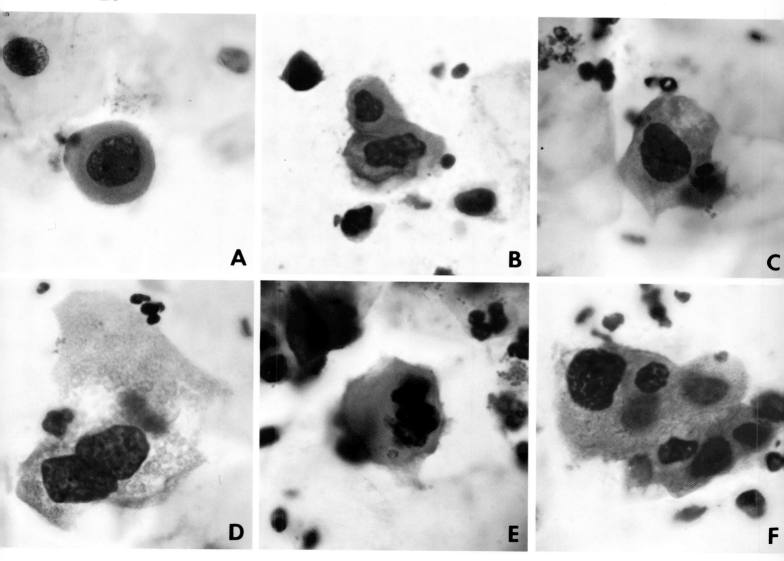

Fig. 26. A and **B**, Sputum 20 months after initial screening. Extreme nuclear irregularity and atypical pearl (**B**) are seen; note nuclear bridge. Considering all material from all specimens (Fig. 24-26), this is diagnostic of cancer. Cell configuration, along with tissue fragments, minimal inflammatory background, and absence of tumor necrosis, strongly suggests in situ carcinoma (**A**, x125). **C** and **D**, Tissue sections. Segmental bronchus has heavily keratinizing surface with in situ squamous cell carcinoma on left and glandular involvement on right. Nuclei on surface of malignant epithelium (**D**) are pyknotic and markedly hyperchromatic, with keratinization and pearl formation. (Hematoxylin and eosin; **C**, x56.)

26

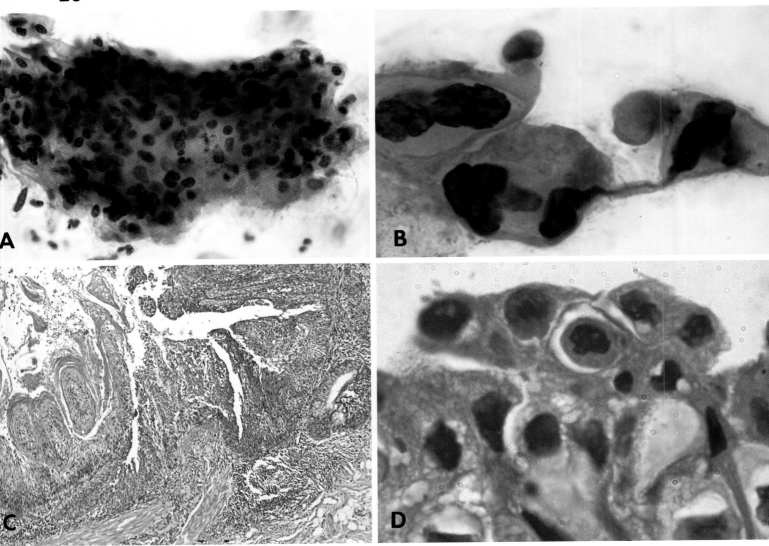

Case 7 (Fig. 27)

Moderate atypia persisted without essential change during frequent cytologic examinations over 20 months. Chest x-rays have been negative.

Fig. 27. A through **H**, Rounded cells with hyperchromasia, moderate nuclear membrane undulation, and irregularity of chromatin pattern (**C**, **H**). Small tissue fragment is seen (**A**) with degenerated and pyknotic nuclei. Most cells show apparent squamous differentiation of keratinizing cytoplasm, with suggestion of tail formation that could be either degenerative (**G**) or a distorted columnar cell (**H**). Columnar cell is also suggested by cytoplasmic vacuolation (**E**).

27

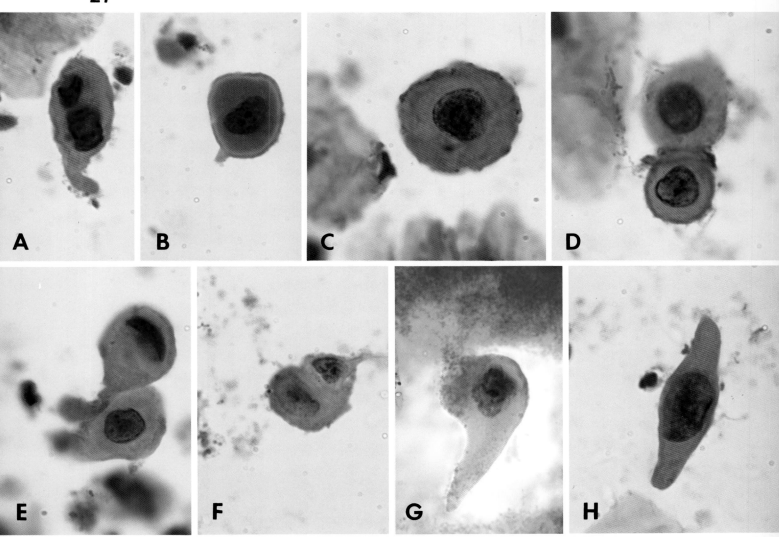

Case 8 (Fig. 28 and 29)

Moderate atypia persisting without essential
change during frequent cytologic
examinations over 38 months. Chest x-rays
have remained negative.

Fig. 28A through **F** and **29A** through **E**. Nuclei are
basically round. Moderate hyperchromasia, undulation,
and chromatin granularity are present (Fig. 28; 29**C**).
There is definite tail formation, with ecto-endoplasm
and Herxheimer's spiral (Fig. 29**E**), which indicates

28

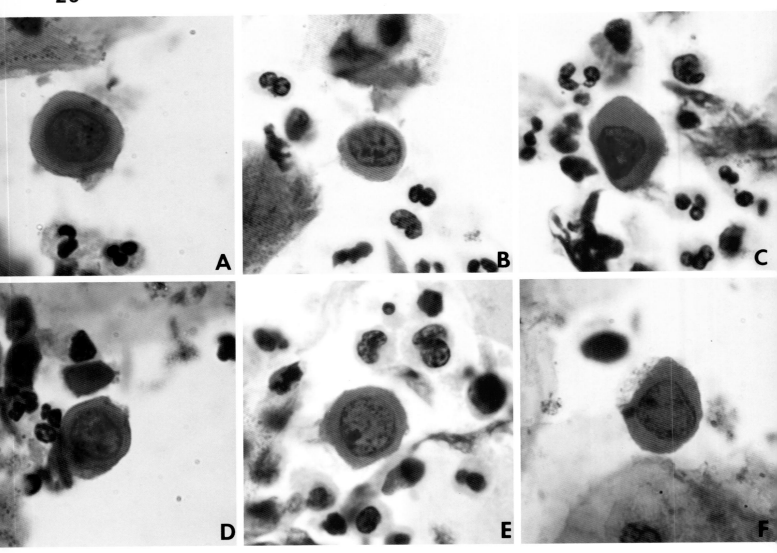

squamous differentiation. Nucleoli (Fig. 28**D**, **E**; 29**B**, **C**) and abortive tailing (Fig. 29**A**, **B**, **D**) suggest columnar cell. Background is inflammatory and somewhat necrotic.

29

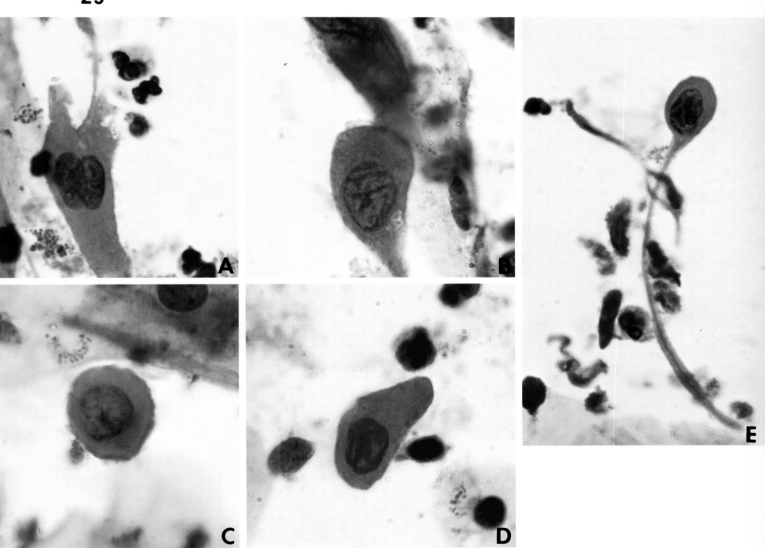

Case 9 (Fig. 30)

Slight atypia was persistent without essential change during 3 years of periodic cytologic examinations. Chest x-ray was repeatedly negative.

Fig. 30. A through **F**, Cells are basically smaller than preceding ones, with high nucleo-cytoplasmic ratios. There is hyperchromasia but with pronounced chromatinic degeneration. Abortive tailing (**C**) may be degenerative. Prominent nucleoli (**A-C**, **E**) suggest columnar cell. Background is inflammatory.

30

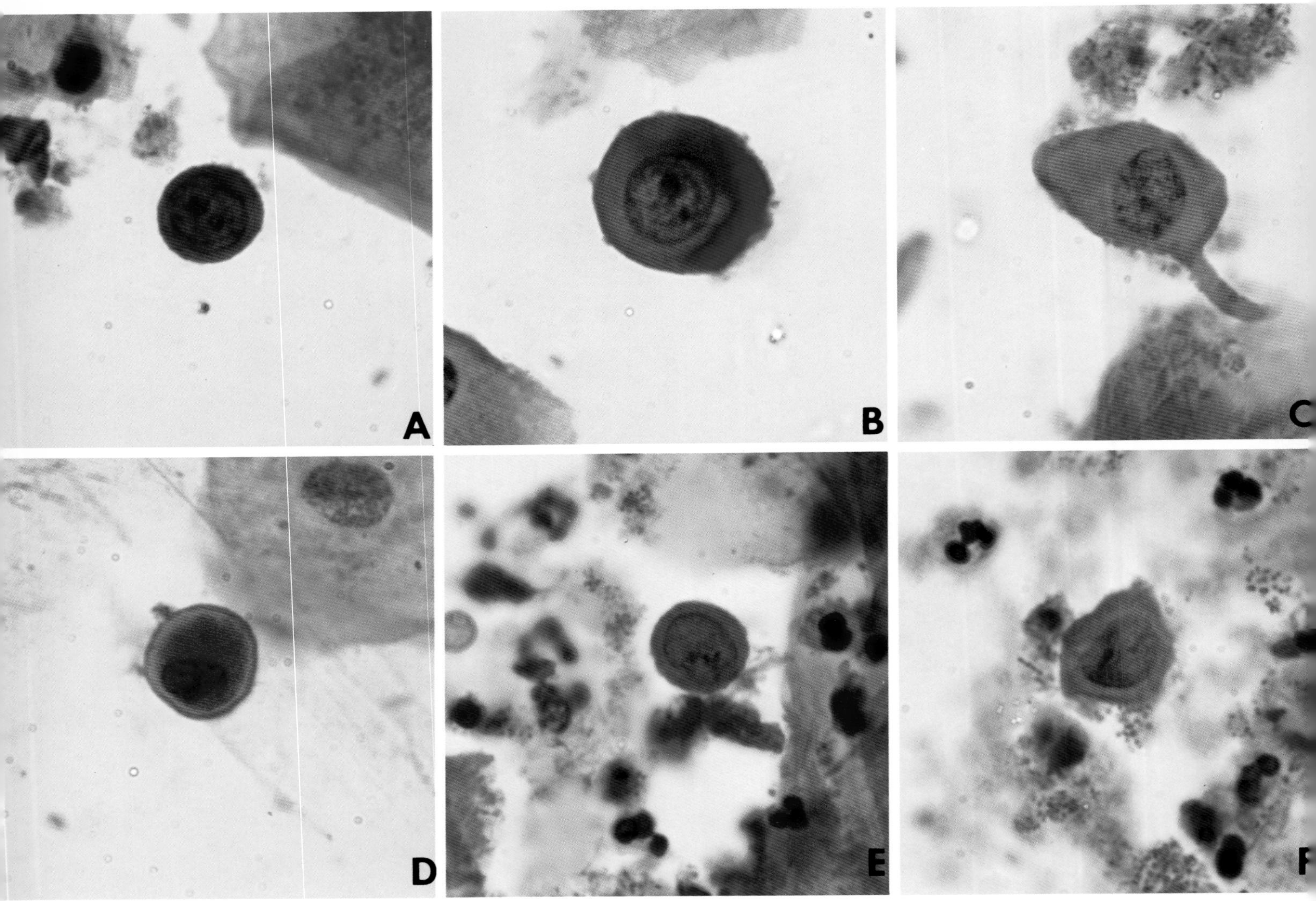

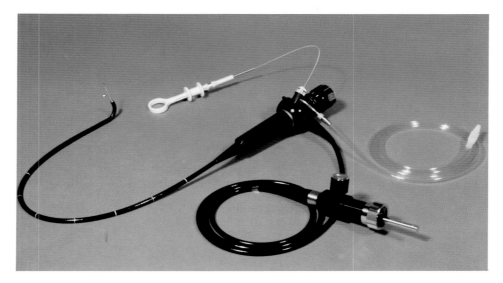

BRONCHOSCOPY

Bernard R. Marsh, M.D.

David R. Sanderson, M.D.

Nael Martini, M.D.

Fig. 1. Fiberoptic bronchoscope. (Courtesy of Olympus Corporation of America, New Hyde Park, New York.)

The challenge of discovering the source of cancer cells in the sputum of patients with negative chest radiographs has long interested bronchoscopists. Until recently, however, such lesions could often not be found until after months or even years of observation and study. Only since 1970 in the United States have instruments and techniques become available which allow successful localization of nearly all such tumors, which are almost invariably of the squamous cell type.

The dramatic impact of the flexible fiberbronchoscope (Fig. 1) has clearly been demonstrated, and nowhere more importantly than in the study of "occult" bronchogenic carcinoma.

This section will summarize some of the more important aspects of the endoscopic search for these tumors, with illustrations of their location and appearance.

Technique

Any investigation of radiographically inapparent tumors is incomplete without a careful search of the upper respiratory tract. Asymptomatic lesions of the nasopharynx, larynx, and even esophagus may exfoliate malignant cells into the sputum. Bronchoscopy in these patients often yields no carcinoma cells, yet the postbronchial sputum remains "positive."

Anesthesia for bronchoscopy may be either local or general. The more detailed studies may be time-consuming, and therefore general anesthesia is desirable both for the patient's comfort and to allow the retrieval of "uncontaminated" cytologic specimens from numerous areas.

A view of the trachea and major bronchi with open-tube instruments should quickly rule in or out the presence of significant lesions in these areas and thereby determine the need for detailed segmental studies with flexible instruments.

The preferred method for introducing the fiberscope is via a 9- or 10-mm endotracheal tube with a "T" adapter attached to its proximal end (Fig. 2). This system allows for simultaneous administration of oxygen and any anesthetic agents desired. Other advantages include better specimen retrieval, an unhurried procedure, and ready access to the lens of the scope for cleaning.

Observations

A detailed, systematic study of every bronchial segment is then undertaken. Each segmental bronchus is explored as far distally as possible. Usually, the subsegmental bronchi and the subsubsegmental bronchial spurs can be identified.

Radiographically occult cancers cover a spectrum from large and friable tumors involving major bronchi to invisible areas of in situ carcinoma within tiny subsegmental bronchi (Cases, 1-23). Between these extremes are tumors exhibiting the following characteristics: (1) slight mucosal pallor, capillary irregularity, or hyperemia; (2) slight mucosal roughening or localized friability;

2

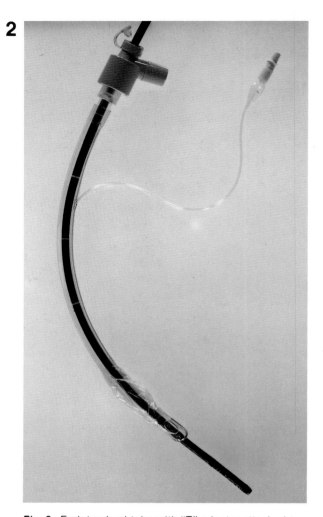

Fig. 2. Endotracheal tube with "T" adapter attached to proximal end of tube and distal inflatable "cuff." Flexible fiberoptic bronchoscope has been inserted through the tube.

(3) slight thickening of a spur, especially segmental or subsegmental; and (4) slight narrowing or even stenosis of an orifice.

With more advanced tumors, one may find an endobronchial mass with bronchial obstruction and ulceration.

3

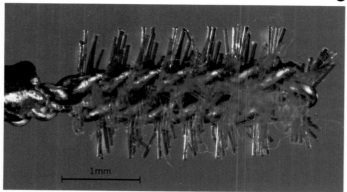

Fig. 3. Distal end of brush for use with fiberscope. (Markings below figure indicate millimeters.)

4

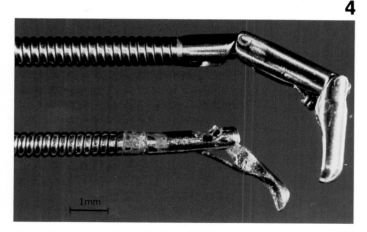

Fig. 4. Distal ends of double-hinged (**Upper**) and single-hinged (**Lower**) endobronchial curettes.

5

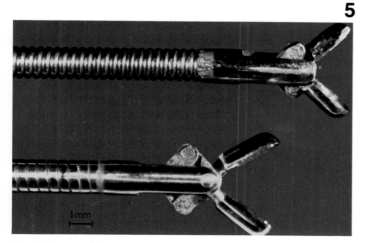

Fig. 5. Types of flexible fiberoptic biopsy forceps.

Many occult cancers are found in the upper lobes, where the flexible bronchoscope provides not only access to the area but also the illumination and magnification necessary to allow appreciation of subtle changes that are not otherwise apparent.

An advanced lesion may be found in a few moments, but a careful search of **all** bronchial segments is essential, because there may be another lesion elsewhere. In a series of 50 patients with occult primary bronchogenic carcinomas, 7 were found to harbor two or more noncontiguous lesions.

Specimens

The visual examination is completed before specimens are obtained. If a definite lesion is found, it is left until last to be brushed and biopsied. This reduces the problem of cross-contamination when multifocal disease is being searched for, and it postpones troublesome bleeding until the visual study has been completed.

If no tumor is visible, sequential brushings are obtained from all segments and subsegments in each lobe of the lungs (Fig. 3). The bronchoscopic channel is first cleaned by aspirating balanced salt solution through it. A brush is then inserted into the channel and the bronchoscope is placed within a lobar bronchus. The brush is passed out of the instrument and into all visible bronchi. The brush is then brought back to the bronchoscope and both are carefully removed. The specimen is dislodged and the brush is removed. The instrument channel is again cleaned and a new brush is put in place before the next lobe is studied. Such a detailed study may not be required in every case, but it is clearly useful in detecting endoscopically inapparent squamous cell carcinoma in situ.

After the brushing procedure, curettings and biopsy specimens are obtained. These specimens help to confirm the localization. More recently introduced curettes are much larger than previously available instruments and provide material of excellent quality for cytologic examination (Fig. 4).

Large biopsy forceps have been introduced which yield superior specimens (Fig. 5).

Biopsy specimens are obtained from all suspicious areas and may also be taken from random segments if necessary. Multiple specimens from brush, curette, and biopsy forceps greatly improve the diagnostic yield in these procedures when large surface areas must be studied.

Repeated observations have shown that in situ carcinoma may extend from a small segmental tumor well into a lobar or even into a main-stem bronchus. Neoplastic changes may be so subtle that they escape the eye of the bronchoscopist, and biopsy specimens should be obtained from the lobar spur and even from the tracheal bifurcation to aid in determining safe margins for bronchial resection. Currently available microforceps are not entirely suitable for this purpose, but better instruments will become available in the future, as larger instrument channels are provided. Open-tube bronchoscopes currently provide the best specimens for this purpose.

Legends—Cases

In each of the 23 cases that follow, the tracheobronchial diagrams are oriented as though the patient were standing and facing the viewer. The arrows in the diagrams indicate the position and direction of view of the distal tip of the bronchoscope. The endoscopic photographs and sketches depict the field of vision and the salient observations from the point of each arrow.

Case 1

A 46-year-old man was referred after repeated bronchoscopy failed to establish the source of carcinoma cells in his sputum. The chest x-ray was normal. Note the smooth, reflective surface of the right middle-lobe spur contrasted with the roughened, slightly thickened spur of the bronchus to the superior segment of the lower lobe (RB6), where a biopsy demonstrated squamous cell carcinoma in situ.

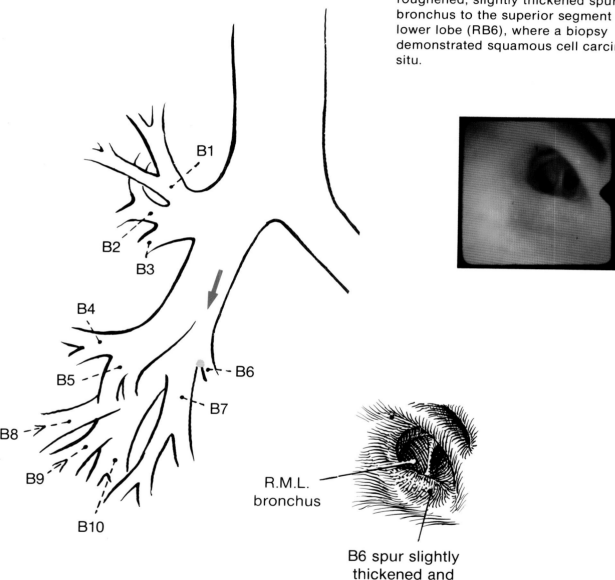

B1

B2

B3

B4

B5

B6

B7

B8

B9

B10

R.M.L. bronchus

B6 spur slightly thickened and roughened

Case 2

A 54-year-old patient had sputum-diagnosed squamous cell carcinoma but no tumor was evident on the chest x-ray. A detailed fiberoptic study revealed only a slightly thickened and nodular apical-posterior segmental spur (LB1-2) which proved to represent squamous cell carcinoma in situ. (From Marsh BR, Frost JK, Erozan YS, et al: Flexible fiberoptic bronchoscopy: Its place in the search for lung cancer. Ann Otol Rhinol Laryngol 82:757-764, 1973. By permission of Annals Publishing Company.)

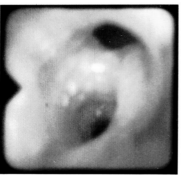

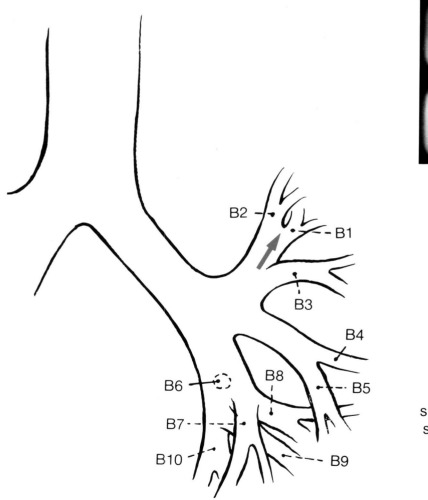

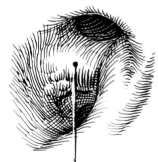

Slightly thickened spur with cobblestone surface — carcinoma in situ

Case 3

A 47-year-old man had carcinoma cells in his sputum, but a chest x-ray did not reveal a lesion. At fiberbronchoscopy, a tiny, friable lesion was found at the subsegmental level within the bronchus to the anterior segment of the left upper lobe (LB3). Note the thickened spur. Biopsy demonstrated squamous cell carcinoma.

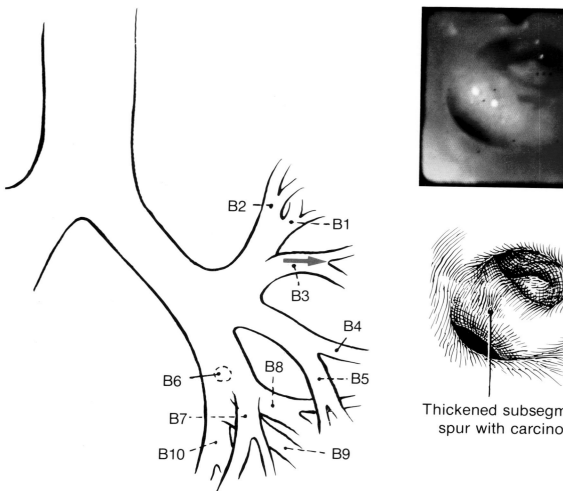

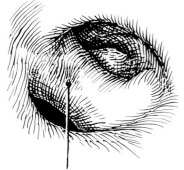

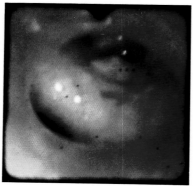

Thickened subsegmental spur with carcinoma

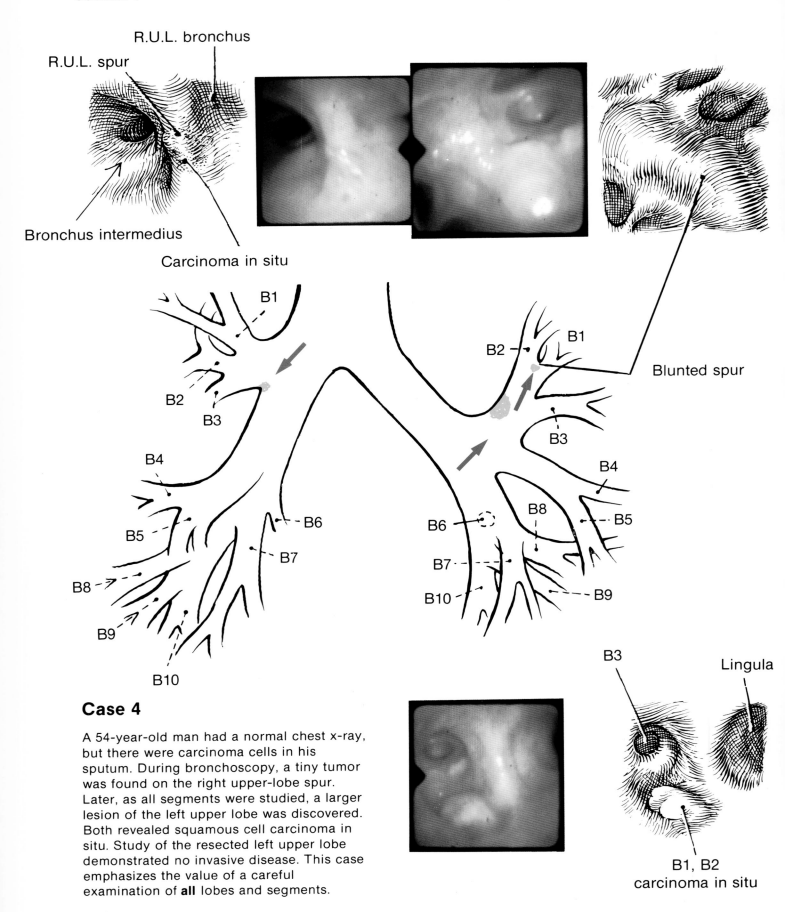

R.U.L. spur

R.U.L. bronchus

Bronchus intermedius

Carcinoma in situ

Blunted spur

B1

B2

B3

B4

B5

B6

B7

B8

B9

B10

B1

B2

B3

B4

B5

B6

B7

B8

B9

B10

B3

Lingula

B1, B2
carcinoma in situ

Case 4

A 54-year-old man had a normal chest x-ray, but there were carcinoma cells in his sputum. During bronchoscopy, a tiny tumor was found on the right upper-lobe spur. Later, as all segments were studied, a larger lesion of the left upper lobe was discovered. Both revealed squamous cell carcinoma in situ. Study of the resected left upper lobe demonstrated no invasive disease. This case emphasizes the value of a careful examination of **all** lobes and segments.

Case 5

A 54-year-old man underwent bronchoscopy because of a negative chest x-ray and sputum containing squamous carcinoma cells. No tumor was observed, but slight pallor of the right lateral and posterior basilar bronchial region was noted. Biopsy from this spur (B9-10) showed squamous cell carcinoma in situ. Lobectomy was

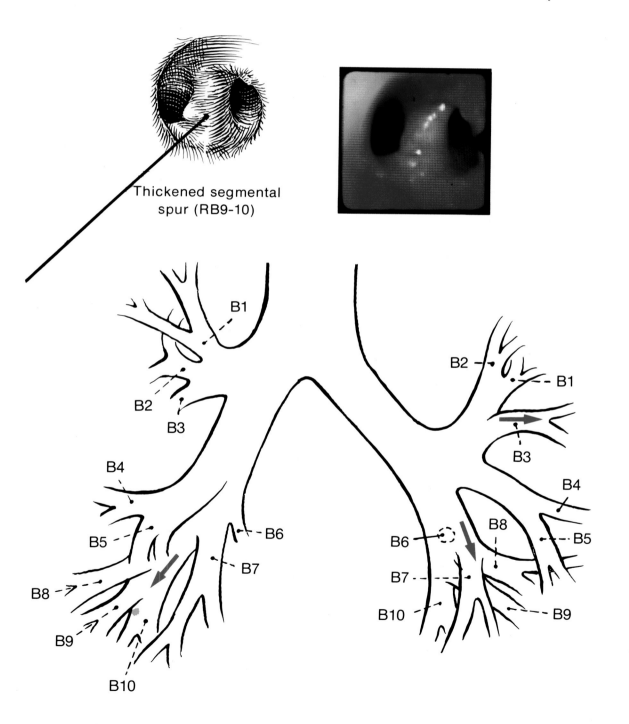

Thickened segmental
spur (RB9-10)

performed, and a 2-mm invasive squamous cancer was found, together with two additional, noncontiguous sites of carcinoma in situ. The patient returned to cigarette smoking, and 4 years later his sputum again was positive for carcinoma cells. At bronchoscopy, biopsy of a thickened, subsegmental spur in the anterior segment of the left upper lobe (LB3) disclosed squamous cell carcinoma. Carcinoma in situ was also detected in a biopsy specimen from the left anteromedial basal bronchial spur (B7-8). (From Marsh BR, Frost JK, Erozan YS, et al: Flexible fiberoptic bronchoscopy: Its place in the search for lung cancer. Ann Otol Rhinol Laryngol 82:757-764, 1973. By permission of Annals Publishing Company.)

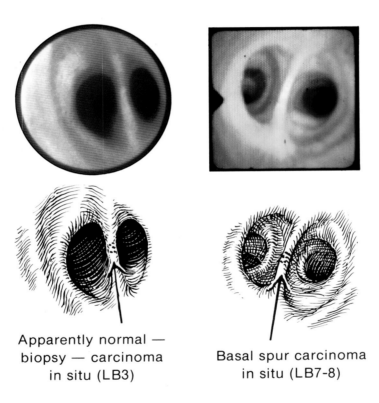

Apparently normal —
biopsy — carcinoma
in situ (LB3)

Basal spur carcinoma
in situ (LB7-8)

Case 6

A 64-year-old man underwent bronchoscopy because squamous carcinoma cells were observed in his sputum. A partial left upper lobectomy (LB1&2, 3) had been performed 4 years previously because of squamous cell carcinoma. At that time the margin of the resected bronchus showed carcinoma in situ. No new lesion was seen on the current chest x-ray. At bronchoscopy, the stump of the left upper-lobe bronchus appeared unremarkable, but the nonresected lingular bronchus (B4,B5) was narrowed and at its subsegmental level was nearly occluded by a friable mass. The surgical specimen demonstrated only squamous cell carcinoma in situ.

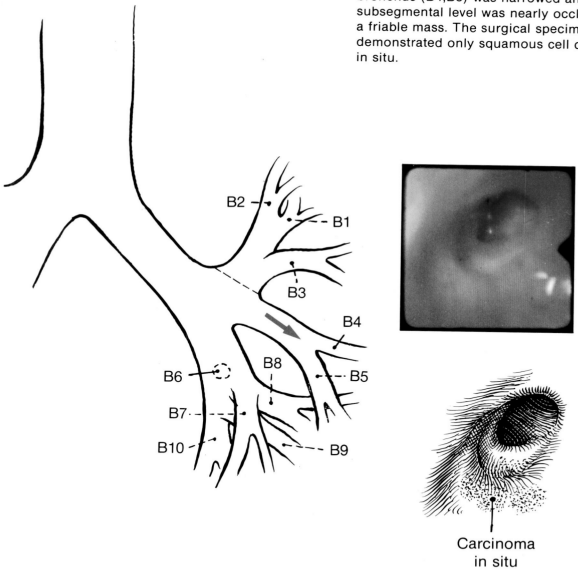

Carcinoma
in situ

Case 7

A man underwent bronchoscopy because squamous carcinoma cells had been detected in his sputum. His chest radiograph was negative. At bronchoscopy, a granular, friable mass was found in the apical and posterior bronchial segments of the right upper lobe (RB1,2). The surgical specimen demonstrated both extensive in situ squamous cell carcinoma and a small area of invasion.

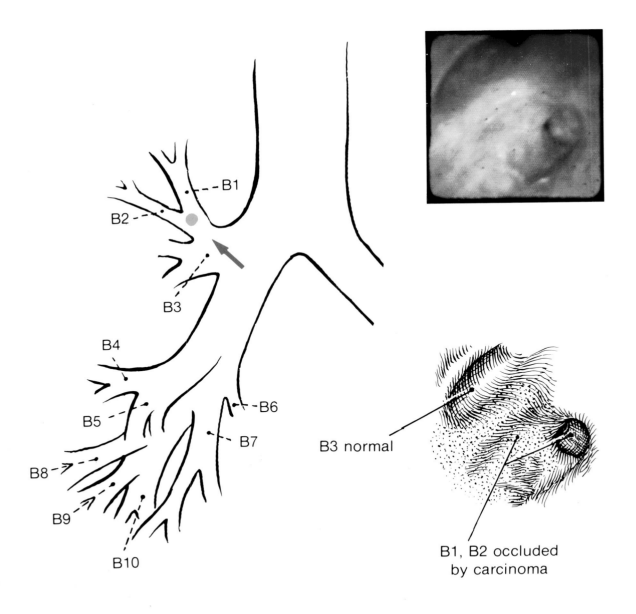

B3 normal

B1, B2 occluded by carcinoma

Case 8

A 56-year-old man had a negative chest x-ray, but there were squamous carcinoma cells in his sputum. At bronchoscopy, a lesion was demonstrated at the trifurcation level of the right upper lobe. Note the flecks of tantalum persisting from a preceding bronchogram.

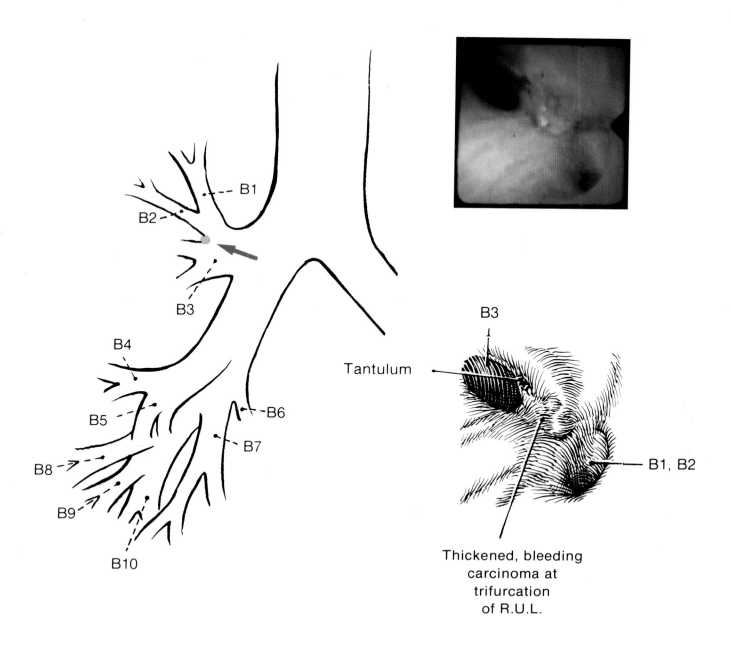

B1

B2

B3

B4

B5

B6

B7

B8

B9

B10

B3

Tantulum

B1, B2

Thickened, bleeding
carcinoma at
trifurcation
of R.U.L.

Case 9

A 54-year-old man had carcinoma cells in the sputum and a negative chest radiograph. At bronchoscopy the lingula (LB4, 5) was stenotic although patent. This large cell undifferentiated carcinoma proved unresectable because of mediastinal involvement. The case is unusual becuase large cell bronchogenic cancers seldom present as radiographically inapparent tumors.

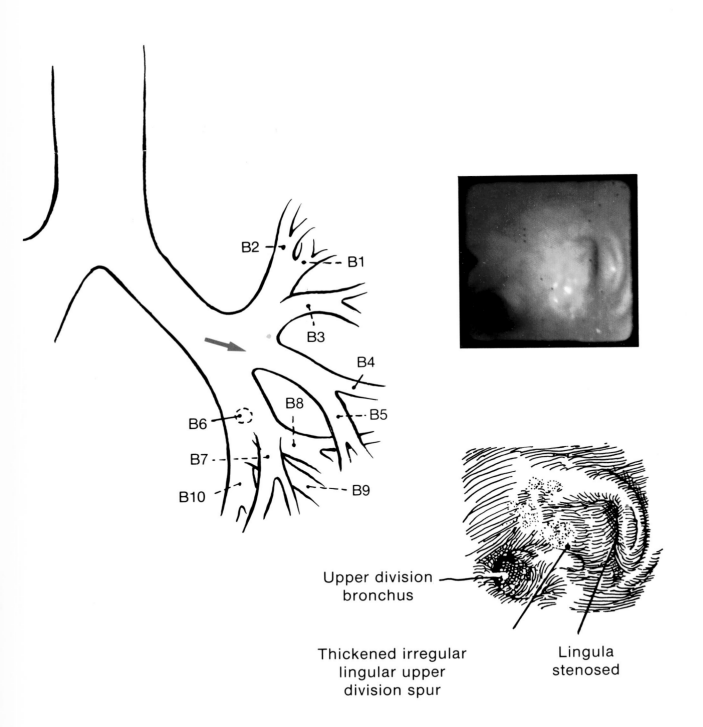

B2

B1

B3

B4

B8

B6

B5

B7

B10

B9

Upper division
bronchus

Thickened irregular
lingular upper
division spur

Lingula
stenosed

Case 10

A 63-year-old man with a history of tuberculosis was examined because a change had been observed in the region of the left hilus on chest radiography. At bronchoscopy, the upper-division bronchus on the left (LB1 & 2, 3) was nearly occluded by squamous cell carcinoma. Additional examination revealed another squamous cell carcinoma in the region of the spur of the right upper-lobe bronchus. This case demonstrates once again the value of careful, detailed inspection of the tracheobronchial tree.

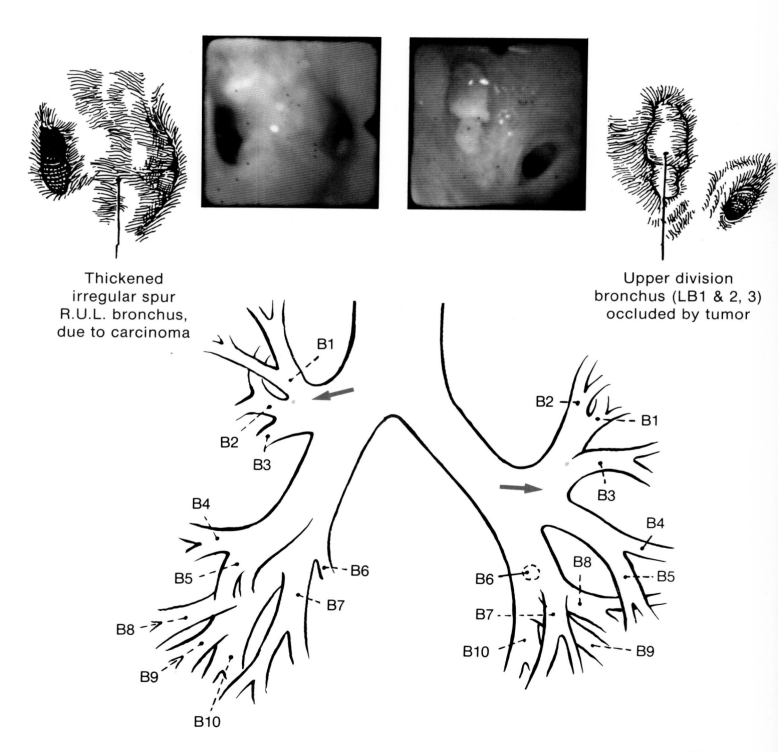

Thickened irregular spur R.U.L. bronchus, due to carcinoma

Upper division bronchus (LB1 & 2, 3) occluded by tumor

Case 11

A 66-year-old man presented with bloody sputum containing squamous cancer cells. At bronchoscopy a large tumor was observed that nearly occluded both the left upper and the left lower-lobe bronchial orifices. The original fiberbronchoscopic specimen from this large lesion did not demonstrate cancer cells. However, a tiny "in situ" squamous cell cancer was found in the right lower lobe (not photographed). A large biopsy specimen was required to prove that the tumor of the left lung was cancerous.

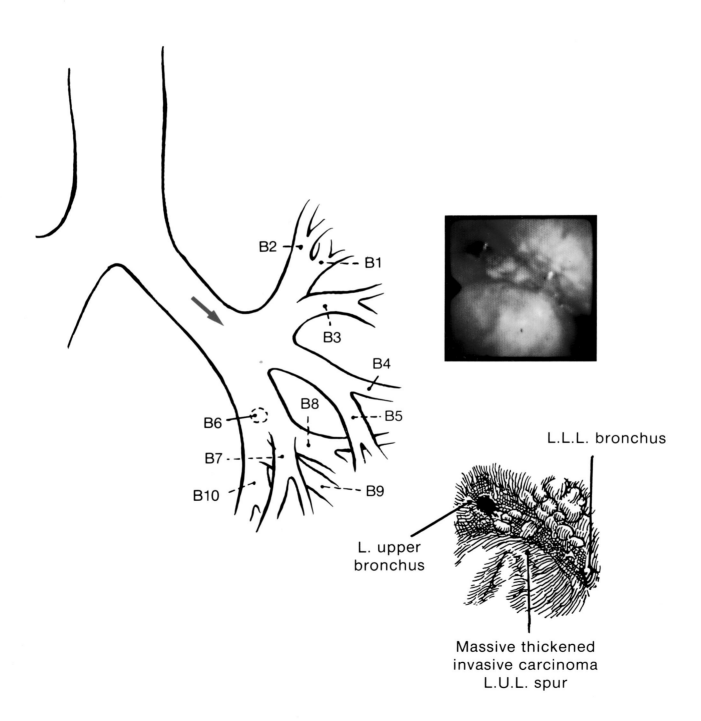

B2

B1

B3

B4

B8

B6

B5

B7

B10

B9

L.L.L. bronchus

L. upper bronchus

Massive thickened invasive carcinoma L.U.L. spur

Case 12

A 57-year-old man's chest x-ray disclosed no abnormality to suggest a source for the squamous cancer cells that were found in his sputum. Detailed bronchial brushings and biopsies identified a squamous cell carcinoma in situ involving the spur between the apical-posterior and anterior segmental bronchi of the left upper lobe (LB1 & 2-3) and extending into the LB1 & 2 segmental bronchus.

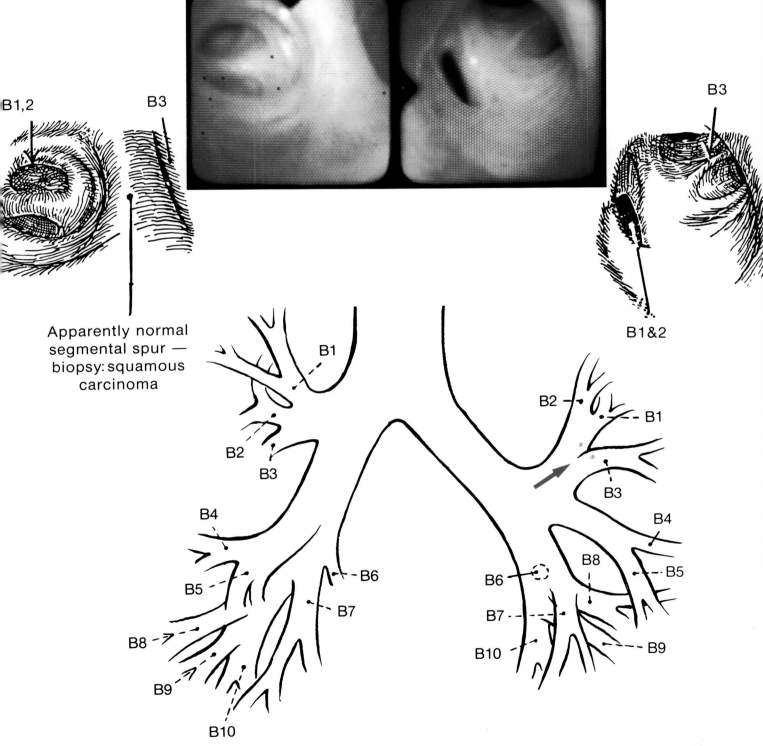

B1,2

B3

Apparently normal
segmental spur —
biopsy: squamous
carcinoma

B3

B1&2

B1

B2

B3

B4

B5

B6

B7

B8

B9

B10

B2

B1

B3

B4

B8

B5

B6

B7

B9

B10

Case 13

A 50-year-old man had had a previous right upper-lobe lobectomy for squamous cell carcinoma. Subsequently, carcinoma cells were again noted in his sputum. The posteroanterior and lateral chest x-ray films revealed no obvious new lesion, but bronchograms demonstrated a constriction in the bronchus to the anterior segment of the left upper lobe (LB3). At bronchoscopy, a friable squamous cell cancer was found at the subsegmental level in this bronchus.

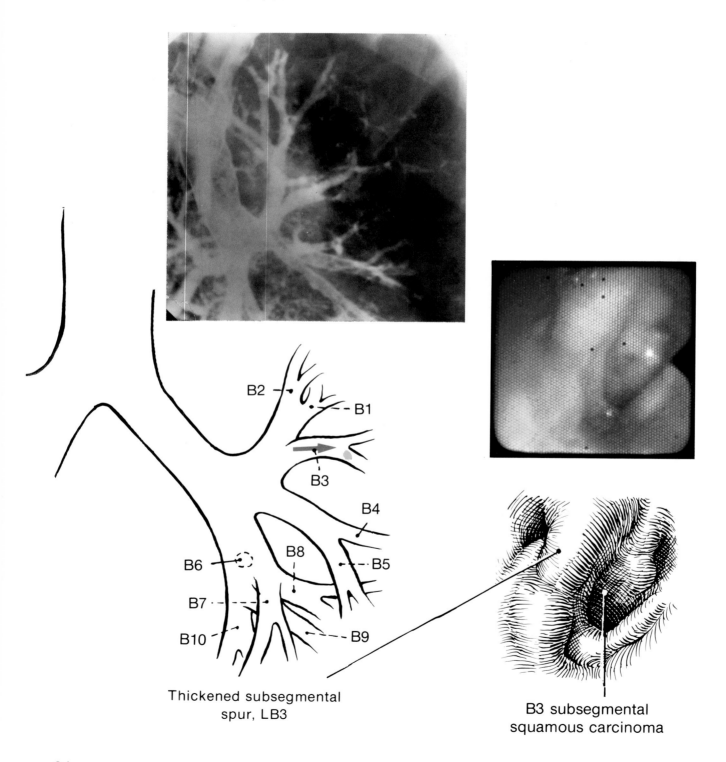

Thickened subsegmental spur, LB3

B3 subsegmental squamous carcinoma

Case 14

A 60-year-old man had squamous cancer cells in his sputum, but no lesion was evident on chest radiography. At bronchoscopy, a friable endobronchial squamous cell cancer was found at the subsegmental level in the anterior segment of the left upper lobe (LB3). This case is remarkably similar to the preceding one. Radiographically inapparent lung cancers tend to arise in the upper-lobe bronchi.

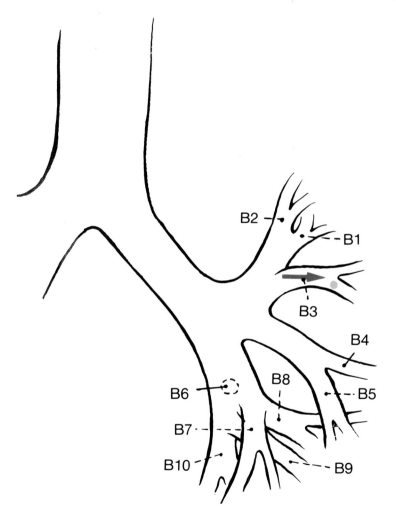

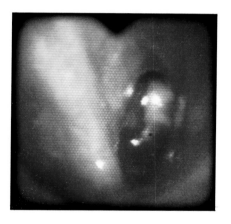

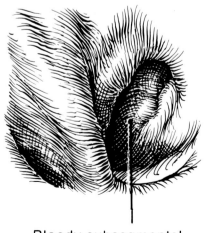

Bloody subsegmental carcinoma, LB3

Case 15

A 70-year-old man had sputum-diagnosed squamous cell carcinoma, but his chest x-ray and a bronchogram were both unrevealing. At bronchoscopy, there was mild narrowing of the right upper-lobe bronchus, but no definite tumor was evident. Brushing and biopsy of the right upper-lobe spur were both positive for squamous cell carcinoma.

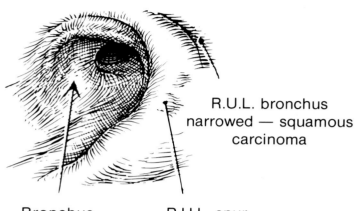

R.U.L. bronchus narrowed — squamous carcinoma

Bronchus intermedius

R.U.L. spur — squamous carcinoma

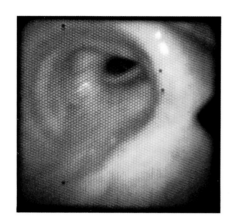

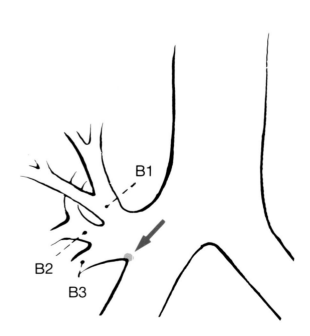

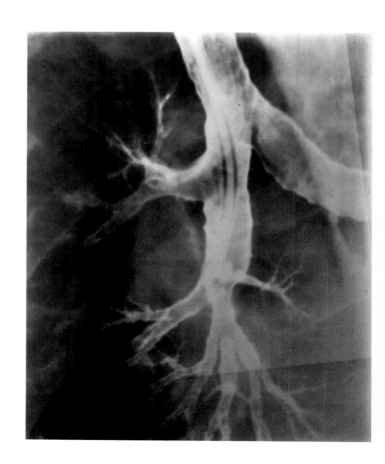

Case 16

A 62-year-old man had sputum that repeatedly disclosed markedly atypical squamous cells. His chest x-ray was unrevealing. At bronchoscopy, a slightly thickened, friable subsegmental spur was observed in the right lower lobe at the level of the anterior basal segmental bronchus

(B8 [a-b]). Also, there was a granular, friable area involving the left upper-lobe bronchus just distal to its origin from the left mainstem bronchus. Bronchoscopic biopsies proved both lesions to be squamous cell carcinoma.

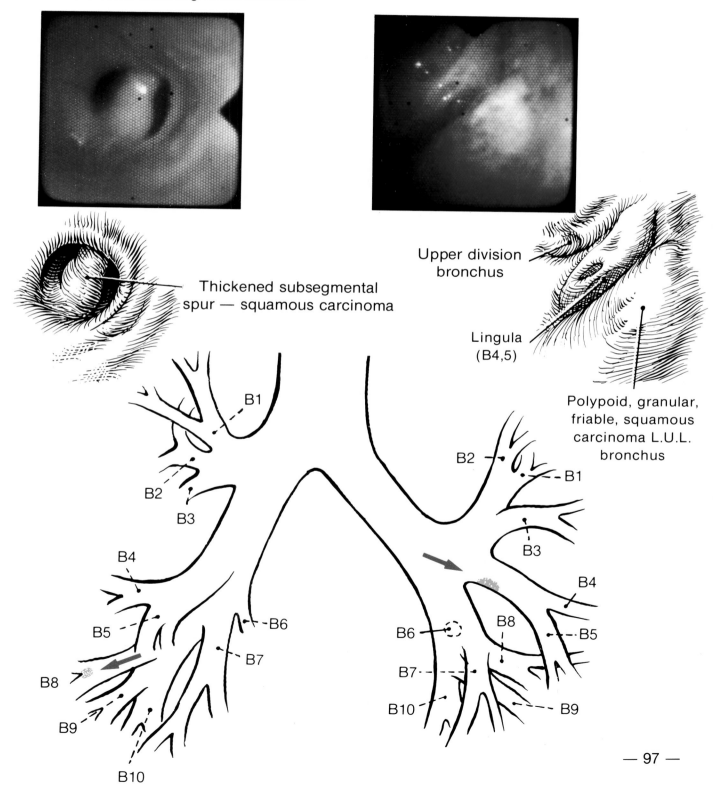

Thickened subsegmental spur — squamous carcinoma

Upper division bronchus

Lingula (B4,5)

Polypoid, granular, friable, squamous carcinoma L.U.L. bronchus

B1

B2

B3

B4

B5

B6

B7

B8

B9

B10

B2

B1

B3

B4

B5

B6

B8

B7

B10

B9

Case 17

A 68-year-old man had a past history of laryngectomy for squamous cell carcinoma. His chest x-ray was negative, but his sputum examination revealed squamous carcinoma cells. At bronchoscopy, there was a small but clearly visible, slightly polypoid tumor just proximal to the segmental spur of the lingular bronchus (LB4-5). Biopsy disclosed squamous cell cancer.

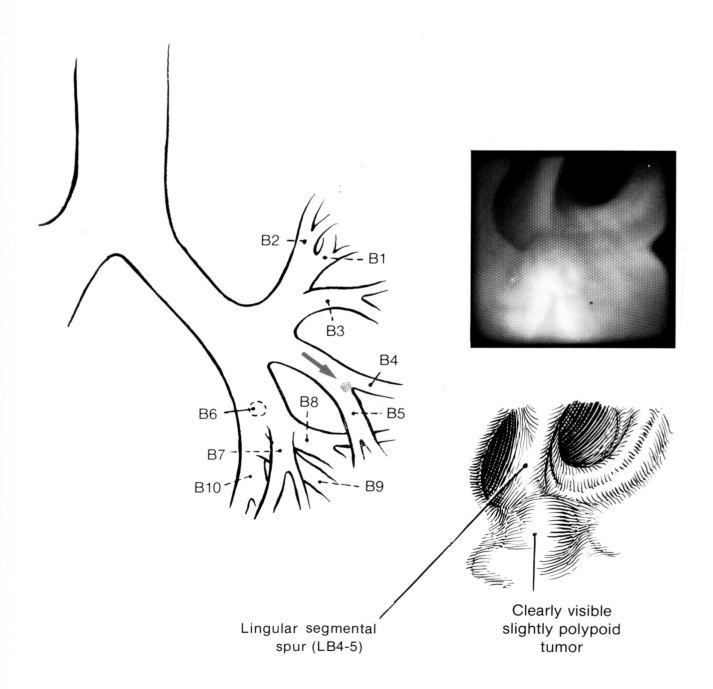

Lingular segmental spur (LB4-5)

Clearly visible slightly polypoid tumor

Case 18

A 53-year-old man had a sputum cytologic examination that revealed markedly atypical squamous cells. His x-ray was unrevealing. At bronchoscopy, there was a 1-mm, white, pimple-like elevation just inside the right upper-lobe bronchus. This was surrounded by approximately 1 cm of slightly reddened mucosa that interrupted the normal longitudinal markings of the bronchial wall. Biopsy revealed squamous cell carcinoma in situ, which was subsequently confirmed at thoracotomy.

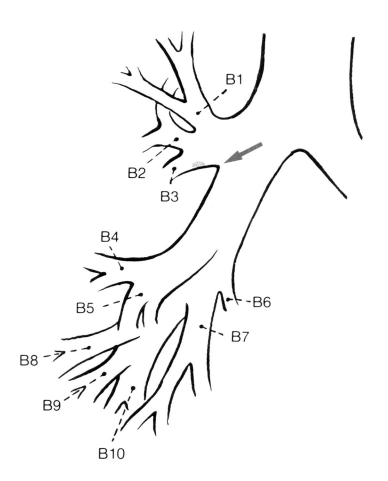

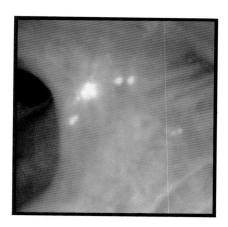

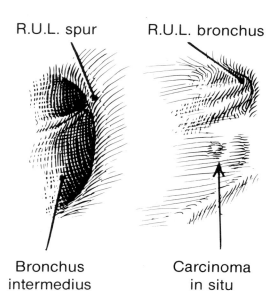

R.U.L. spur   R.U.L. bronchus

Bronchus intermedius   Carcinoma in situ

Case 19

A 53-year-old man had sputum showing squamous carcinoma cells but an x-ray that was considered negative. At bronchoscopy, no lesion was seen, but brushings from the left lower lobe were positive for squamous carcinoma cells. At a follow-up bronchoscopy, careful search of the left lower lobe (A) demonstrated no lesion, but in the anterior subsegment (LB8) of the anteromedial basal segment bronchus (LB8 & 9) an area of slight roughening was discovered (B) which proved on biopsy and subsequent surgical resection to be squamous cell carcinoma in situ.

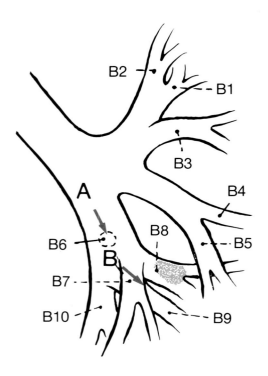

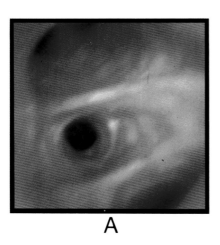

A

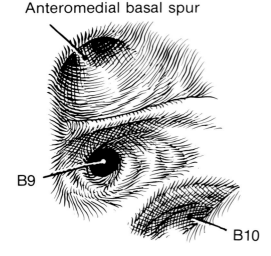

Anteromedial basal spur

B9

B10

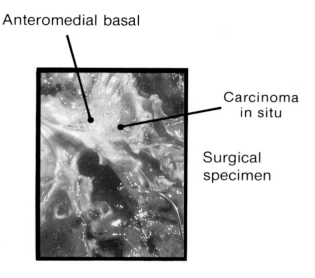

Anteromedial basal

Carcinoma
in situ

Surgical
specimen

Small focus of carcinoma
in situ interrupting
long folds

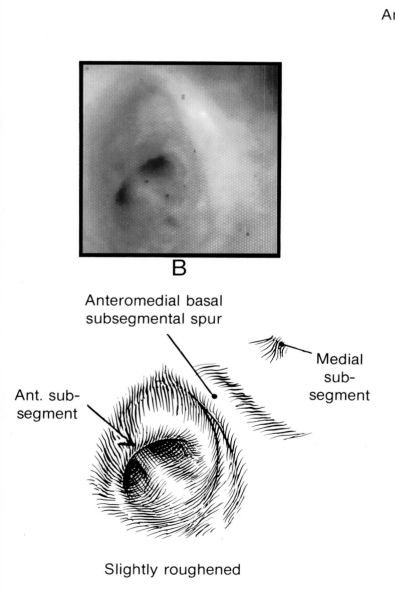

B

Anteromedial basal
subsegmental spur

Medial
sub-
segment

Ant. sub-
segment

Slightly roughened

Case 20

A 63-year-old man had a negative chest x-ray, but his sputum was positive for squamous carcinoma. In the bronchus to the anterior segment of the left upper lobe, there was blunting of the LB3 (a-b) spur with adjacent granular mucosa. The lobectomy specimen revealed squamous cell carcinoma in situ.

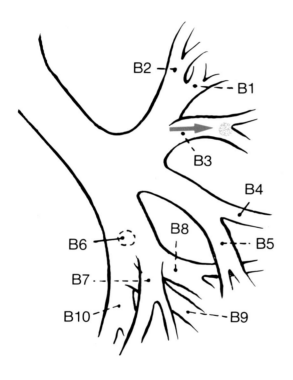

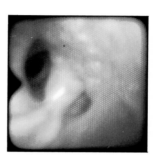

Carcinoma
in situ

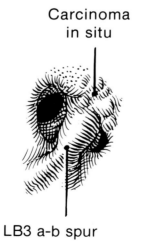

LB3 a-b spur

Case 21

A 58-year-old man had sputum that contained squamous carcinoma cells. At bronchoscopy, a polypoid tumor was found within the bronchus leading to the apical-posterior segment of the left upper lobe (LB1 & 2). Left upper lobectomy demonstrated squamous cell carcinoma in situ.

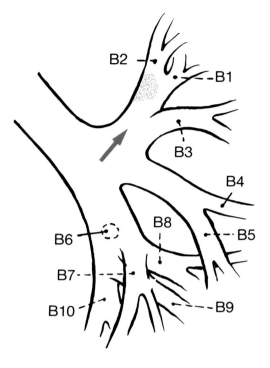

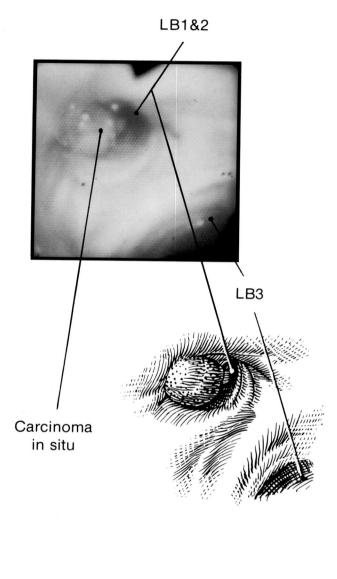

LB1&2

LB3

Carcinoma
in situ

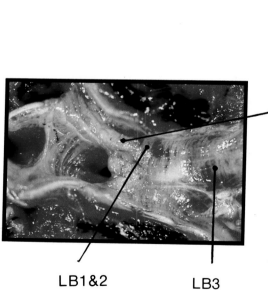

LB1&2   LB3

Case 22

A 76-year-old cigarette smoker had squamous carcinoma cells in the sputum. At bronchoscopy, a tumor was suspected in the apical segment bronchus of the right upper lobe (RB1).

Brushings and biopsy specimens were positive for carcinoma. A right upper lobectomy revealed squamous cell carcinoma in situ involving an area 1 by 0.6 cm.

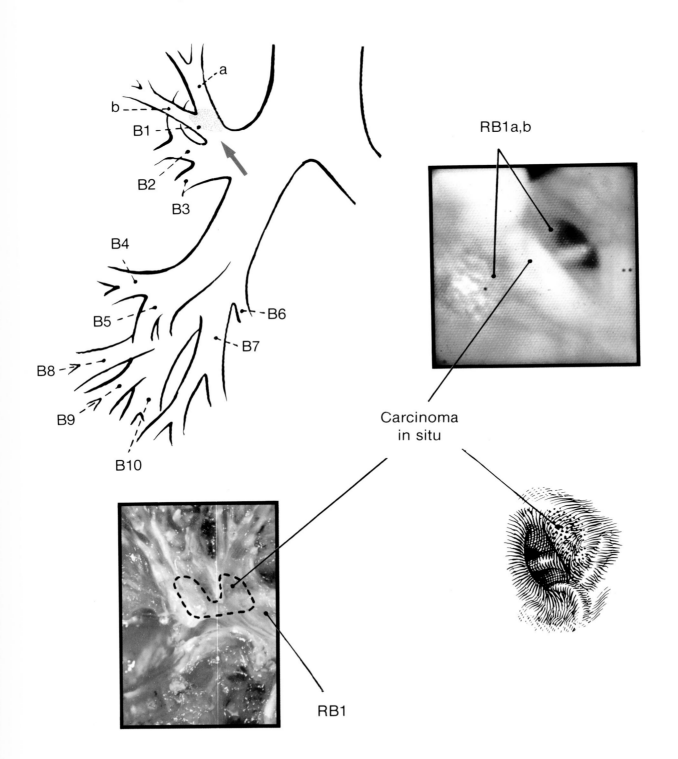

RB1a,b

Carcinoma in situ

RB1

Case 23

A 53-year-old patient had been a smoker since the age of 13. The sputum was positive for squamous carcinoma cells, but the chest radiograph was negative. At bronchoscopy, no tumor was seen, but selective brushings from the bronchus to the anterior segment of the right upper lobe (RB3) were positive on two separate occasions for squamous carcinoma. A right upper-lobe lobectomy was done. The surgical specimen revealed a well-differentiated squamous cell carcinoma in situ in RB3 measuring 1.2 by 0.8 cm.

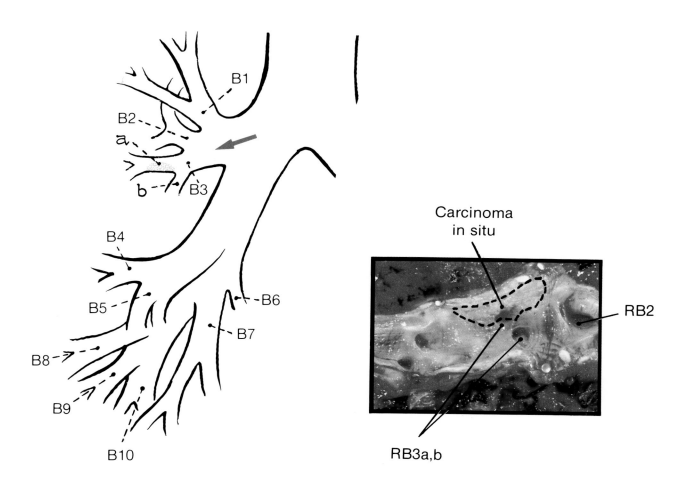

Section 5

PATHOLOGY OF CANCERS DETECTED CYTOLOGICALLY

Lewis B. Woolner, M.D.

Introduction

The cytologic and radiologic screening programs of the Cooperative Early Lung Cancer Group have permitted detection of bronchogenic carcinomas at a relatively early stage. Sputum cytology testing and chest radiography, as screening procedures, tend to be complementary in effectiveness. The roentgenologic manifestations and pathologic findings of early lung cancers detected radiologically are presented in the next Section.

Cytologic screening and bronchoscopic localization have made possible the surgical resection and pathologic documentation of radiographically inapparent, or "occult," cancers. These are mainly intrabronchial squamous cell cancers of the hilar type, and as a rule they are still in the in situ or microinvasive stage when detected.

Examination and processing of the surgical specimen of radiographically occult cancer calls for special handling by the pathologist. A number of procedures are necessary. The first of these is immediate frozen sectioning of the bronchial wall at the line of surgical resection to determine the adequacy of the bronchial margin. Next, the resected portion of the bronchial tree is carefully opened, inspected, and photographed. Later, after formalin fixation, the open bronchi are meticulously mapped, and serial block sectioning is carried out. The serial blocking should include all the visible carcinomatous area, along with a generous portion of adjacent, normal-appearing mucosa.

In the cases of occult cancer detected by the screening programs, the remainder of the opened bronchial tree is also serially blocked and is examined histologically. In the series of cases to be described, Case 1 is a typical example of occult lung cancer processed and sectioned according to the Cooperative Early Lung Cancer Group protocol.

The final pathologic report on resected specimens of occult cancers which have been processed as described includes detailed measurements of the size and location of each tumor, with a description of gross mucosal changes, if such are present. Carcinomas that are limited to surface bronchial epithelium, with or without involvement of ducts or acini of mucous glands, are classified as carcinoma in situ. Those in which the in situ surface changes are accompanied by microinvasion of the bronchial wall are classified as carcinoma in situ with microinvasion, and the depth of infiltration of the bronchial wall is indicated.

Carcinomas that are predominantly infiltrative and that have inconspicuous or absent in situ components are included under the heading "invasive carcinoma."

Mucosal abnormalities other than in situ or invasive carcinoma may be detected on complete serial block sectioning of the resected bronchi. These, including basal cell hyperplasia, squamous cell metaplasia, and focal squamous cell atypia, are listed on the final pathology report, along with the site and extent of the abnormality. The above methods and criteria were used in categorizing a series of 41 surgically resected occult cancers detected by screening. Seventeen cancers were totally in situ, 16 also demonstrated microinvasion, and 8 were frankly invasive.

All resected occult carcinomas in this series were of the squamous cell type or were squamous cell cancers with a prominent large cell undifferentiated component. There were no occult small cell cancers. All of the tumors were intrabronchial "hilar type" carcinomas with sites of origin anywhere from the tracheal bifurcation to the sub-subsegmental bronchi. The size of the occult cancers in the series varied considerably, but the majority of in situ or microinvasive cancers were very small.

Occult tumors that are entirely in situ tend to be difficult to detect on bronchoscopic inspection. In general, the more infiltrative the lesion, the more likely that it will be visible to the bronchoscopist and grossly visible to the pathologist. Data on size and visibility of the 41 resected occult tumors in the series are tabulated below.

Size and Visibility of Occult Bronchogenic Carcinoma in 41 Resected Cases

| | | Lesions visible to | | | |
| | | Pathologist | | Bronchoscopist | |
Degree of invasion	Mean diameter (range), cm	No.	(%)	No.	(%)
In situ	1.0 (0.5 - 2)	7/17	(41)	5/17	(29)
With microinvasion	2.5 (0.5 - 6)	15/16	(94)	11/16	(69)
Invasive	3.3 (2 - 4.5)	8/8	(100)	8/8	(100)

Illustrative Cases

The spectrum of pathologic findings encountered in radiographically occult bronchogenic carcinoma is illustrated by the cases that follow. The method of processing the surgical specimen is demonstrated in Case 1. The other cases show, in logical sequence, the entire diagnostic and pathologic workup, including numbers of diagnostic specimens required. Typical sputum cytologic findings on which recommendation for localizing bronchoscopy was based are demonstrated. Similarly, the brushing or biopsy data by which localization of the lesion was accomplished is presented, along with a summary of the bronchoscopic findings. The extent of surgical resection and the detailed pathologic findings in each case complete the picture.

Case 1

A 69-year-old man had left upper lobectomy 10 years previously for T1 N0 M0 stage I (AJC) squamous cell carcinoma. The postoperative follow-up chest radiograph was stable, and sputum cytology tests were negative as recently as 1 year ago.

Sputum Cytology

Tests were now positive for squamous carcinoma cells.

Localizing Bronchoscopy

No tumor was visualized. Bronchial brushings and biopsy near the line of previous surgical resection were positive for squamous cell carcinoma.

Surgery

Left lower lobectomy was performed (completion of pneumonectomy).

Pathology

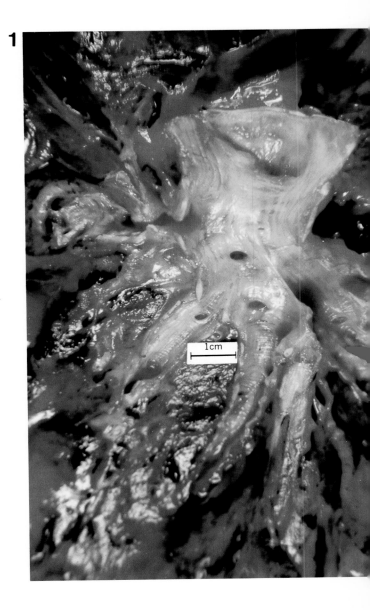

Fig. 1. Resected left lower lobe showing lower-lobe bronchus and its opened basal subdivisions. Surgical line of resection passes through left main bronchus just above fissure—site of left upper lobectomy 10 years before.

2

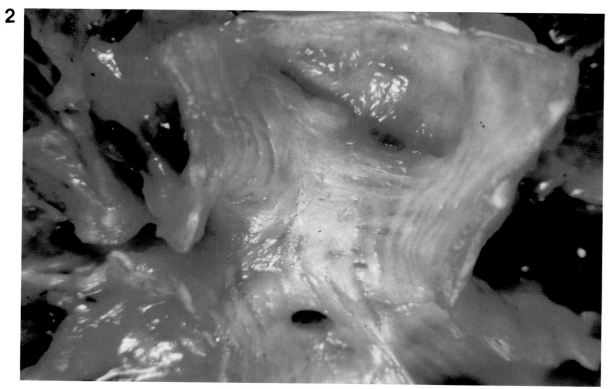

Fig. 2. Close-up view of fissure and adjacent main and lower-lobe bronchi. Biopsy site is visible just proximal to fissure. Remainder of mucosa appears normal.

3

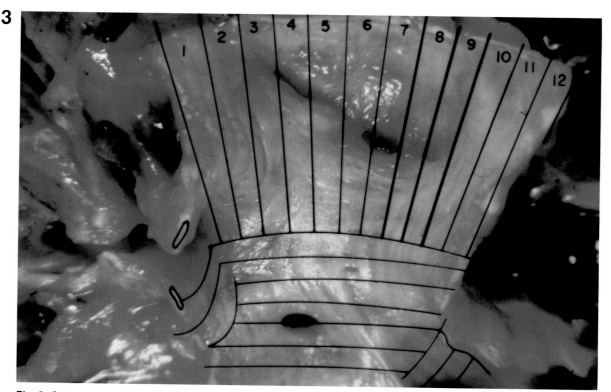

Fig. 3. Serial block sectioning of left main bronchus and area of fissure was carried out as in diagram. Remainder of bronchial tree was mapped and sectioned. Abnormal findings (see below) were limited to blocks 8 and 9.

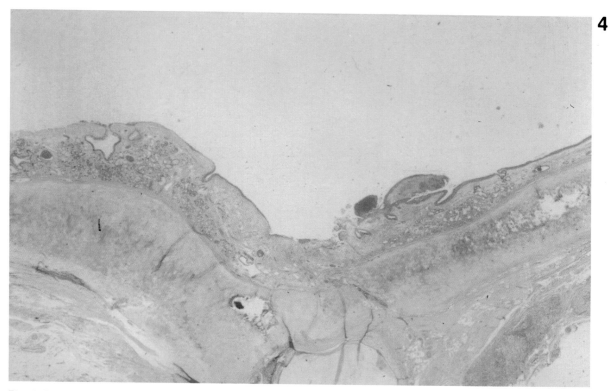

4

Fig. 4. Block 8 (see diagram) shows biopsy site with granulation tissue formation and polypoid mucosal abnormality.

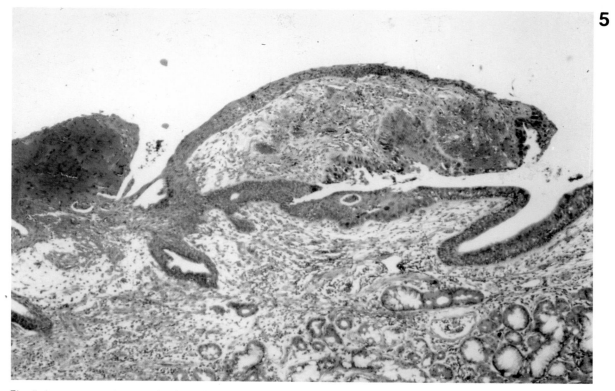

5

Fig. 5. Low-power microscopic view of same area as in previous figure shows focal cytologic change in surface epithelium.

6

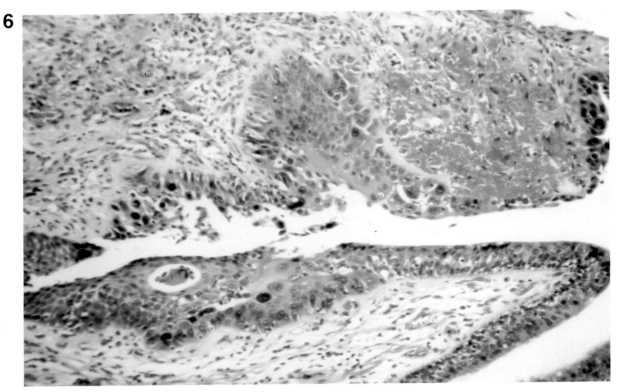

Fig. 6. High-power magnification of same area as in previous two figures shows focal carcinoma in situ.

7

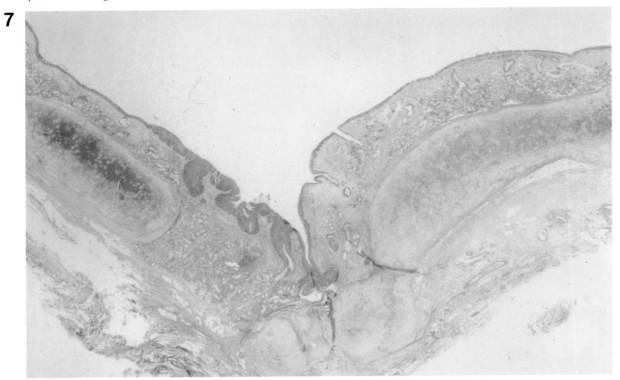

Fig. 7. Block 9 (see diagram) shows mucosal abnormality involving fissure and adjacent surface epithelium 0.45 cm in length.

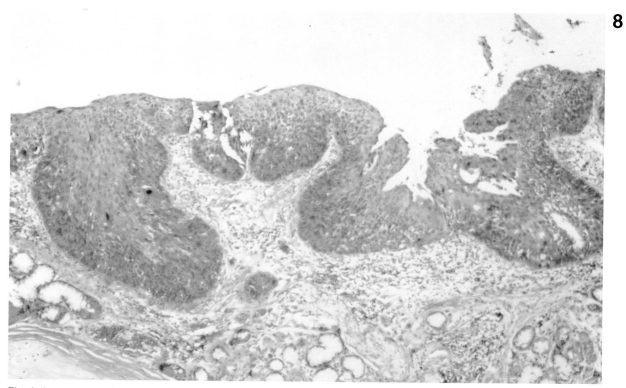

8

Fig. 8. Low-power microscopic field includes almost entire area of mucosal abnormality.

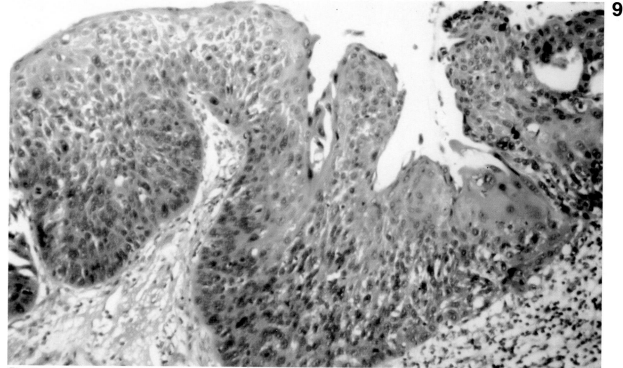

9

Fig. 9. High-power view of same area as in previous figure shows carcinoma in situ involving surface epithelium.

10

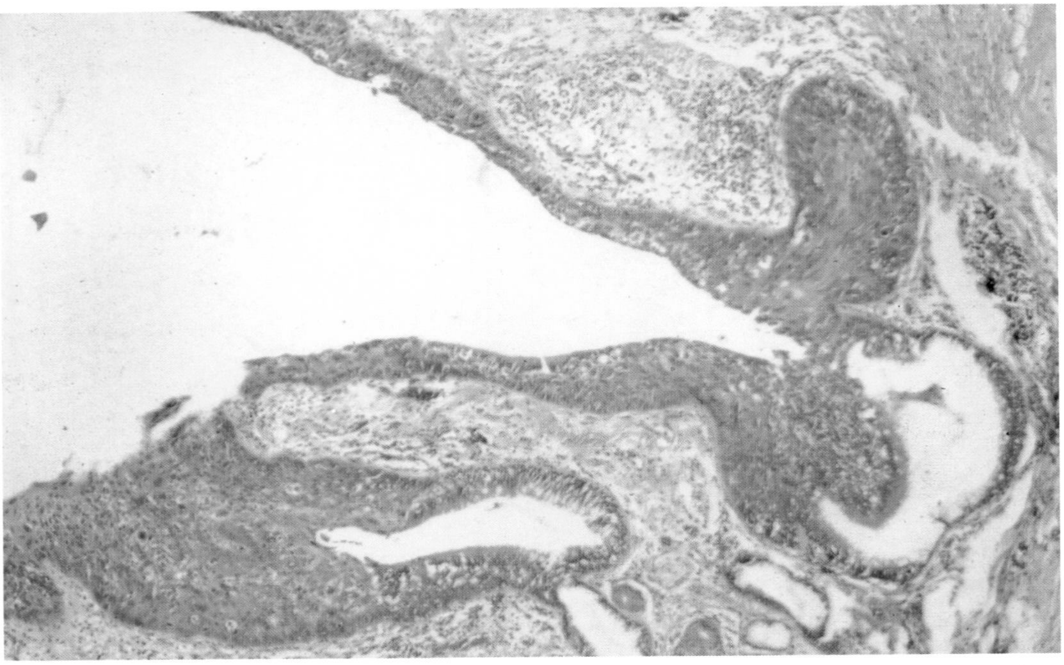

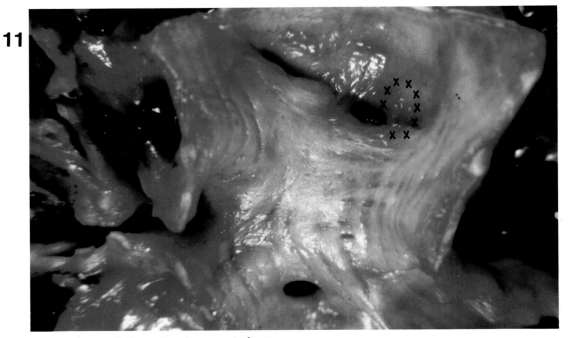

Fig. 10. Depth of fissure and cytologic change on either side are seen, with extension of in situ carcinoma into ducts.

11

Fig. 11. Gross specimen showing extent of cancer.

Summary

The gross specimen shows the actual size of the carcinoma in situ, 0.5 by 0.4 cm (enclosed by X's), situated in the mucosa of the left upper-lobe bronchus near the fissure (site of left upper lobectomy 10 years before). The biopsy site is visible, but the lesion was not seen by the bronchoscopist and was not visible grossly on pathologic examination. Histologically, the lesion is squamous cell carcinoma in situ limited to the surface epithelium and the ducts of mucous glands.

Case 2

A 47-year-old obese male accountant had moderately severe chronic obstructive pulmonary disease.

Sputum Cytology

The initial and follow-up screening sputum specimens were negative for 1 year. Then moderately atypical metaplastic squamous cells were detected (Fig. 1A and B), and repeat specimens were requested. The first repeat study showed moderate atypia, and a second repeat study revealed marked atypia (Fig. 1C and D). Induced-sputum specimens were obtained, and both the initial fresh and the delayed postinduction preparations disclosed marked squamous

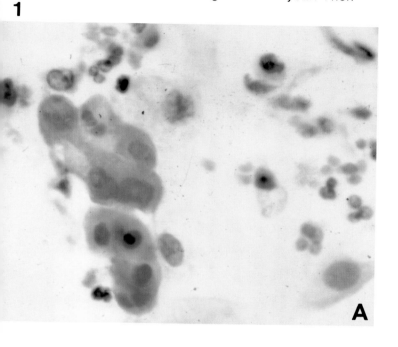

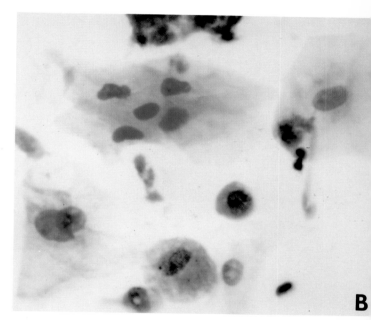

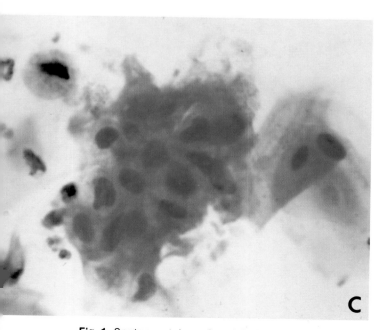

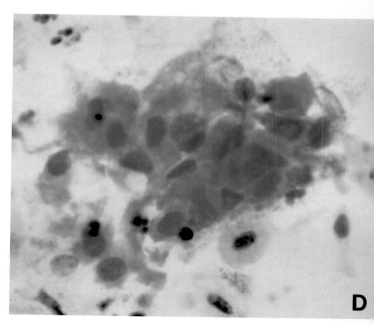

Fig. 1. Sputum cytology. **A** and **B**, First abnormal specimen shows moderate squamous cell atypia. **C** and **D**, Later specimens show marked atypia. (Papanicolaou; x540.)

cell atypia. Localization was recommended on this basis.

Localizing Bronchoscopy

Examination was performed 4 months after the first abnormal sputum test, and the results were negative except for chronic bronchitis.

The initial "differential" bronchial secretions were negative on the left side but were positive for squamous carcinoma cells on

the right. Subsequent "pooled" bilateral secretions were also positive.

Bronchial brushings from the right superior segmental bronchus (RB6) showed markedly atypical squamous cells (Fig. 2A). All others were negative.

Bronchial biopsy specimens from the spur between RB6 and the bronchus intermedius showed squamous cell carcinoma (Fig. 2B). Others either showed normal mucosa or were judged inadequate.

2

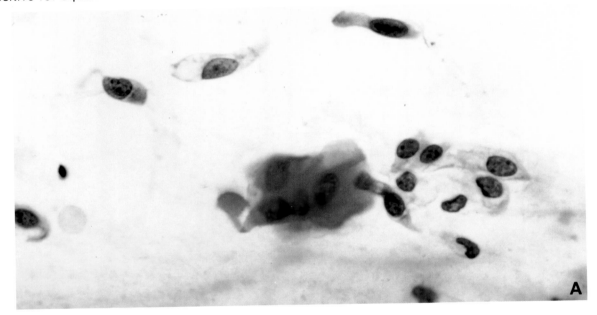

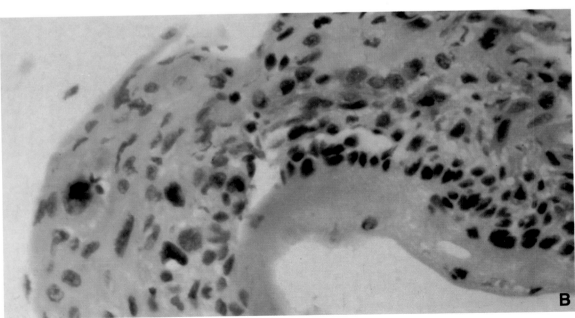

Surgery

Operation was carried out 10 days after bronchoscopy. No tumor could be palpated. A right middle and lower bilobectomy was performed. Fresh frozen sections from the margin of the resection disclosed no tumor.

Fig. 2 (opposite page). **A**, Bronchial brush (RB6). Markedly atypical squamous cells are seen with bronchial epithelial cells in background (Papanicolaou stain). **B**, Bronchial biopsy (RB6-bronchus intermedius spur). Keratinized squamous cell carcinoma is present (small biopsy specimen).

Pathology

Fig. 3. Resected right middle and lower lobes showing surgical line of resection through bronchus intermedius, opened RB6, and middle-lobe bronchi, as labeled. Spur between RB6 and bronchus intermedius represents positive biopsy site (**arrow**).

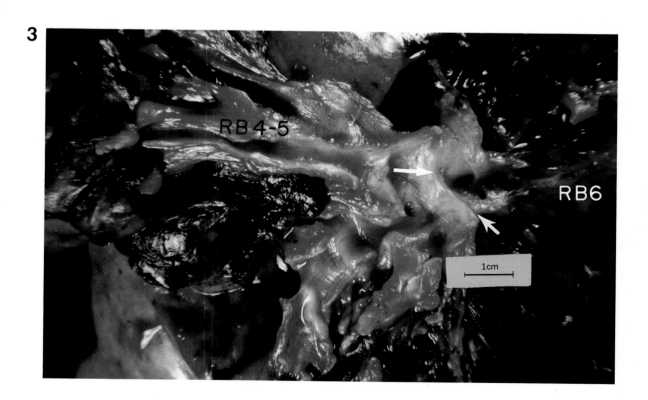

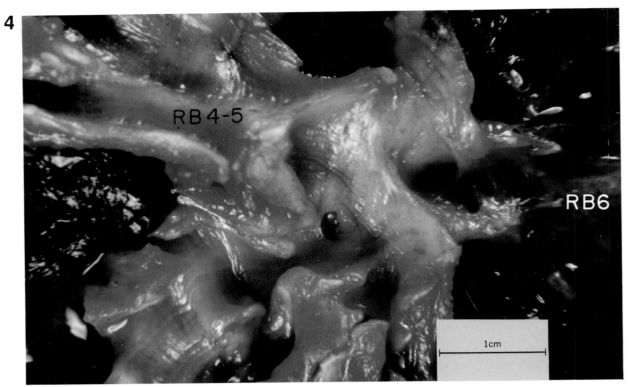

Fig. 4. Closer view of bronchus intermedius, spur, and opened RB6. Biopsy site is visible on spur. Mucosa of RB6 near orifice appears somewhat whitish and more opaque than normal. Remainder of bronchial mucosa is essentially normal.

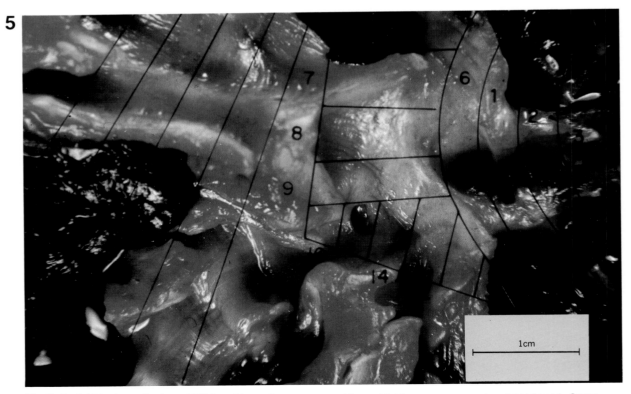

Fig. 5. Serial block sectioning of RB6 and bronchus intermedius was carried out as in diagram. Remainder of bronchial tree was mapped and sectioned. Cross sections of RB6 are shown below.

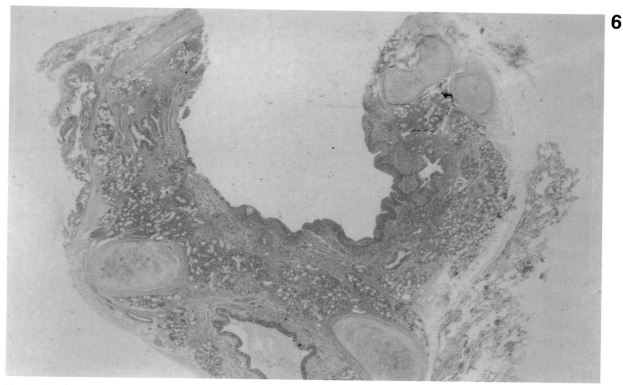

6

Fig. 6. First cross section through proximal RB6 near spur. Approximately two-thirds of circumference of bronchus shows surface epithelial alteration.

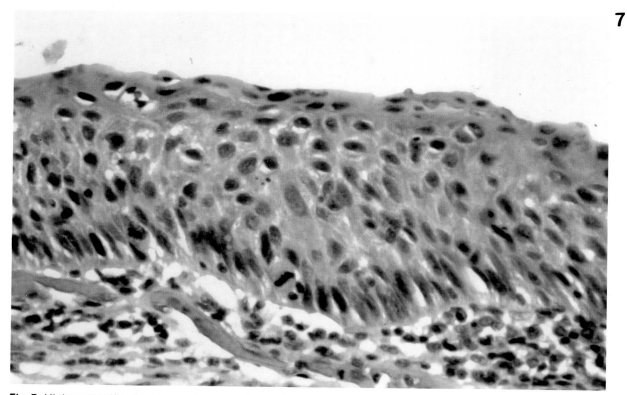

7

Fig. 7. Higher magnification demonstrates carcinoma in situ with slight surface maturation.

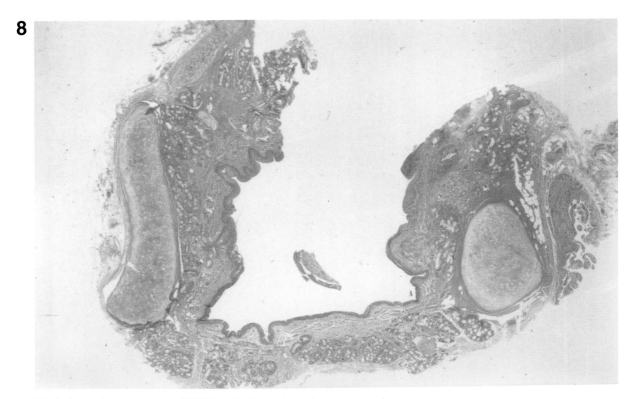

Fig. 8. Second cross section of RB6. In situ change is again apparent in surface epithelium.

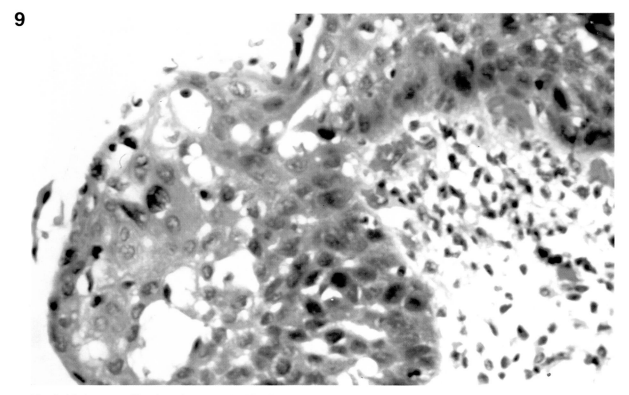

Fig. 9. Higher magnification shows marked in situ carcinomatous change with much nuclear variation.

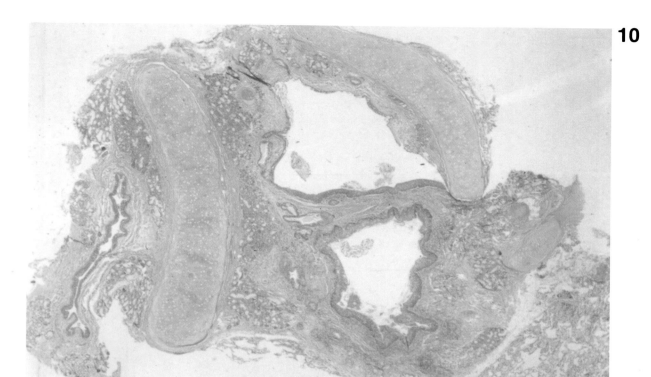

Fig. 10. Fourth cross section of RB6. In situ change continues along two subsegmental branches. More distal blocks are negative.

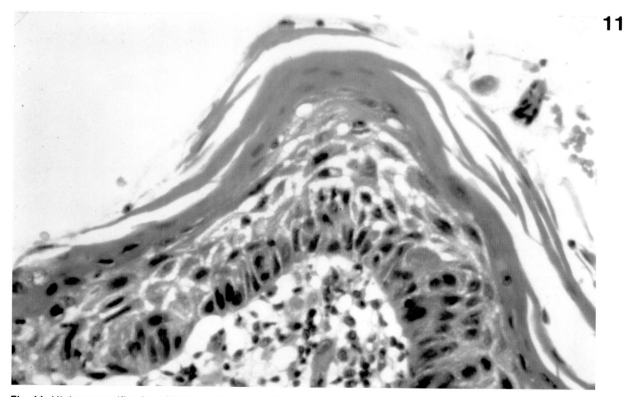

Fig. 11. Higher magnification shows carcinoma in situ with highly keratinized superficial zone.

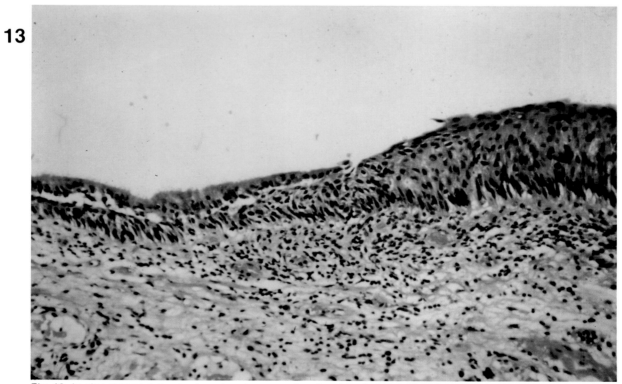

12

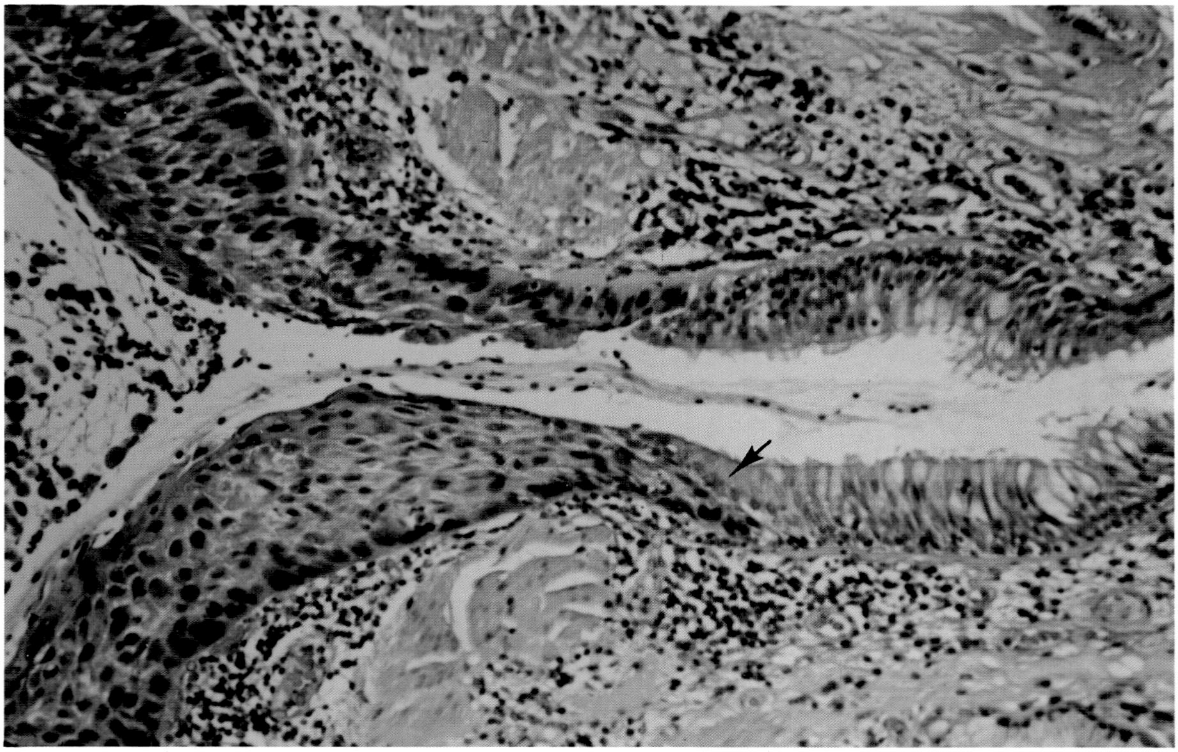

Fig. 12. Extension of in situ change into ducts of mucous glands. Note acute angle at junctional zone (**arrow**).

13

Fig. 13. In situ change extends along basal zone and undermines benign ciliated surface cells, with "slit formation" between the two.

14

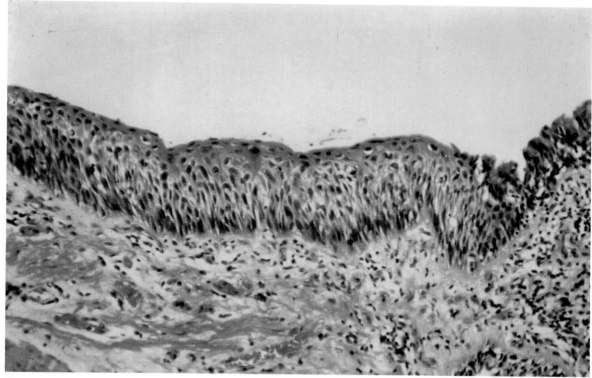

Fig. 14. In situ change extends to bronchus intermedius (section 8 in Fig. 5), with abrupt transition to normal epithelium.

15

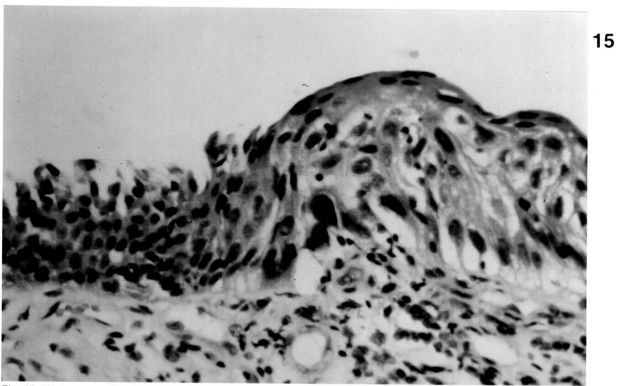

Fig. 15. Higher magnification of transitional zone.

16

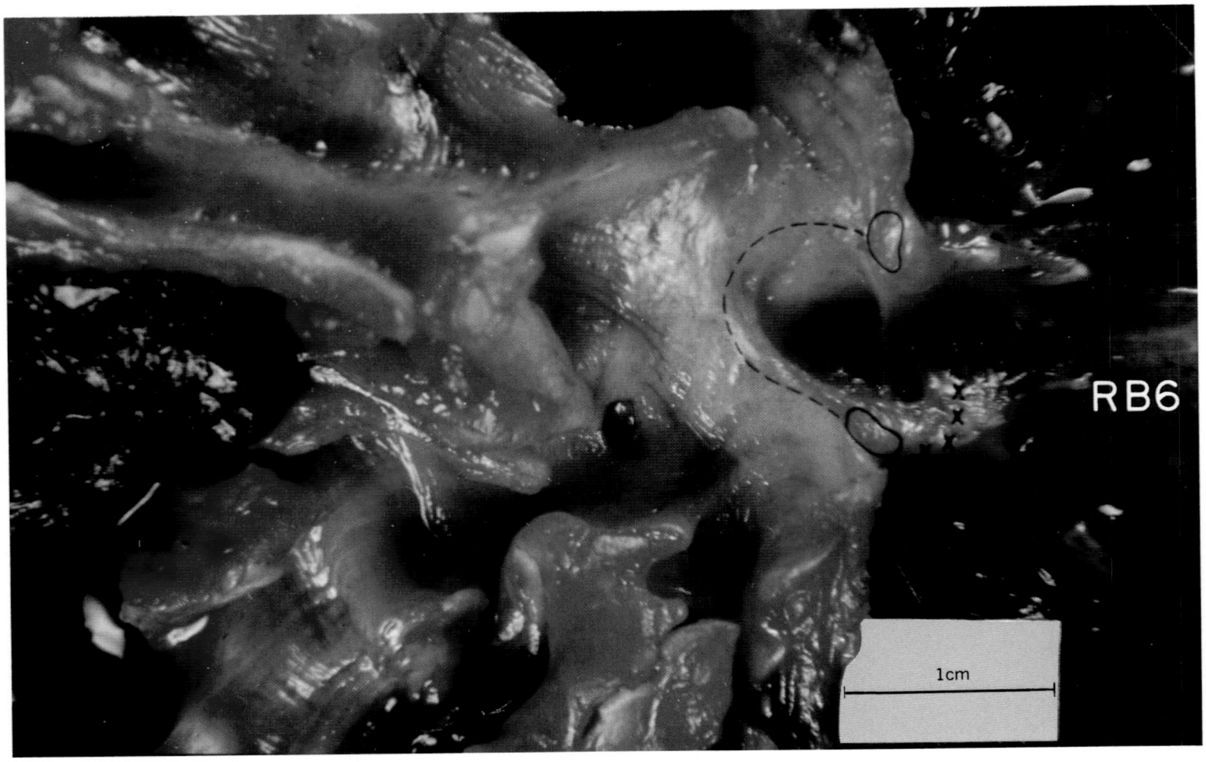

Fig. 16. Gross specimen showing extent of tumor.

Summary

The gross specimen shows the extent of the carcinoma in situ (as marked). The area of involvement includes the proximal 0.9 cm of RB6, the spur, and the mucosa of the adjacent bronchus intermedius over an area approximately 0.2 cm by 0.8 cm. The lesion was not seen by the bronchoscopist and was barely visible to the pathologist on gross examination. Histologically, the lesion is squamous cell carcinoma in situ limited to the surface epithelium and the ducts of mucous glands.

Case 3

A 67-year-old retired truck driver had moderate chronic obstructive pulmonary disease.

Sputum Cytology

The initial sputum specimen was positive for cancer cells of squamous type (Fig. 1A and

B). A repeat specimen was also positive. Induced specimens were obtained. The aerosol-induced, directly prepared specimen revealed squamous carcinoma cells (Fig. 1C and D). The delayed postinduction collection disclosed markedly atypical squamous cells. Localizing bronchoscopic examination was recommended.

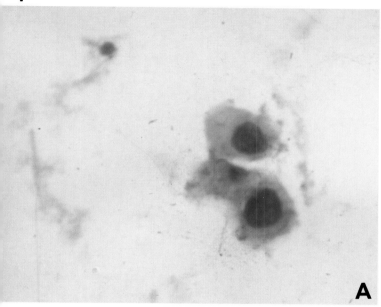

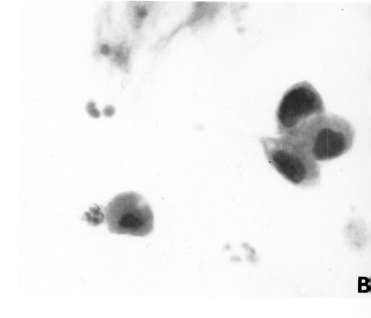

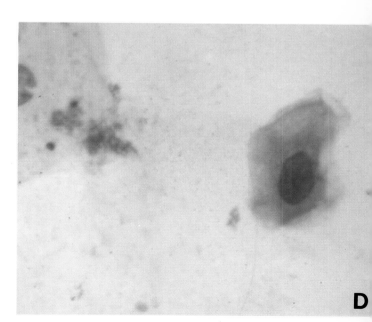

Fig. 1. Sputum cytology. **A** and **B**, Initial specimen shows carcinoma cells of squamous type. **C** and **D**, Induced sputum. Single squamous carcinoma cells are shown. (Papanicolaou stain.)

Localizing Bronchoscopy

The first fiberbronchoscopic examination was conducted 5 days after the initial positive sputum cytology test. It was cursory and results were negative. A detailed examination with the patient under general anesthesia was performed 3 weeks later. There was evidence of diffuse chronic bronchitis but no tumor. The middle-lobe orifice (RB4,5) was narrowed, and there was a suggestion of granularity of the LB2-3 spur.

Bronchial brushings from the right upper-lobe segmental bronchi (RB1,2,3) showed carcinoma cells of the squamous type (Fig. 2A). All others were negative.

Bronchial biopsy specimens from the RB1-2 spur revealed in situ squamous cell carcinoma (Fig. 2B). Other sites showed

2

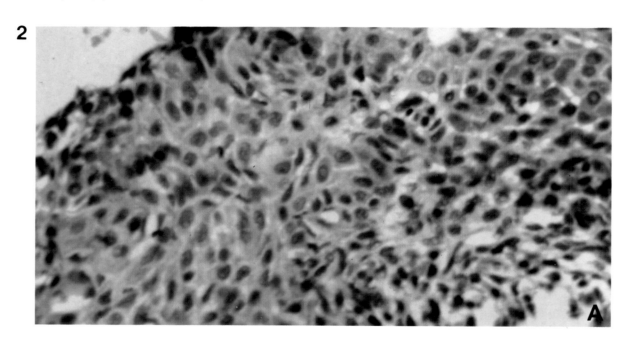

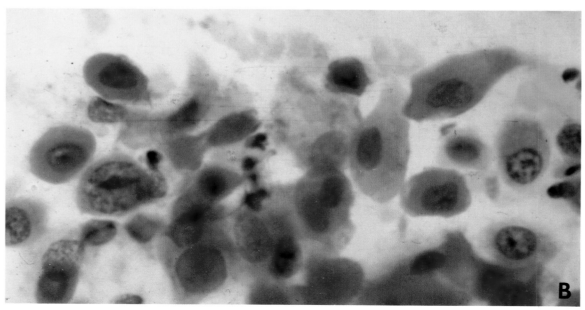

normal bronchial mucosa or squamous metaplasia.

Surgery

At operation 2 weeks after the second bronchoscopy, no grossly palpable tumor was evident. Right upper lobectomy was performed. The margin of resection was found to be free of cancer on frozen-section study.

Fig. 2 (opposite page). **A,** Bronchial brush (RB1,2,3). Squamous carcinoma cells in cluster showing marked nuclear abnormalities and abundant eosinophilic cytoplasm. (Papanicolaou stain.) **B,** Bronchial biopsy (RB1-2). Squamous cell carcinoma is seen. (Hematoxylin and eosin stain.)

Pathology

Fig. 3. Resected right upper lobe showing three segmental bronchi, as labeled, together with subsegmental divisions of each. RB1-2 spur represents positive biopsy site (**arrow**).

3

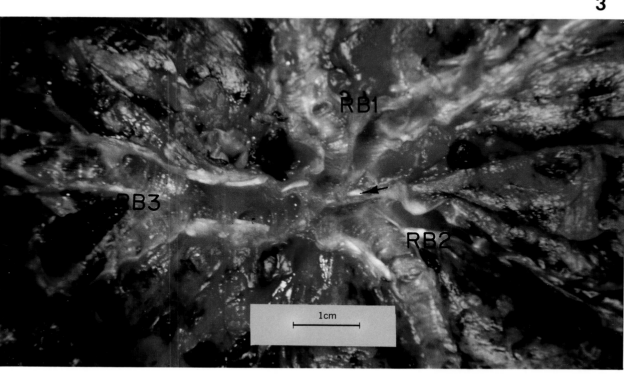

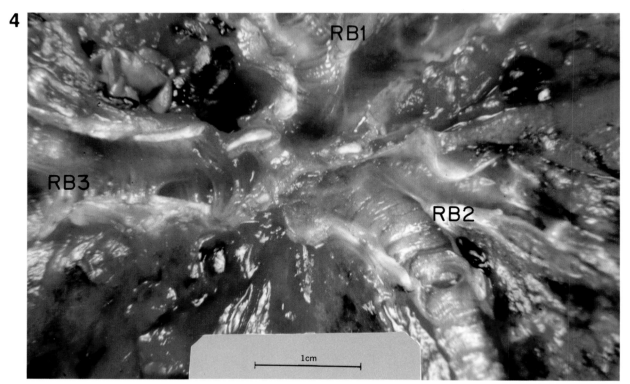

Fig. 4. Closer view of trifurcation area. RB1-2 spur appears slightly thickened; also, mucosa of adjacent RB2 is granular, with loss of transverse striations. Remainder of mucosa is grossly normal.

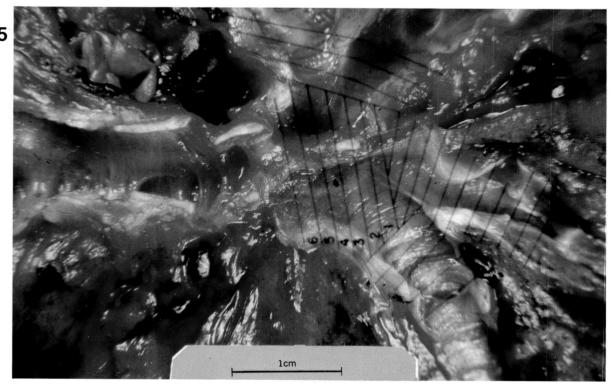

Fig. 5. Serial block sectioning of RB1-2 spur and proximal portions of RB1 and RB2 was carried out as diagramed. Remainder of bronchial tree was mapped and sectioned. Abnormal findings were limited to blocks 4, 5, and 6 (see below).

6

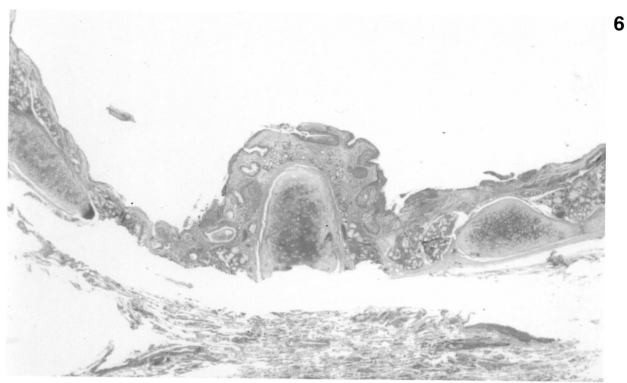

Fig. 6. Block 6 represents cross section of RB1-2 spur and adjacent bronchial walls (see Fig. 5). Mucosal change is confined to spur and adjacent RB2.

7

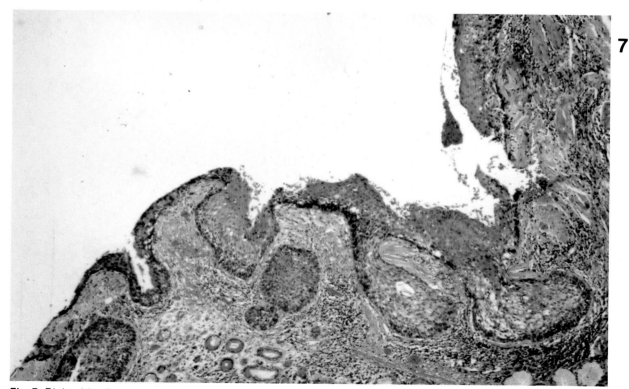

Fig. 7. Right side of spur shows carcinoma in situ that involves surface epithelium and ducts of mucous glands.

8

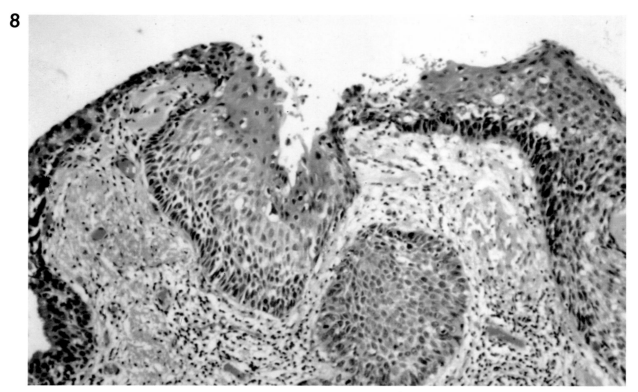

Fig. 8. Higher magnification of same area shows surface keratinization and duct involvement. No penetration of basement membrane is seen.

9

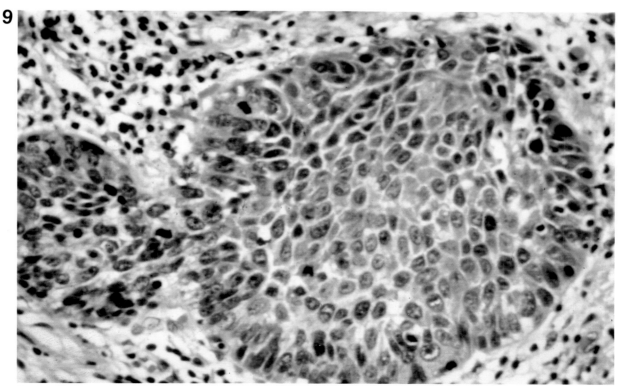

Fig. 9. Cellular detail shows well-differentiated carcinoma in situ within duct of mucous gland. Numerous mitotic figures are seen.

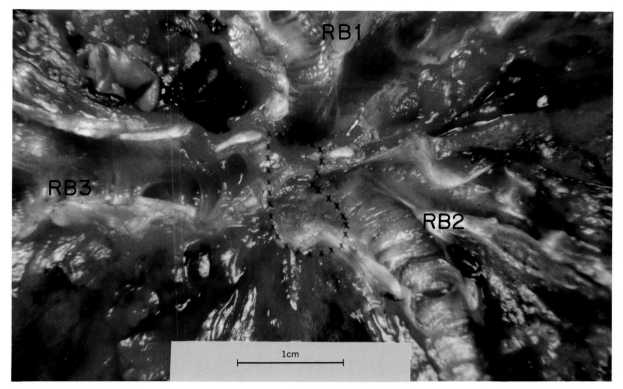

Fig. 10. Gross specimen showing extent of tumor.

Summary

The gross specimen shows the extent of the carcinoma in situ, 0.7 by 1 cm (enclosed by X's), which involves the orifice of RB2 and the RB1-2 spur. The lesion was not seen by the bronchoscopist but was grossly visible on pathologic examination (slight thickening of spur and granularity of adjacent mucosa). Histologically, this is a very well-differentiated carcinoma in situ limited to the surface epithelium and the ducts of mucous glands.

Case 4

A 50-year-old man had cystectomy, prostatectomy, and creation of an ileal conduit 3 years previously as treatment for localized transitional cell carcinoma of the bladder. There was no evidence of recurrence.

Sputum Cytology

The initial sputum specimen showed metaplastic squamous cells with marked atypia (Fig. 1A and B). Repeat specimens were requested immediately. On the first repeat study, marked atypia was again seen. A second repeat study produced a scanty specimen that disclosed only slight atypia. Nevertheless, with two specimens showing marked squamous atypia, localizing bronchoscopy was advised. Before this, two more repeat specimens and induced specimens were studied. The third repeat study showed marked atypia once more, and the fourth showed carcinoma cells of the squamous type (Fig. 1C and D). Induced sputum, both fresh direct and postinduction delayed specimens, were positive for squamous cancer cells.

1

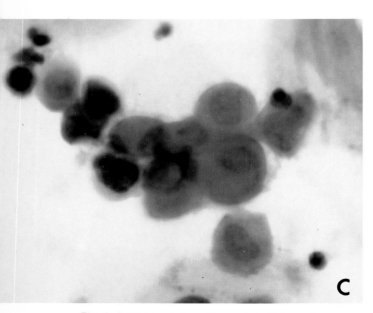
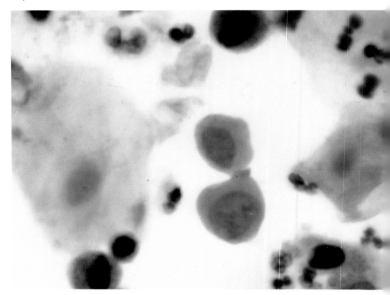
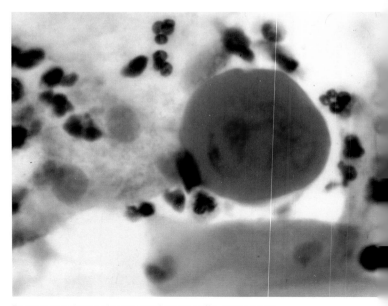

Fig. 1. Sputum cytology. **A** and **B**, Initial specimen shows markedly atypical squamous cells. **C** and **D**, Repeat specimen shows carcinoma cells, squamous type. (Papanicolaou stain.)

Localizing Bronchoscopy

Fiberoptic bronchoscopy was performed 2 months after the first abnormal sputum test. In the right upper-lobe bronchus, the inferior margin of RB1 was blunted and the RB1-2 spur appeared thickened.

"Pooled" bilateral bronchial secretions were positive for squamous carcinoma cells.

Bronchial brushings from the right upper lobe (RB1,2,3) revealed a few moderately atypical squamous cells (Fig. 2A). Other brushings were negative.

Bronchial biopsy specimens from the RB1-2 spur and the right upper-lobe spur showed squamous cell carcinoma (Fig. 2B). Specimens from other areas showed either normal bronchial epithelium or squamous metaplasia with slight atypia.

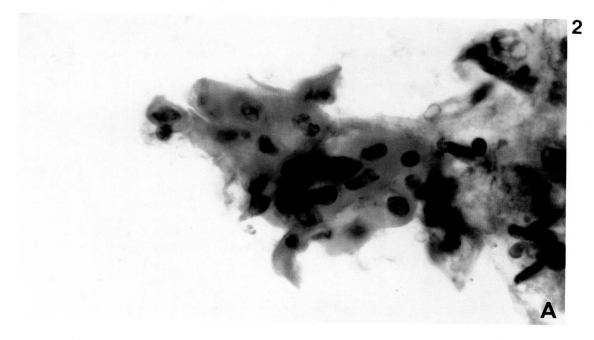

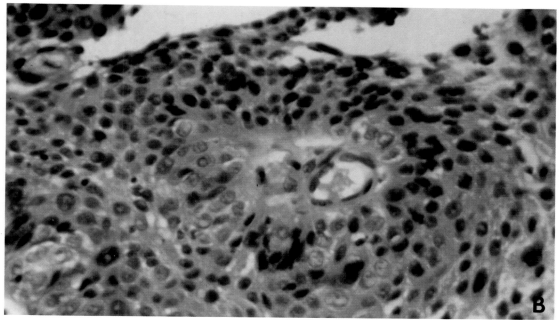

Fig. 2. A, Bronchial brush (right upper-lobe bronchus). Clump of moderately atypical squamous cells is shown. (Papanicolaou stain.) **B**, Bronchial biopsy specimen (RB1-2 spur) shows squamous cell carcinoma. (Hematoxylin and eosin stain.)

Surgery

At operation 2 weeks after fiberoptic
bronchoscopy, no abnormality was palpated.
Right upper lobectomy was carried out. The
margin of resection was free of tumor (fresh
frozen sectioning).

Pathology

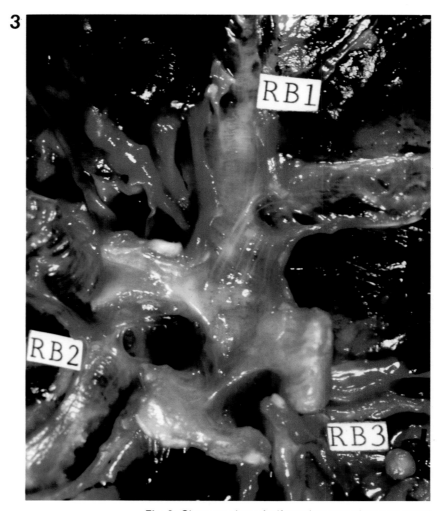

Fig. 3. Close-up view of trifurcation area shows mucosal
thickening involving orifice of RB1 and adjacent right
upper-lobe bronchial wall.

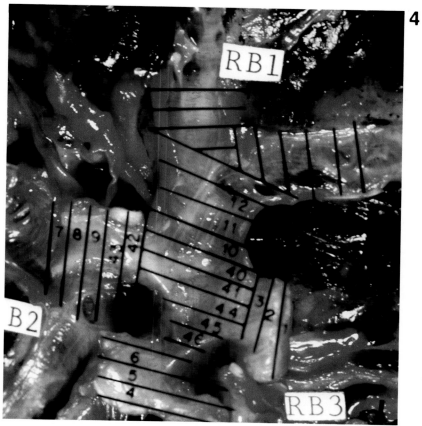

Fig. 4. Serial block sectioning of specimen was carried out as on diagram. Abnormal findings were limited to blocks 3, 5, and 6, and 40 through 46.

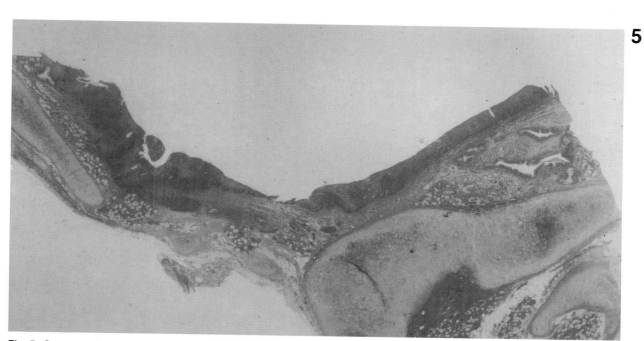

Fig. 5. Cross section of block 41 (see diagram). Entire mucosa shows alteration of surface epithelium with pronounced thickening.

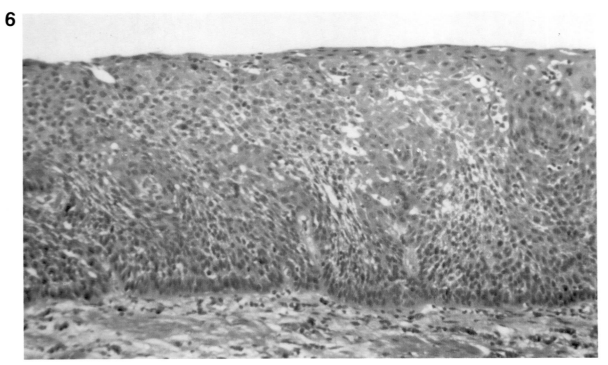

Fig. 6. Higher magnification of mucosa (right side of block 41) demonstrates squamous cell carcinoma in situ with slight surface maturation.

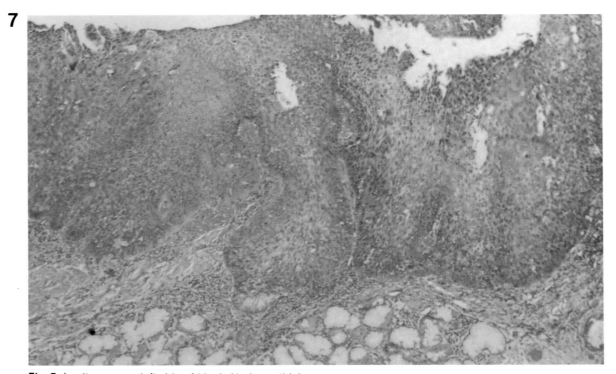

Fig. 7. In situ area on left side of block 41 shows thick carcinomatous zone.

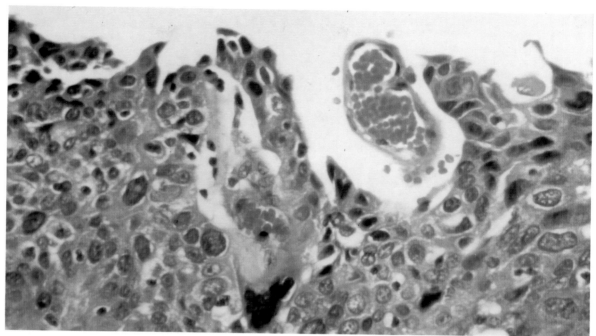

Fig. 8. High-power magnification of surface of same area as in previous figure shows marked cytologic carcinomatous change.

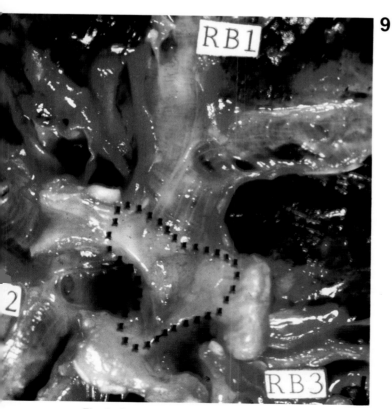

Fig. 9. Gross specimen with outline of tumor.

Summary

The area of involvement of this carcinoma in situ, approximately 1.7 by 1.2 cm (X's), includes the distal right upper-lobe bronchus and the adjacent trifurcation, with extension to the orifices of RB1 and RB2. The lesion was visible to the bronchoscopist and was also clearly visible on pathologic examination. Histologically, the lesion is squamous cell carcinoma in situ limited to the surface epithelium and the ducts of mucous glands.

Case 5

A 52-year-old truck driver had chronic bronchitis and tussive syncope.

Sputum Cytology

The initial sputum specimen and four repeat specimens showed moderately atypical squamous cells (Fig. 1A). Sputum continued to be collected because of persistent moderate atypia. The fifth repeat specimen revealed marked atypia (Fig. 1B and C) and the sixth, carcinoma cells of the squamous type (Fig. 1D). Localization with the fiberoptic bronchoscope was recommended, but before this, additional sputum specimens, including induced preparations, were studied. The seventh repeat specimen again showed squamous cancer cells, as did

1

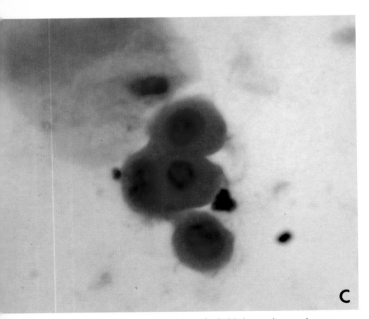

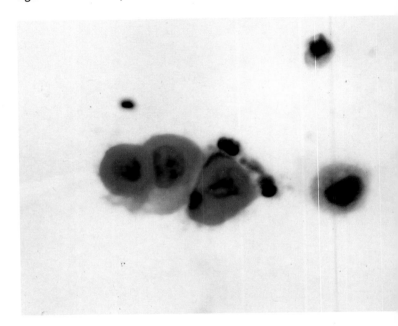

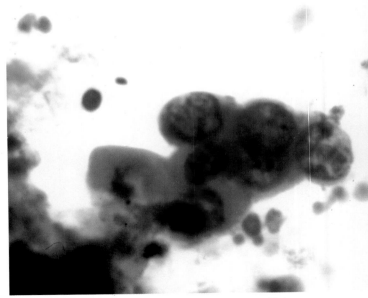

Fig. 1. Sputum cytology. **A**, Initial specimen shows clump of abnormal squamous cells (moderate atypia). **B** and **C**, Repeat specimens show marked atypia. **D**, Final specimen reveals carcinoma cells, squamous type. Note cyanophilic cytoplasm in some cells. (Papanicolaou stain.)

both fresh and delayed "pooled" postinduction preparations.

Localizing Bronchoscopy

This study was performed nearly 6 months after the initial abnormal sputum cytology. It disclosed severe generalized chronic bronchitis. A tiny verrucous area was observed in the left upper-lobe bronchus between the LB1 & 2 and LB3 segmental bronchi.

"Pooled" bilateral bronchial secretions were positive for squamous cancer cells.

Bronchial brushings from LB1,2,3 showed a few atypical squamous cells (Fig. 2A). Brushings from other areas were negative.

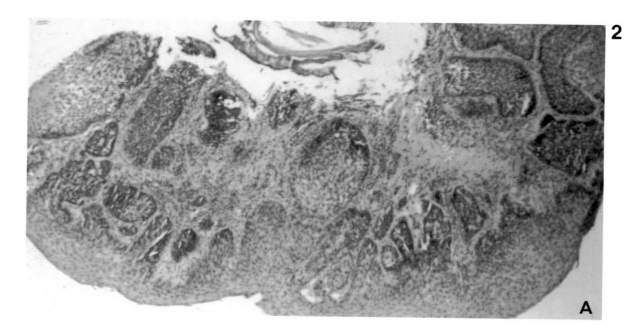

2

A

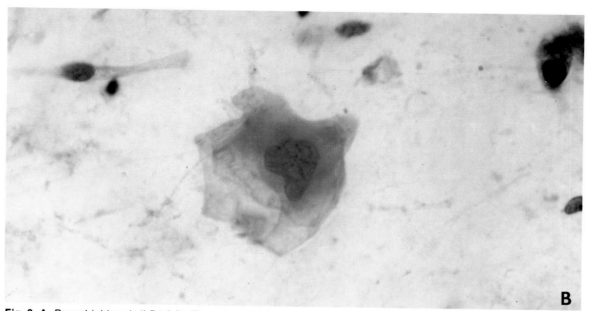

B

Fig. 2. A, Bronchial brush (LB1,2,3). There is a single markedly atypical squamous cell, with bronchial epithelial cells in background. (Papanicolaou stain.) **B**, Bronchial biopsy specimen (LB1 & 2-3 spur) shows in situ and infiltrative squamous cell carcinoma. (Hematoxylin and eosin stain.)

Bronchial biopsy specimens from the LB1 &
2-3 spur revealed squamous cell carcinoma
(Fig. 2B). Other areas showed either
bronchial mucosa or squamous metaplasia.

Surgery

At operation 1 week after fiberoptic
bronchoscopy, no gross abnormality was
palpated. Left upper lobectomy was carried
out. The margin of resection was free of
tumor.

Pathology

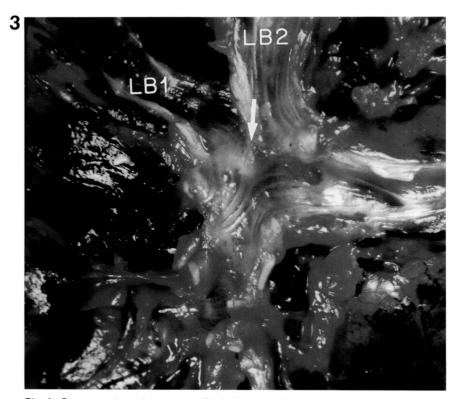

Fig. 3. Close-up view of common LB1 & 2 shows slight
mucosal alteration. Biopsy site is visible just within
orifice of LB1 & 2 (**arrow**).

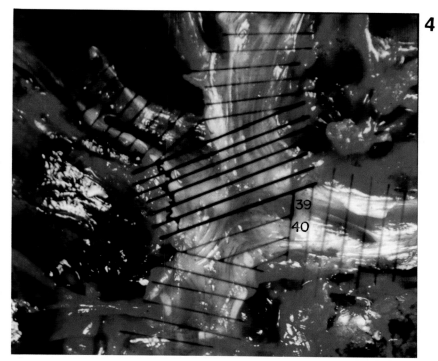

Fig. 4. Serial block sectioning of specimen was carried out as in diagram. Abnormal findings were limited to blocks 1 through 4 (distal to biopsy site) and 39 and 40 (proximal).

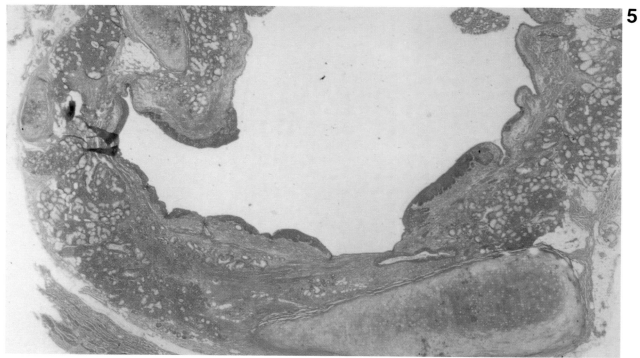

Fig. 5. Cross section through LB1 & 2 just distal to biopsy site. Surface epithelial alteration is present over much of section.

6

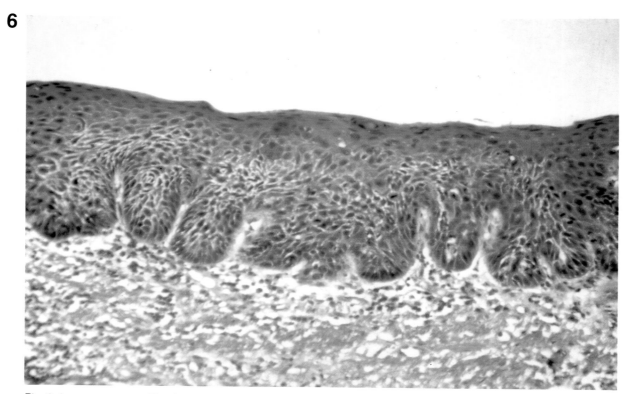

Fig. 6. Low-power magnification demonstrates
carcinoma in situ.

7

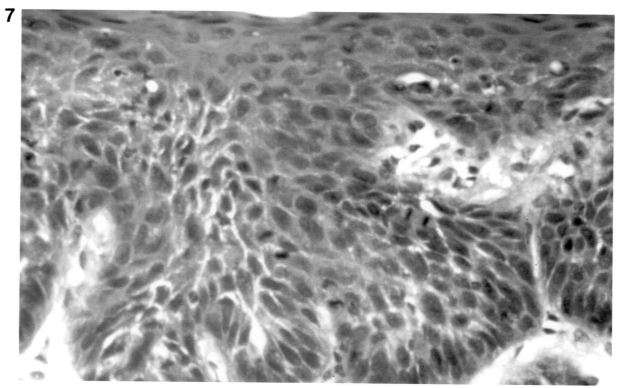

Fig. 7. Higher-power magnification shows considerable
maturation of tumor cells.

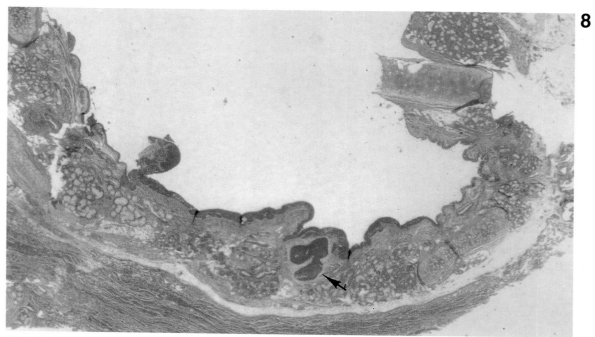

8

Fig. 8. Cross section of next block on LB1 & 2 distal to area in previous figure. Alteration of surface epithelium and focal microinvasion by tumor (**arrow**) are seen.

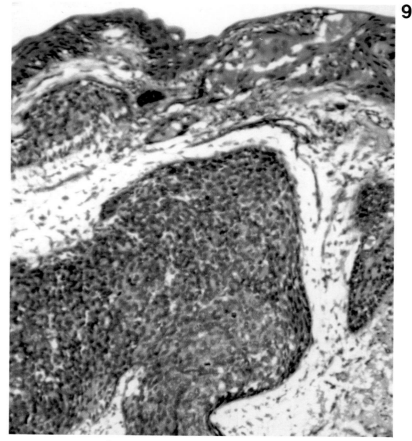

9

Fig. 9. Higher magnification of invasive focus (depth of invasion approximately 0.1 cm).

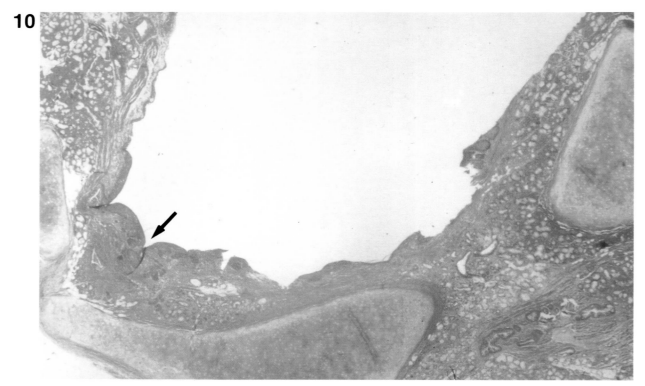

Fig. 10. Cross section of LB1 & 2 at biopsy site. In situ squamous carcinoma and focal microinvasion are present.

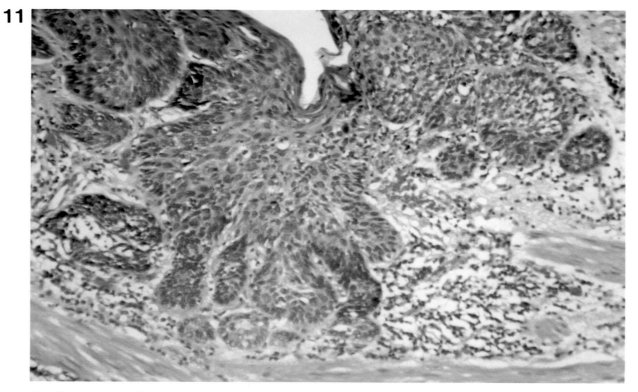

Fig. 11. Higher magnification of microinvasive zone.

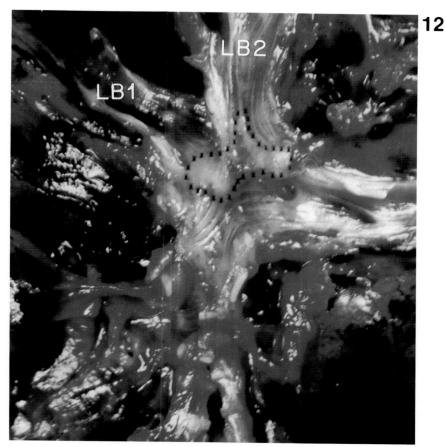

Fig. 12. Gross specimen with area of tumor outlined.

Summary

The area of involvement of this carcinoma in situ includes the common LB1 & 2 bronchus and also the LB1-2 and LB1 & 2-3 spurs. The carcinoma measures 1.4 cm in length and varies in width from 0.1 to 1.0 cm (average 0.6 cm). The lesion was visible to the bronchoscopist and was also visible on pathologic examination. Histologically, the lesion is squamous cell carcinoma in situ with three foci of microinvasion of mucosa, each approximately 0.2 cm in diameter and 0.1 cm in depth.

Case 6

A 50-year-old insurance man had a 1-year history of insulin-dependent diabetes mellitus. There were no significant respiratory symptoms.

Sputum Cytology

Initial and subsequent screening specimens were negative for 3 1/3 years; then a specimen revealed markedly atypical squamous cells (Fig. 1A and B). The first repeat study showed moderate atypia and a second showed only squamous metaplasia. Two more specimens were obtained a month later. One revealed markedly atypical squamous cells. The other was positive for squamous carcinoma cells (Fig. 1C and D). Localization procedures were advised, including induced-sputum specimens. These

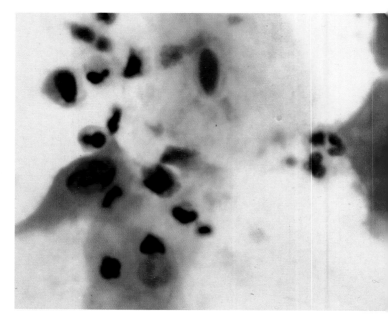

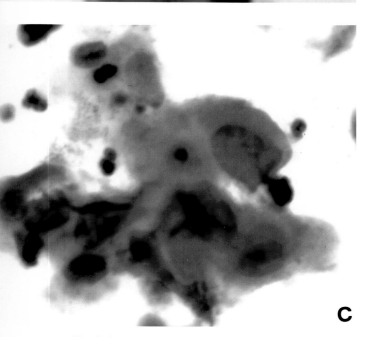

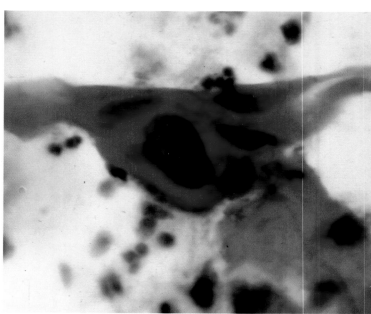

Fig. 1. Sputum cytology. **A** and **B**, First abnormal specimen shows markedly atypical squamous cells. **C** and **D**, Repeat specimens reveal clumps of carcinoma cells, squamous type. (Papanicolaou stain.)

also were positive for squamous cancer cells.

Localizing Bronchoscopy

Fiberoptic bronchoscopy disclosed a small but definitely suspicious area in the left upper lobe on the spur separating the lingula (LB4 and LB5) and LB3. The remainder of the examination was negative except for chronic bronchitis.

"Pooled" bronchial secretions from both sides were positive for squamous cancer cells.

Bronchial brushings from the left upper lobe were positive (Fig. 2A), and those from all other sites were negative.

Bronchial biopsy specimens from the LB3-4 spur showed infiltrative squamous cell

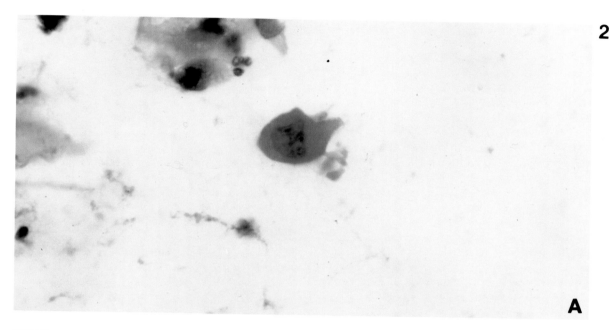

2

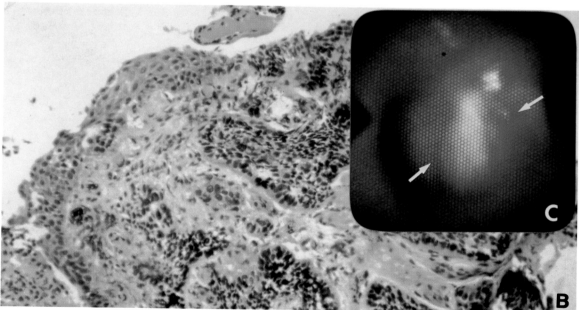

Fig. 2. A, Bronchial brush (left upper-lobe bronchus). Single squamous carcinoma cell is shown, with bronchial epithelial cells in background. (Papanicolaou stain.) **B**, Bronchial biopsy (LB3-4 spur). In situ and infiltrative squamous cell carcinoma are present. (Hematoxylin and eosin stain.) **C**, Fiberbronchoscopic view shows tumor at LB3-4 spur (**arrows**).

carcinoma (Fig. 2B). Others showed normal or metaplastic mucosa.

Surgery

At operation 4 months after the first abnormal sputum specimens and 1 month after localization had been recommended, no tumor was palpable. Left upper lobectomy was performed. The resected margin was free of tumor (fresh frozen section).

Pathology

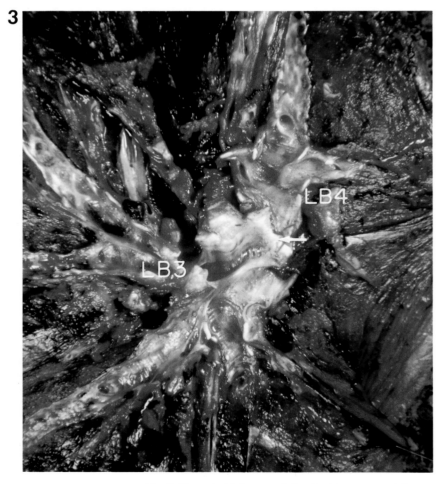

Fig. 3. Resected left upper lobe showing segmental bronchi, as labeled. LB3-4 spur (**arrow**) represents site of positive biopsy.

4

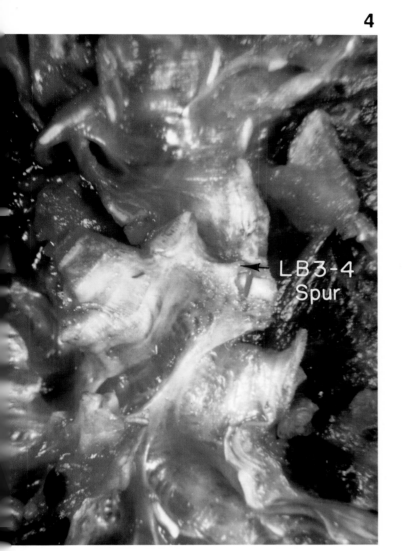

Fig. 4. Closer view of LB3-4 spur (**arrow**). No gross abnormality is visible at this time. Biopsy site is not visible.

5

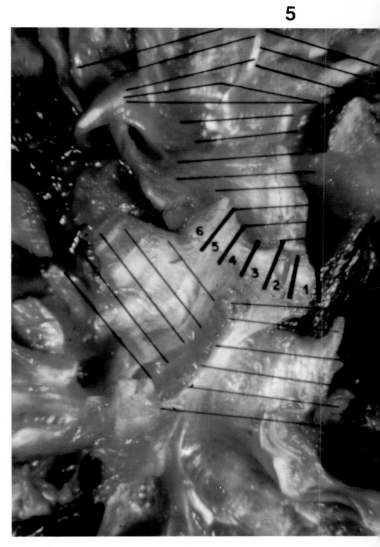

Fig. 5. Serial block sectioning of LB3-4 spur was carried out as in diagram. Remainder of bronchial tree was also sectioned. Abnormal findings were limited to block 1.

6

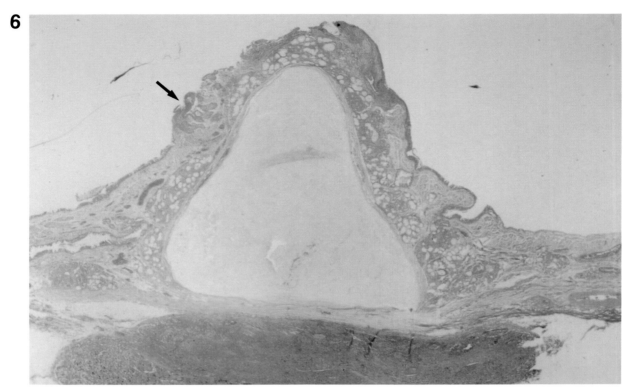

Fig. 6. Cross section of block 1 on LB3-4 spur (see Fig. 5). Infiltrative tumor is present near summit of spur (**arrow**).

7

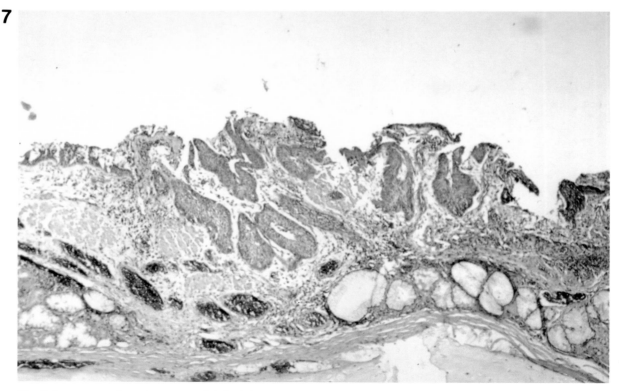

Fig. 7. Low-power view shows superficially infiltrative squamous cell carcinoma on one aspect of spur.

8

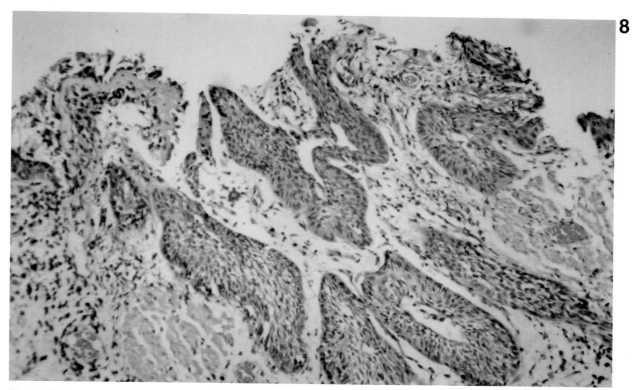

Fig. 8. Higher magnification of same area as in previous figure.

9

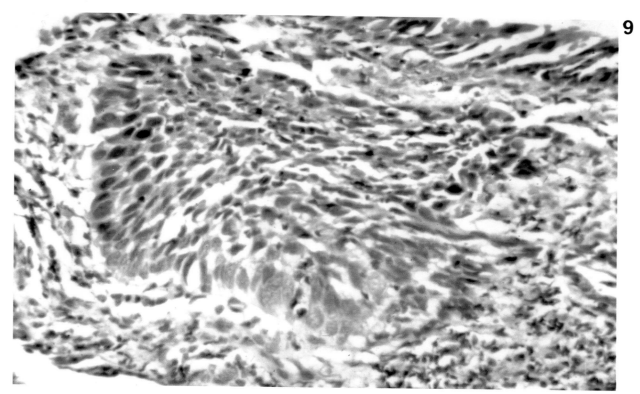

Fig. 9. In situ squamous cell carcinoma is present on opposite side of spur near summit.

10

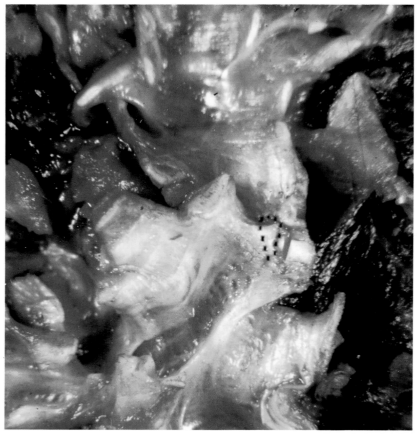

Fig. 10. Gross specimen showing extent of tumor.

Summary

The gross specimen shows the site and approximate size of a squamous cell carcinoma on the summit of the LB3-4 spur. The residual carcinoma measures 0.5 by 0.2 cm (as marked), with microinvasion of the mucosa. (A polyploid portion of the tumor approximately 0.4 by 0.2 cm was removed by bronchoscopic biopsy.) The lesion was visible to the bronchoscopist, but no residual tumor was visible on gross pathologic examination. Histologically, the lesion is an in situ and infiltrative squamous carcinoma extending 0.2 cm into the mucosa.

Case 7

A 56-year-old gas station attendant had chronic obstructive pulmonary disease with recurrent upper respiratory infections.

Sputum Cytology

The initial screening specimen showed moderately atypical squamous cells (Fig. 1A and B). Repeat specimens showed squamous carcinoma cells (Fig. 1C and D). Localization procedures were recommended. These included induced-sputum specimens, which revealed only moderate and slight atypia.

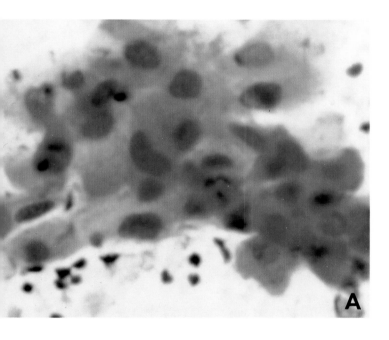
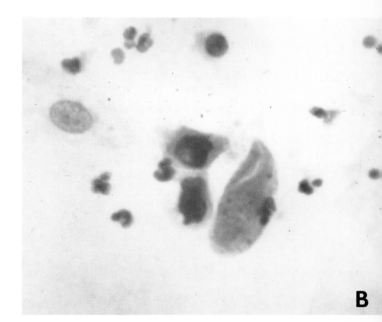
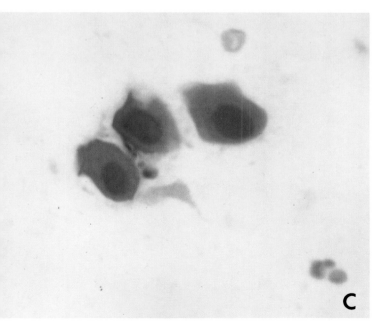
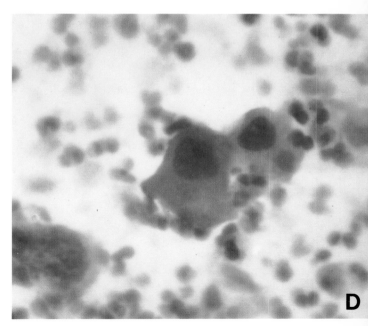

Fig. 1. Sputum cytology. **A** and **B**, Initial screening specimen shows moderately atypical squamous cells. **C** and **D**, Repeat specimen reveals carcinoma cells, squamous type. (Papanicolaou stain.)

Localizing Bronchoscopy

The first bronchoscopy was of limited extent; it was performed under local anesthesia 1 month after the first abnormal sputum. Both rigid and fiberoptic bronchoscopes were used. Bronchoscopy was unsatisfactory because of incessant coughing. Marked chronic bronchitis was present bilaterally, but no tumor was seen. Bronchial secretions showed markedly atypical squamous cells from the left side; results were negative on the right. No brushings or biopsy specimens were obtained.

A second bronchoscopy, 8 days later, was conducted under general anesthesia and with a fiberoptic bronchoscope. Chronic bronchitis was observed but again no tumor.

Bronchial secretions on the left side were positive for squamous carcinoma cells; the right side was negative. Bilateral bronchial brushings were all negative. Multiple (12) bronchial biopsy specimens showed only slight focal squamous metaplasia.

A third bronchoscopy was done 4 weeks after the second and 10 weeks after the first abnormal sputum examination. General anesthesia and the fiberoptic bronchoscope were utilized. No abnormality was seen. Bronchial brushings from LB1 & 2 showed marked atypia (Fig. 2A) and from LB3, moderate atypia. All others were negative. Bronchial biopsy specimens were negative except for the LB1 & 2-3 spur, which showed in situ squamous cell cancer (Fig. 2B).

Fig. 2. **A**, Bronchial brush (LB1-2). Clump of markedly atypical squamous cells is seen, with bronchial epithelial cells in background. (Papanicolaou stain.) **B**, Bronchial biopsy specimen (LB1-2 spur) shows squamous cell carcinoma. (Hematoxylin and eosin stain.) **C**, Fiberbronchoscopic view shows LB1-2 spur (**arrow**).

2

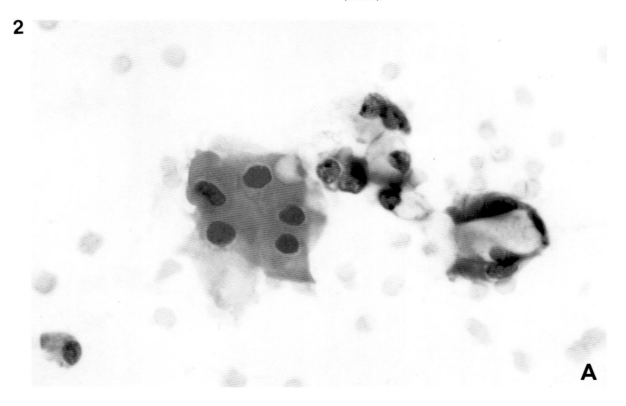

A

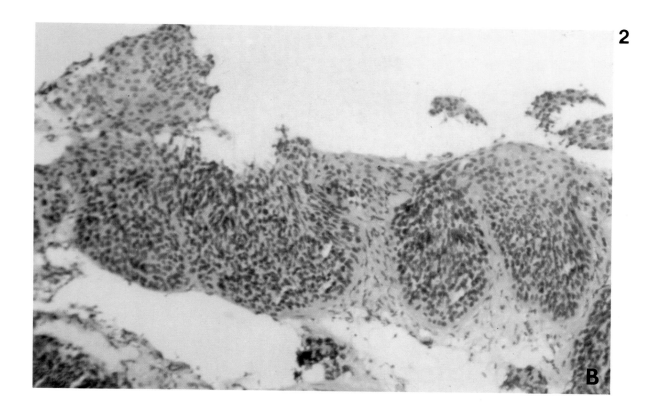

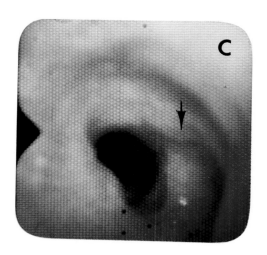

Surgery

At operation 2½ months after the first abnormal sputum, there was no palpable abnormality. Left upper lobectomy was performed. Frozen-section studies showed that the resected margin was free of cancer.

Pathology

3

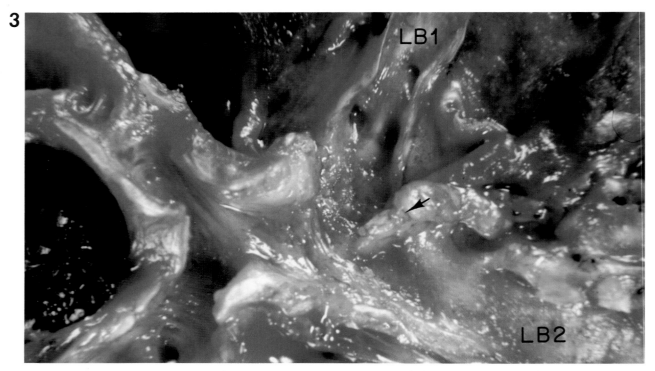

Fig. 3. Close-up view of common LB1 & 2 and its two subdivisions. Spur between LB1 & LB2, site of positive biopsy, is somewhat thickened (**arrow**). Adjacent mucosa of LB1 appears granular. Mucosa of proximal LB2 is whitish and opaque.

4

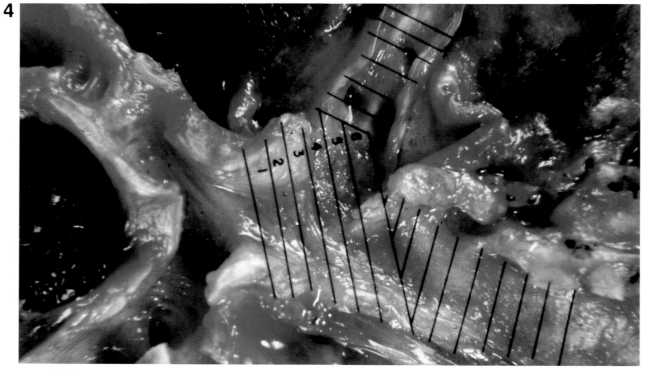

Fig. 4. Serial block sectioning of LB1 & 2 was carried out as in diagram. Remainder of bronchial tree was mapped and sectioned. Abnormal findings were limited to blocks 1 through 6.

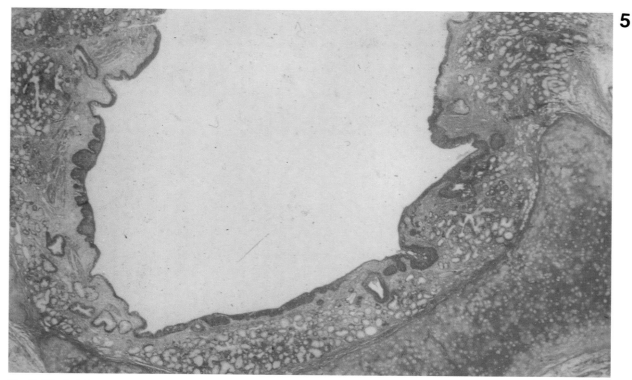

5

Fig. 5. Block 1 (see diagram) represents first cross section of LB1 & 2. Much of the bronchial epithelial lining is thickened and squamoid.

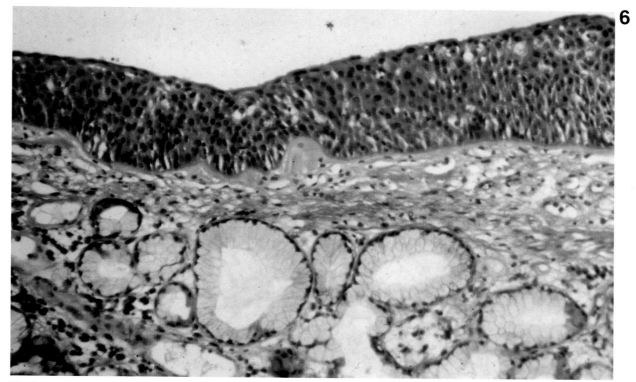

6

Fig. 6. Low-power view of one area of surface epithelium on block 1 shows atypical squamous metaplasia.

7

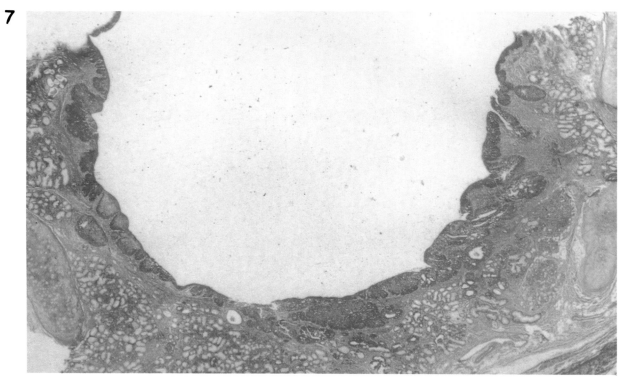

Fig. 7. Block 2 (see diagram) represents second (more distal) section through LB1 & 2. Surface epithelium appears abnormally thickened, with extension of process into ducts of mucous glands.

8

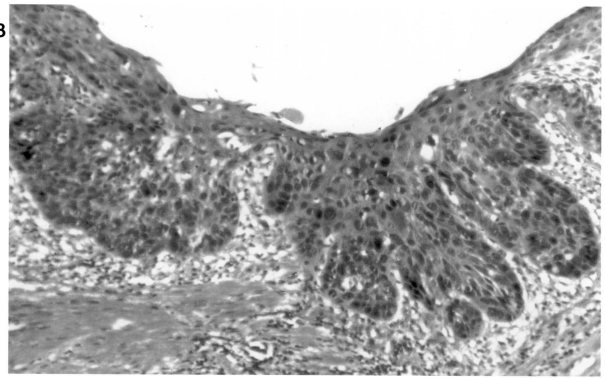

Fig. 8. High-power view of surface epithelium at same level as in previous figure shows carcinoma in situ with marked nuclear variation and hyperchromasia.

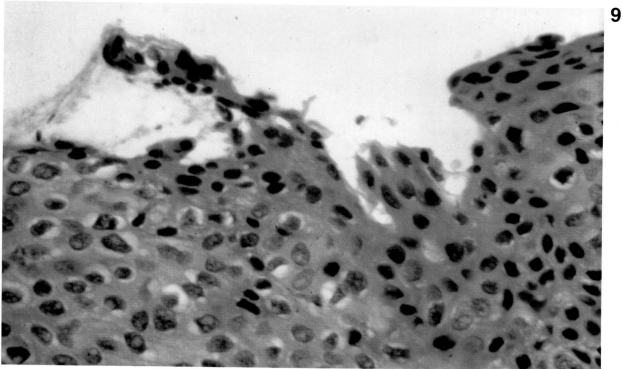

9

Fig. 9. Details of surface change in another area shows carcinoma cells with hyperchromatic nuclei and fairly abundant cytoplasm.

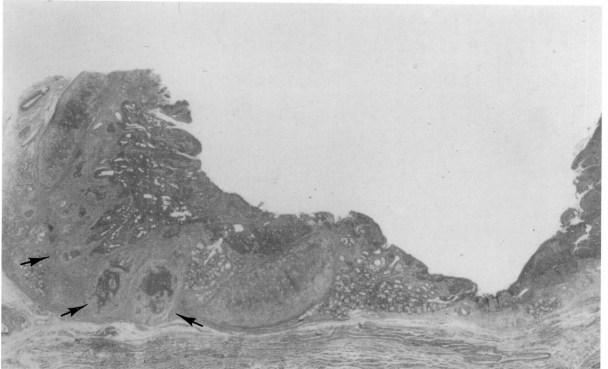

10

Fig. 10. Block 4 (see diagram) represents fourth section through LB1 & 2. Surface in situ change is present as in previous blocks, but focal invasive carcinoma extends deeply into bronchial wall at one point (**arrows**).

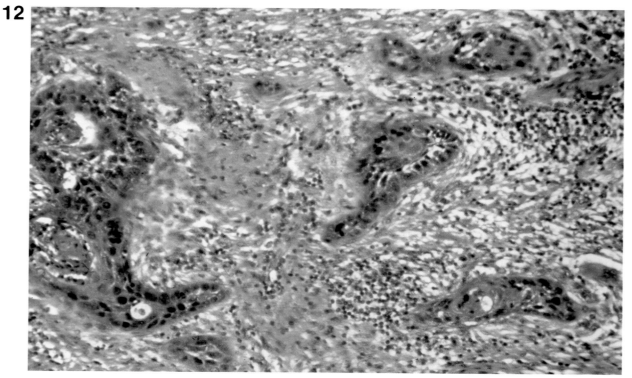

11

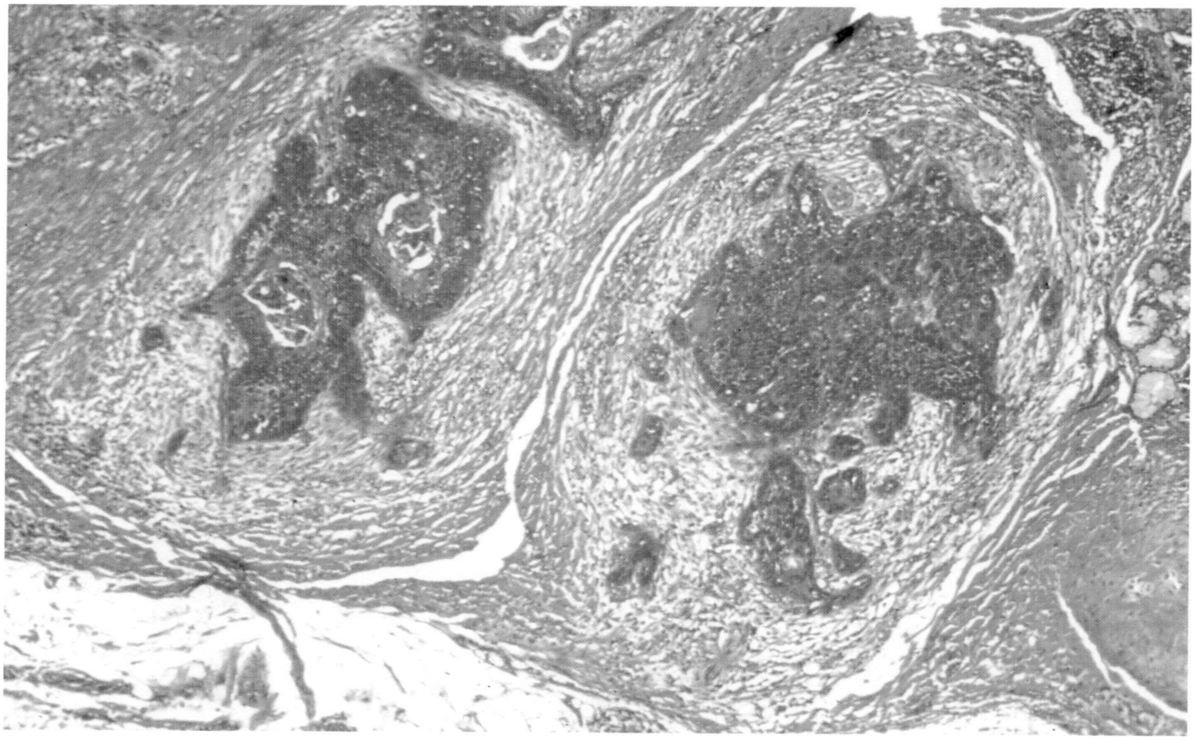

Fig. 11. Focal invasive squamous carcinoma in block 4 (see above) extends deeply into but not through bronchial wall.

12

Fig. 12. High-power magnification shows invasive keratinized squamous carcinoma deep in bronchial wall.

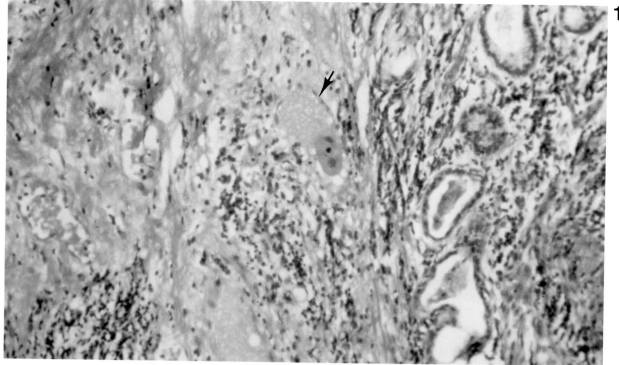

13

Fig. 13. Deeper section through same block as in previous figures shows numerous small capillaries, one of which contains tiny focus of carcinoma (**arrow**).

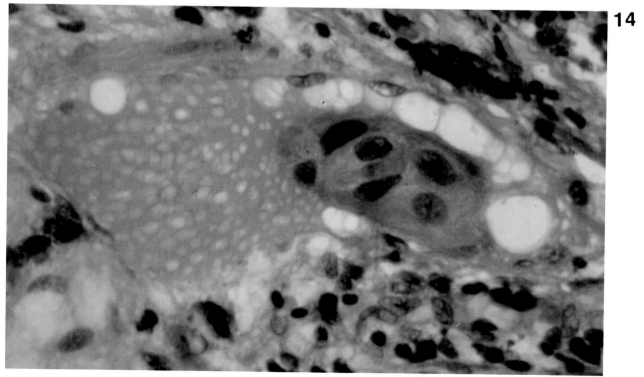

14

Fig. 14. High magnification shows details of capillary vascular invasion by carcinoma.

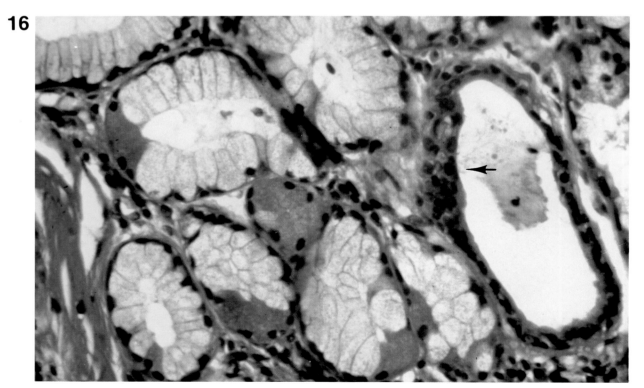

15

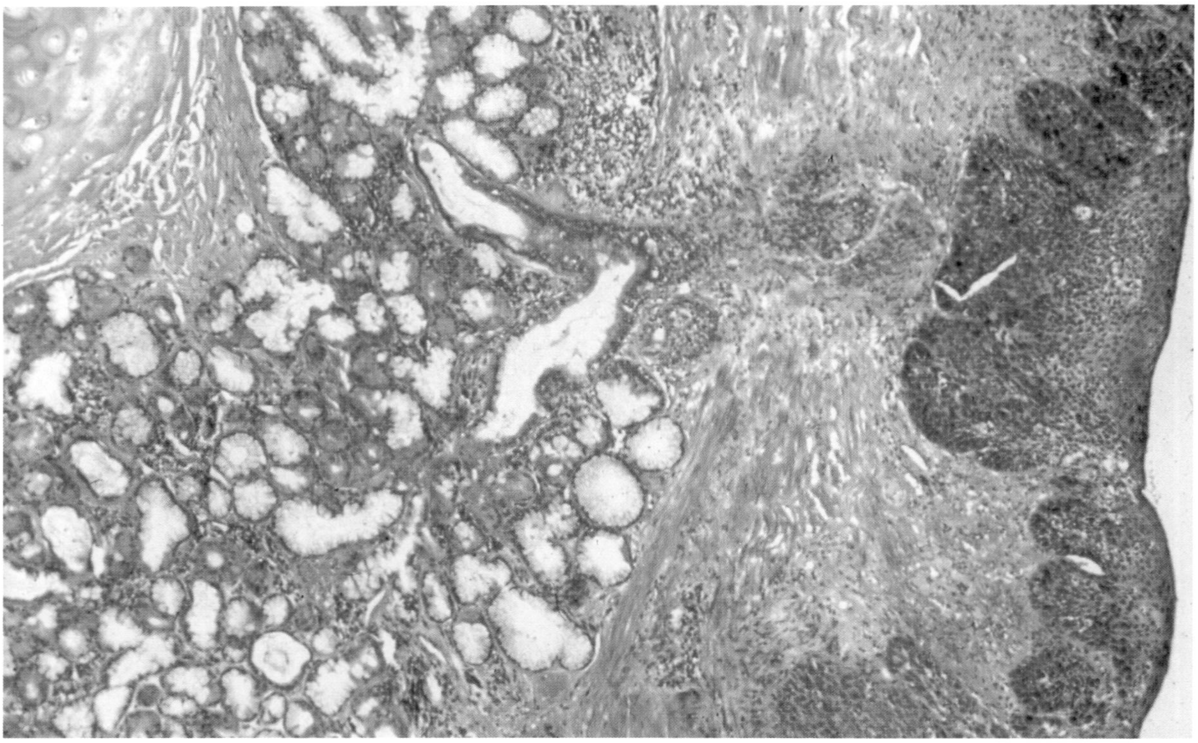

Fig. 15. Block 5 shows surface in situ carcinoma and underlying mucous glands with early ductal involvement.

16

Fig. 16. Block 5 also shows beginning proliferative change (**arrow**) in mucous glands of bronchial wall.

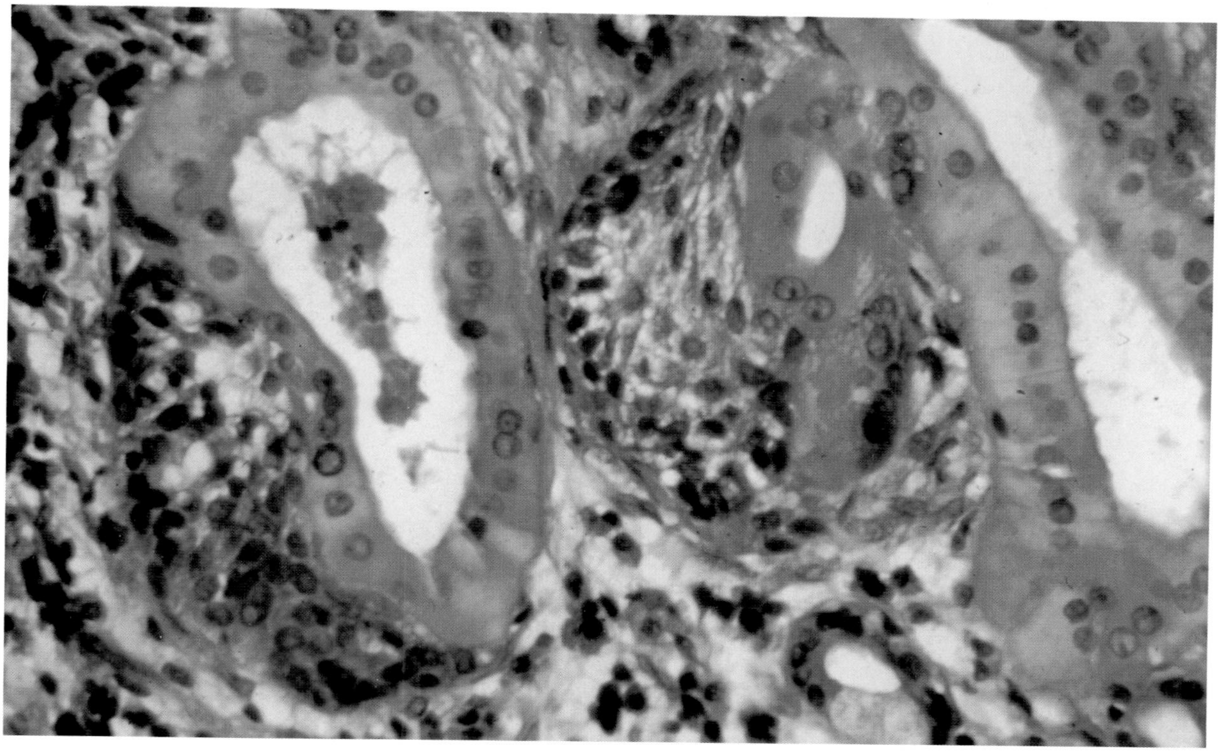

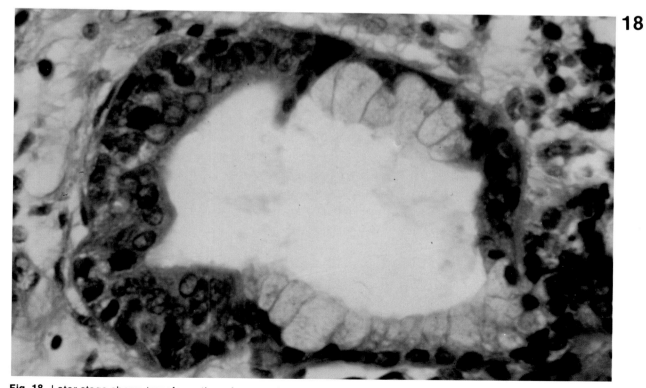

Fig. 17. This is a slightly more advanced stage in involvement of mucous glands.

Fig. 18. Later stage shows transformation of oncocytic glands to in situ carcinoma.

19

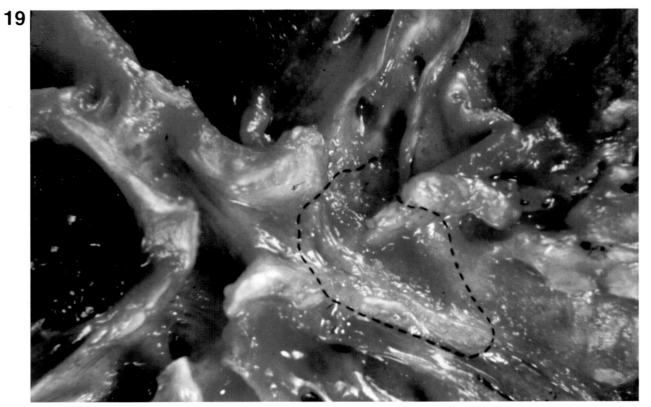

Fig. 19. Gross specimen showing location of tumor.

Summary

This carcinoma in situ involves the common LB1 & 2 bronchus and the orifices of LB1 and LB2 (2.0 by 0.8 cm) as marked. The lesion was not seen by the bronchoscopist but was visible on gross pathologic examination. Histologically, the lesion is squamous cell carcinoma in situ with focal microinvasion extending deeply into but not through the bronchial wall at one point. Vascular invasion by tumor cells was demonstrated in one capillary.

Case 8

A 62-year-old retired male civil service employee had a cerebral infarction 3 years previously and there was slight residual weakness in the left leg.

Sputum Cytology

The initial specimen showed carcinoma cells of the squamous type (Fig. 1A and B). Localizing bronchoscopy was recommended.

Localizing Bronchoscopy

The first bronchoscopy was performed 3 days after the positive sputum test. Results were negative. Postbronchoscopic sputum revealed markedly atypical squamous cells.

A second bronchoscopy 2 weeks later was also negative. Multiple (13) bilateral spur biopsies were negative. The initial postbronchoscopic sputum disclosed metaplastic squamous cells with marked atypia. Two more postbronchoscopic specimens were positive for squamous cancer cells, as were induced-sputum preparations (Fig. 1C and D).

A third bronchoscopy, 3 months after the second one, was also grossly negative. Bronchial brushings from the right upper lobe (RB1,2,3) were positive (Fig. 2A). Others were all negative. Multiple (14) bronchial spur biopsy specimens were negative.

A fourth bronchoscopy 3 days later revealed narrowing of one subdivision of RB2, although no tumor was visualized. Bronchial brushings from RB2 were positive; those from RB3 and RB6 were negative. Surgery was advised.

1

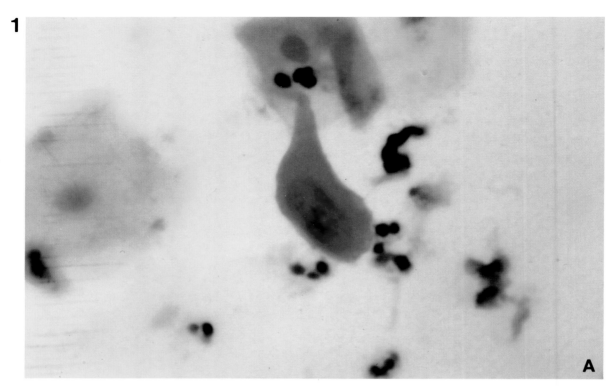

A

Fig. 1. Sputum cytology. **A** and **B**, Initial specimen shows single carcinoma cells, squamous type. **C** and **D** Induced-sputum specimen reveals highly keratinized squamous carcinoma cells. (Papanicolaou stain.)

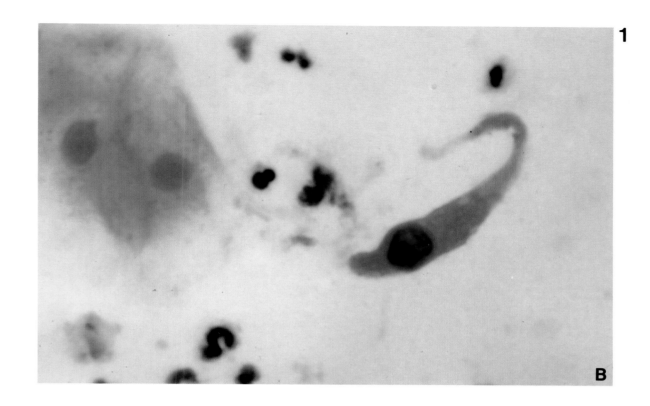

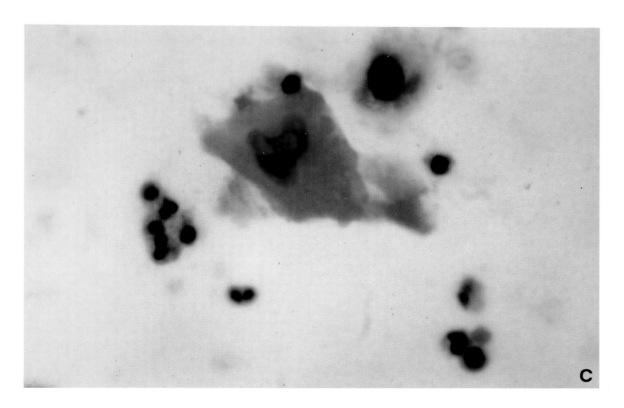

1

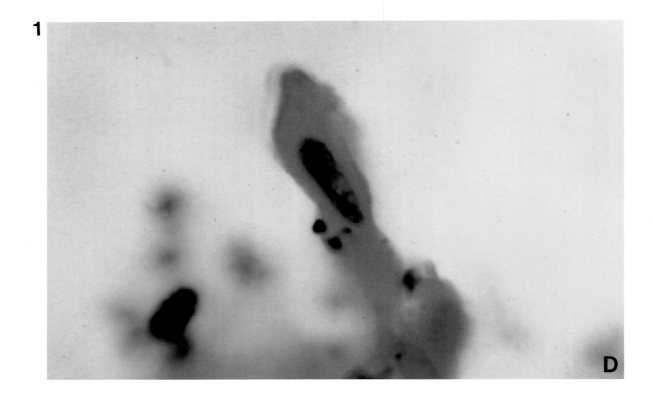

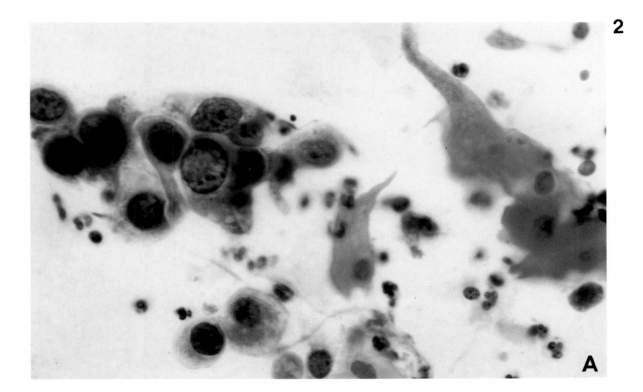

2

Surgery

At operation 1 week after the final bronchoscopy (4 months after first abnormal sputum), the right lung was negative to palpation. Right upper lobectomy was performed. The bronchial margin was free of cancer (fresh frozen sections).

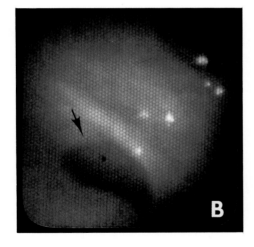

Fig. 2. A, Bronchial brush (RB1,2,3). Carcinoma cells, squamous type, are present, many with cyanophilic cytoplasm. (Papanicolaou stain.) **B,** Fiberbronchoscopic view shows narrowed orifice of RB2 subdivision **(arrow)**.

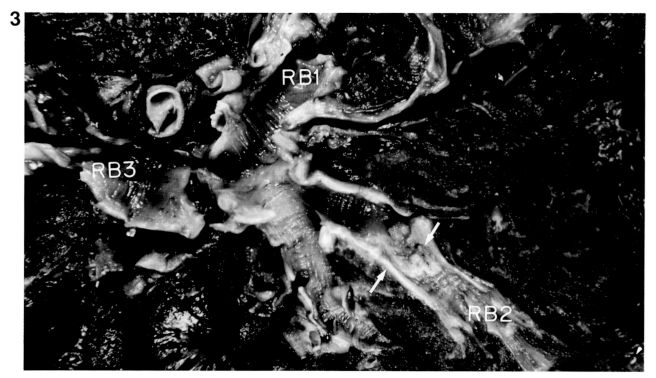

Fig. 3. Resected right upper lobe showing three segmental branches of right upper-lobe bronchus, as labeled. Gross tumor is visible at orifice of second-division branch of RB2 (**arrows**).

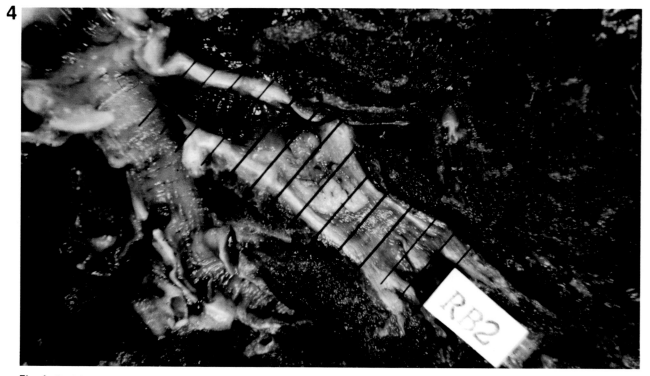

Fig. 4. Serial block sectioning of tumor area was carried out as in diagram. Remainder of bronchial tree was mapped and sectioned. Cross sections of tumor area are shown below.

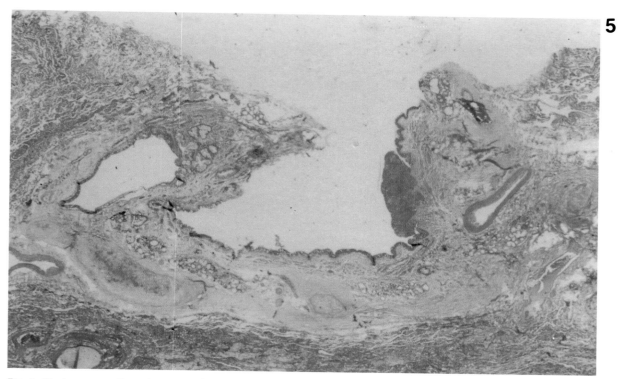

5

Fig. 5. First cross section of tumor (see diagram). Small, raised plaque is seen on one aspect of bronchial wall.

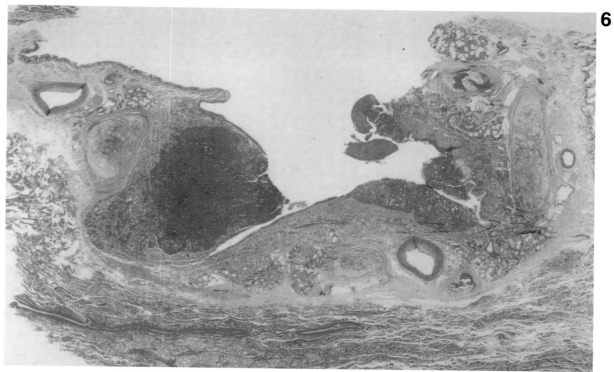

6

Fig. 6. Second cross section of tumor area (distal) shows continuation of in situ squamous cell carcinoma on right. Invasive carcinoma is present at orifice of another, unopened, second-division branch of RB2 on left.

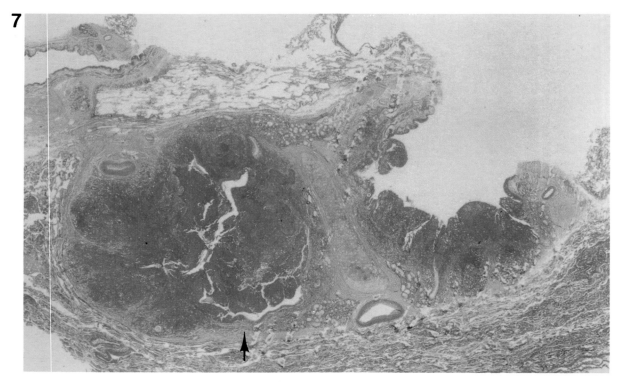

Fig. 7. More distal cross section of tumor area. In situ squamous cell carcinoma continues along opened second-division branch of RB2. Lumen of adjacent, unopened, second-division bronchus appears almost filled with tumor (**arrow**).

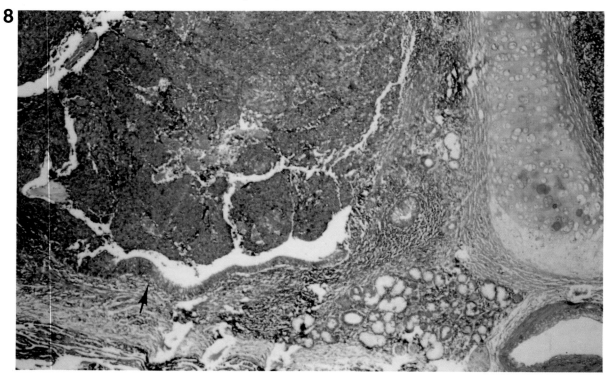

Fig. 8. Higher magnification of unopened branch shows residual ciliated bronchial epithelium merging into undifferentiated carcinoma on left (**arrow**).

9

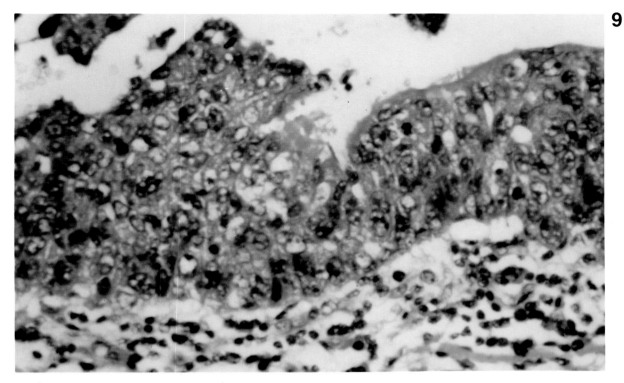

Fig. 9. High magnification of same junctional zone as in previous figure between ciliated bronchial epithelium and undifferentiated large cell carcinoma.

10

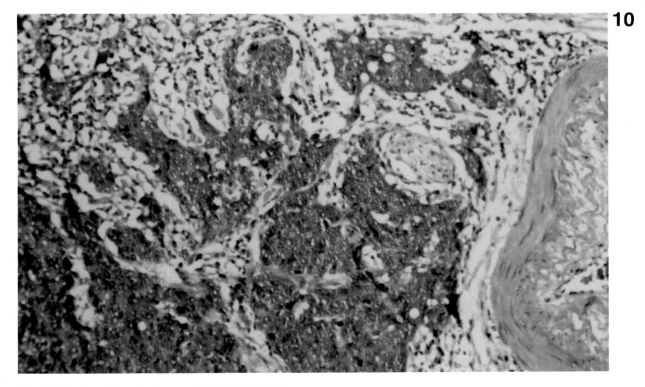

Fig. 10. Margin of invasive large cell undifferentiated carcinoma extends through entire thickness of bronchial wall at this level.

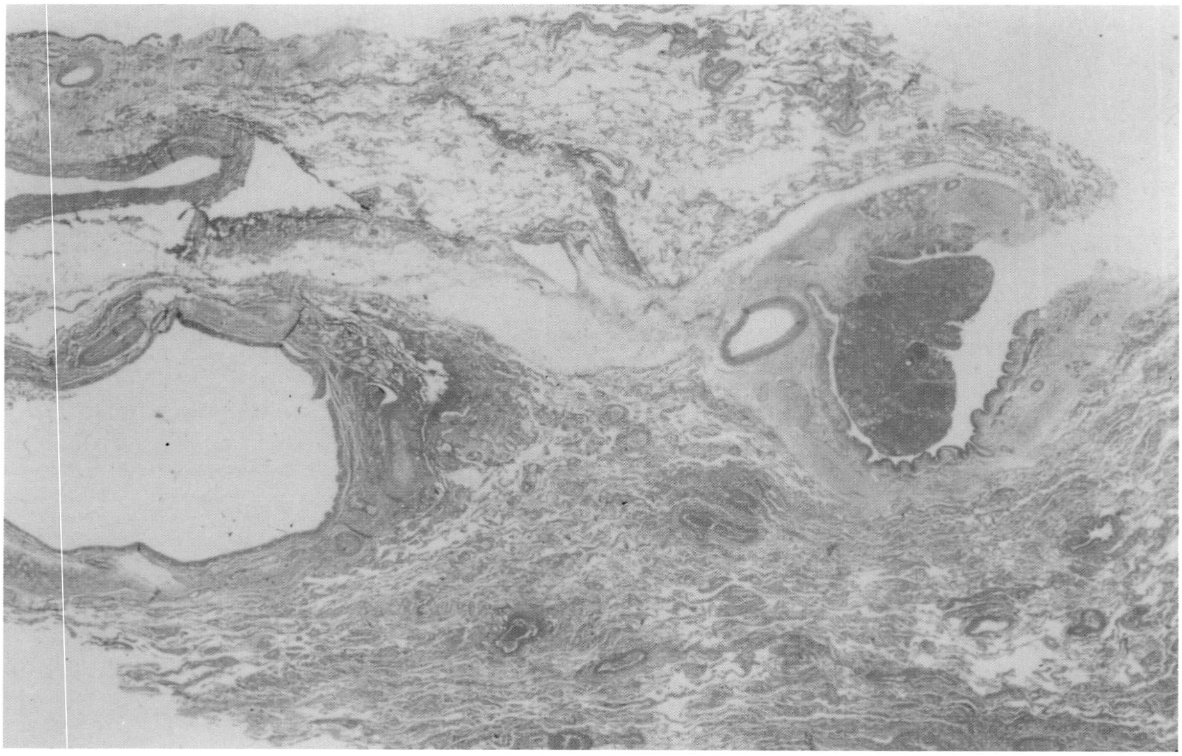

Fig. 11. Most distal tissue block through tumor area (see diagram). Opened second-division branch of RB2 (right) contains polypoid in situ squamous cell carcinoma. Unopened adjacent second-division branch (left) is free of tumor.

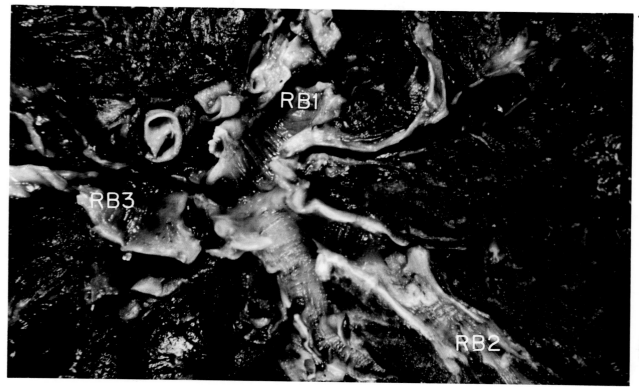

12

Fig. 12. Gross specimen showing tumor (see Fig. 3).

Summary

This in situ and infiltrative carcinoma, 0.9 cm in length, involves the second-division branches of RB2. The tumor was not seen by the bronchoscopist but was grossly visible on pathologic examination. Histologically, the lesion is in situ keratinizing squamous cell carcinoma in one second-division branch of RB2; an invasive nonkeratinizing large cell undifferentiated carcinoma is present in an adjacent second-division branch. The infiltrative carcinoma extends through the entire thickness of the bronchial wall but not into the adjacent pulmonary parenchyma.

Case 9

A 64-year-old retired male clerk had myocardial revascularization (coronary artery bypass) 2½ years previously. Currently there was no dyspnea or angina.

Sputum Cytology

The initial specimen was positive for squamous carcinoma cells (Fig. 1A and B). Induced sputum was obtained. The initial fresh specimen showed moderately atypical squamous cells; a delayed postinduction specimen revealed squamous cancer cells (Fig. 1C and D). Localizing bronchoscopy was recommended.

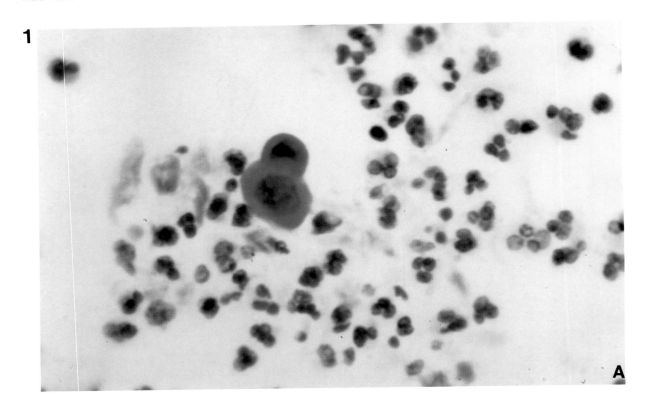

1

A

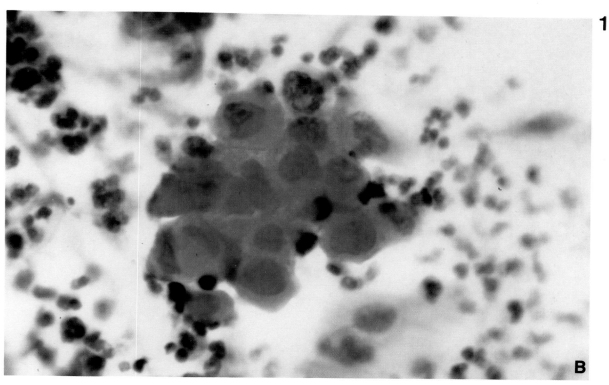

Fig. 1. Sputum cytology. **A** and **B**, Initial specimen shows carcinoma cells, squamous type, with degenerating inflammatory cells in background. **C** and **D**, Delayed sputum reveals carcinoma cells, squamous type, with marked cytoplasmic orangophilia. (Papanicolaou stain.)

1

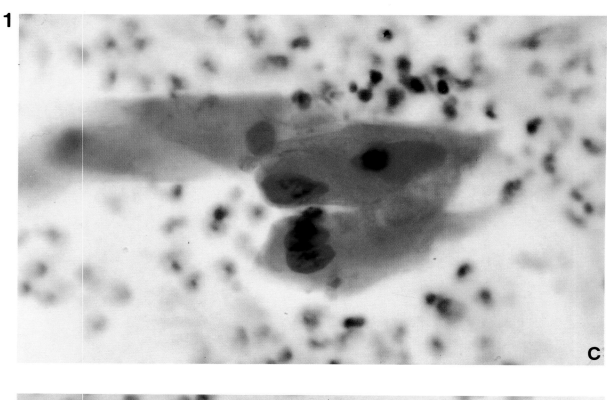

C

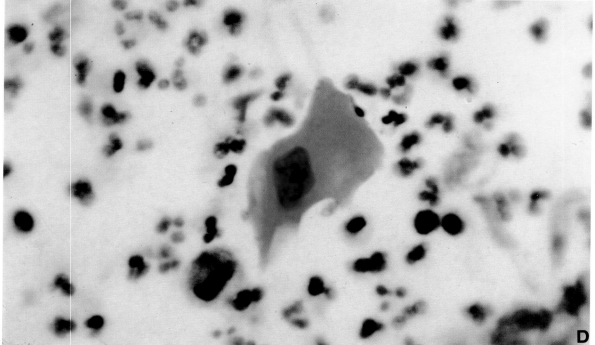

D

2

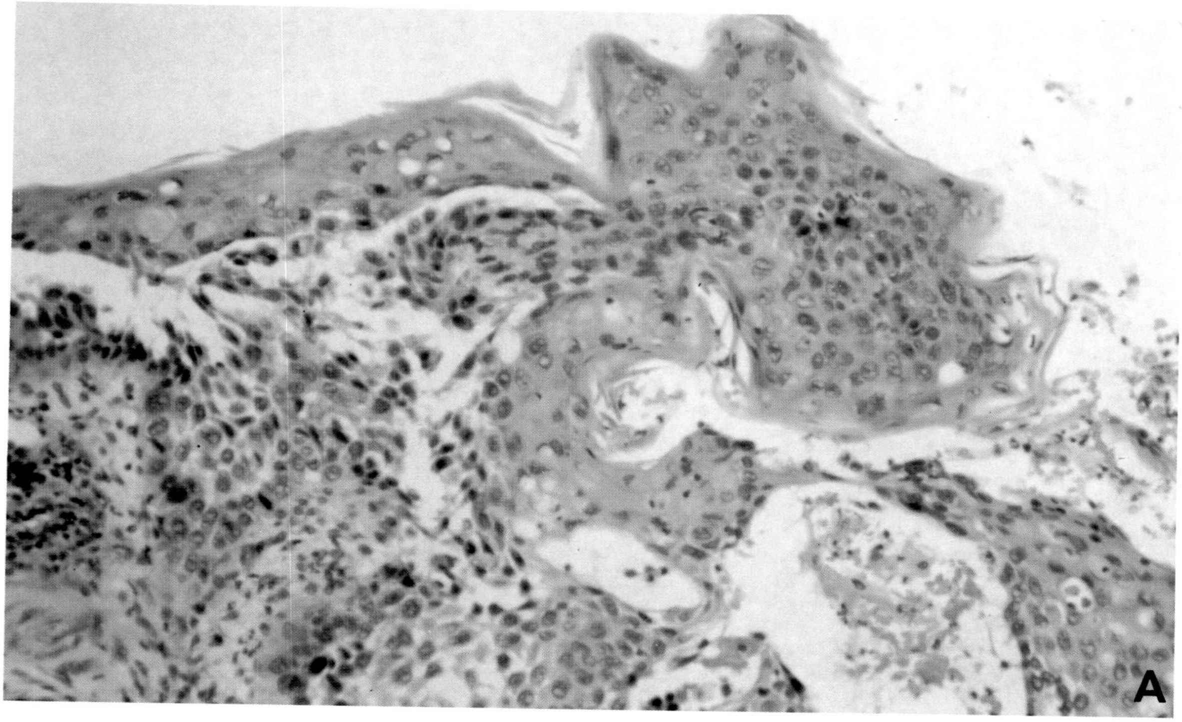

Localizing Bronchoscopy

Fiberoptic bronchoscopy was carried out 10 days after the first positive sputum. The trachea and the right side of the bronchial tree were normal. The mucosa surrounding the bronchus to the superior segment of the left lower lobe (LB6) was irregular and tumor was grossly evident. The left upper lobe appeared normal, but tumor extended very close to its orifice. Bronchial biopsy specimens obtained from the right side, tracheal bifurcation, and left upper lobe were normal. A specimen from the left lower lobe above LB6 disclosed in situ and infiltrative squamous cell carcinoma (Fig. 2A).

Fig. 2. A, Bronchial biopsy specimen (left lower lobe) shows squamous cell carcinoma with surface keratin production. (Hematoxylin and eosin stain.)

2

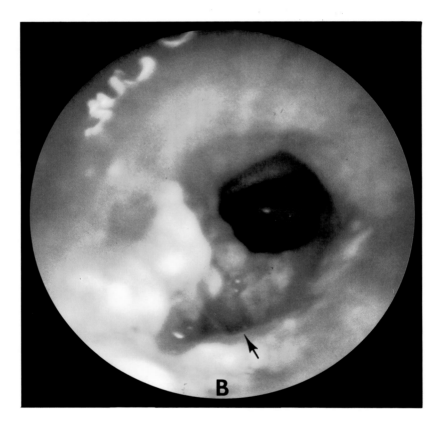

Fig. 2. B, In endobronchial view, orifice of LB6 is surrounded by tumor (**arrow**).

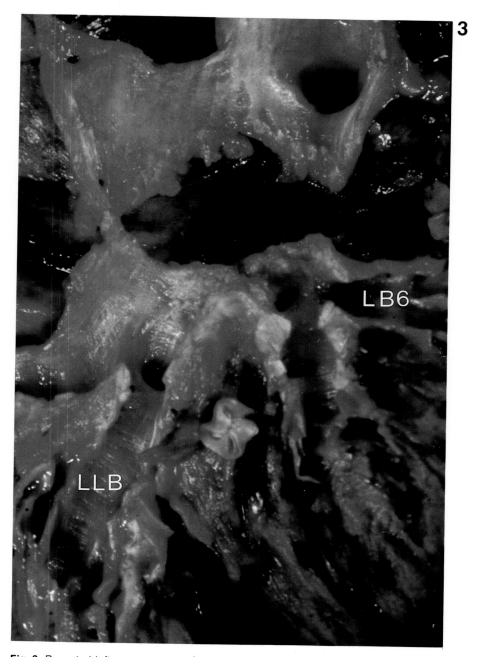

3

Fig. 3. Resected left upper and left lower lobes showing orifice of unopened left upper-lobe bronchus. Warty tumor involves lower-lobe bronchus (LLB) and proximal LB6.

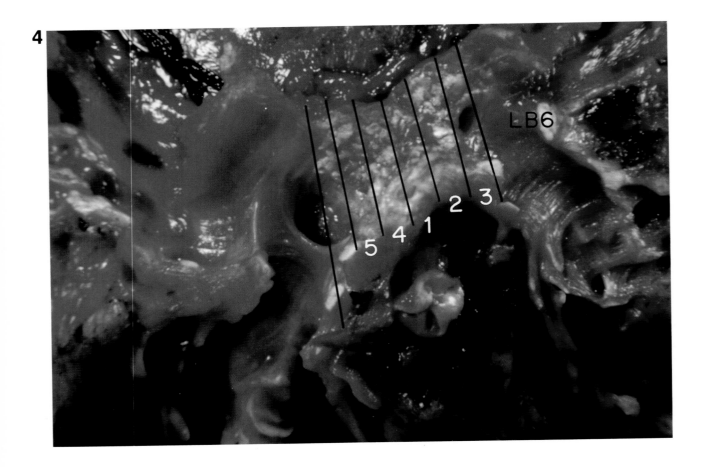

Surgery

At thoracotomy 3½ weeks after initial positive sputum, no gross tumor was palpable. Left lower lobectomy was performed. The margin of resection was involved by tumor, and left pneumonectomy was required.

Fig. 4. Serial block sectioning of entire warty lesion was carried out as in diagram. Remainder of bronchial tree was mapped and sectioned. Cross sections of LB6 are shown below.

5

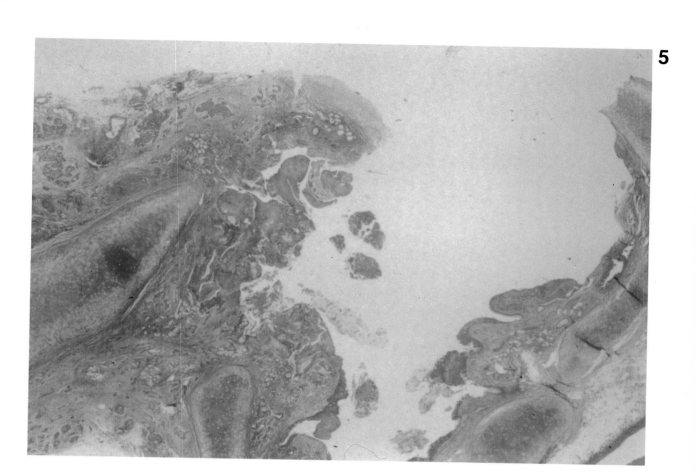

Fig. 5. Block 1 represents first cross section of LB6. Warty papillary tumor involves much of bronchial surface.

6

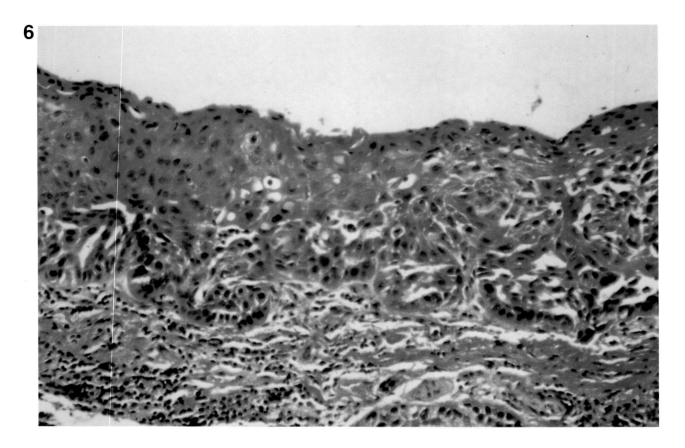

Fig. 6. Carcinoma in situ is seen, with maturation and keratin production at margin of infiltrative tumor.

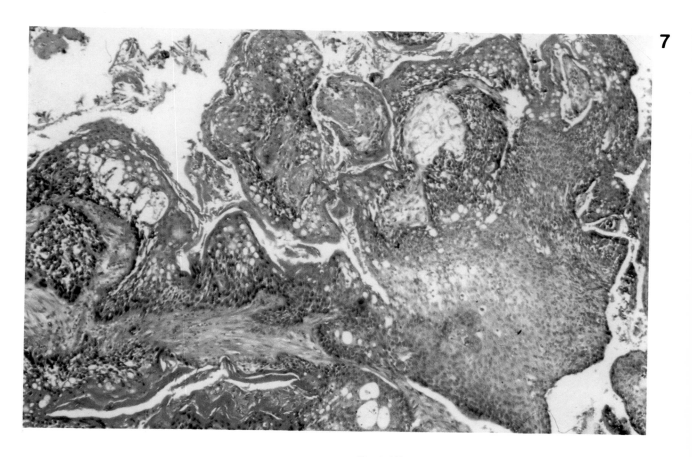

Fig. 7. Warty papillary squamous cell carcinoma projects from bronchial surface.

8

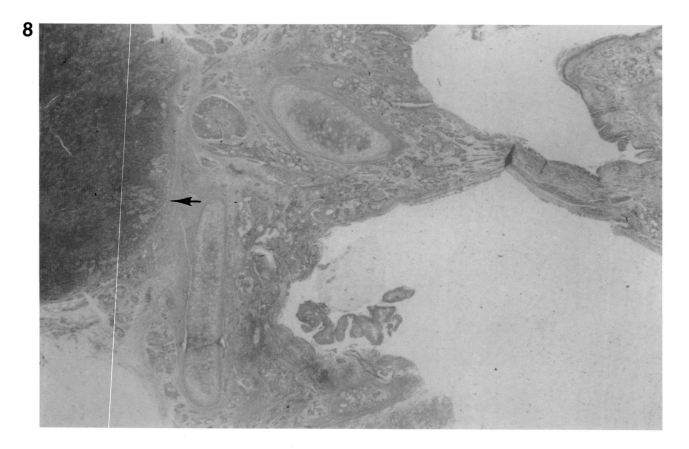

Fig. 8. Block 2 represents second cross section of LB6.
Little surface papillary squamous cell carcinoma is
evident, but there is extensive invasion of bronchial wall
by tumor and also direct invasion of margin of
peribronchial lymph node (**arrow**).

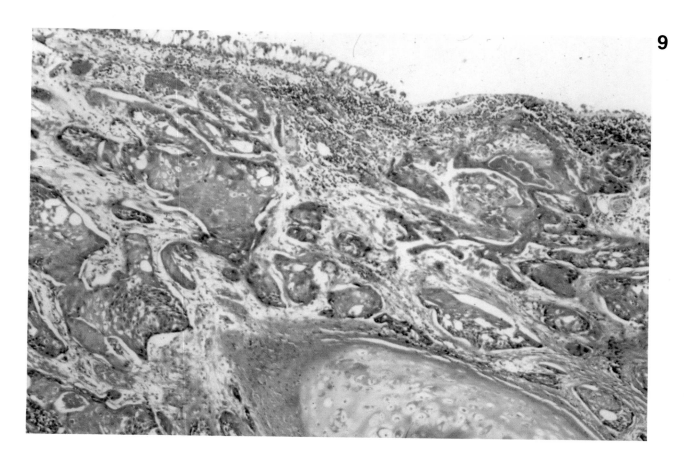

Fig. 9. Invasive squamous cell carcinoma extends deeply into bronchial wall under normal ciliated surface epithelium.

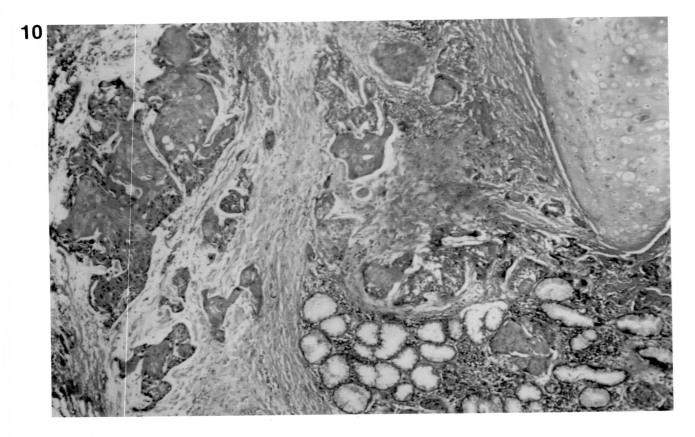

Fig. 10. Invasive squamous cell carcinoma extends
between bronchial cartilages into deeper portions of
bronchial wall.

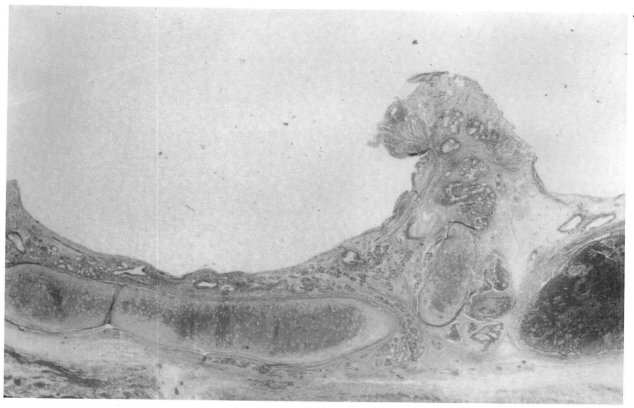

Fig. 11. Block 3 represents third cross section of LB6. Surface is normal, but extensive infiltrative squamous cell carcinoma surrounds bronchial cartilages.

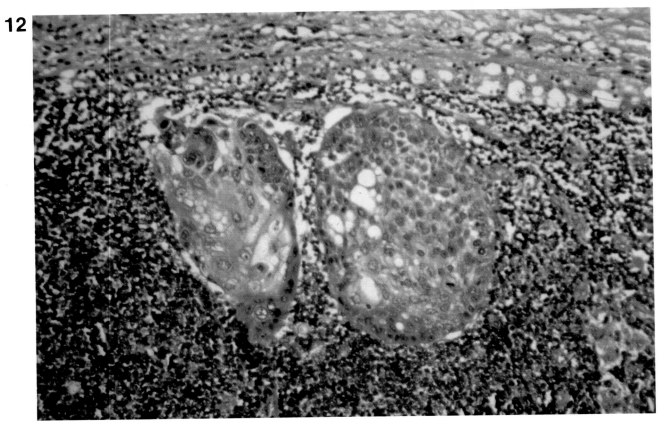

Fig. 12. Island of well-differentiated squamous cell carcinoma is present in peripheral sinus of peribronchial lymph node.

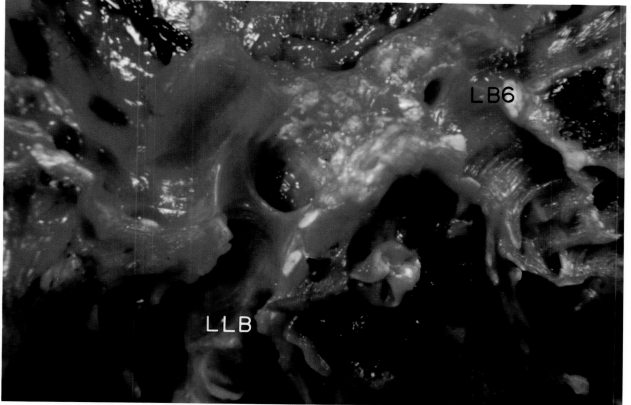

13

Fig. 13. Gross specimen of tumor (see Fig. 4).

Summary

This invasive squamous cell carcinoma with a warty surface component involves the left lower-lobe bronchus and proximal LB6. The lesion was grossly visible to the pathologist and to the bronchoscopist. Serial block sectioning revealed a large, warty, papillary squamous cell carcinoma with a relatively small in situ component. Well-differentiated invasive squamous cell carcinoma infiltrates the entire thickness of the bronchial wall, into the margin of a peribronchial lymph node, and extends along the bronchial wall beyond the gross margins of the tumor for 1.5 cm.

Case 10

A 61-year-old farmer desired a general medical examination. He had a history of hypertension that had been treated for 1 year.

Sputum Cytology

The initial screening specimen was negative. A second specimen obtained 4 months later showed markedly atypical squamous cells (Fig. 1A). Two repeat specimens were obtained, both of which showed marked atypia. Localization procedures were recommended. Induced-sputum preparations were positive for carcinoma cells of the squamous type (Fig. 1B, C, and D).

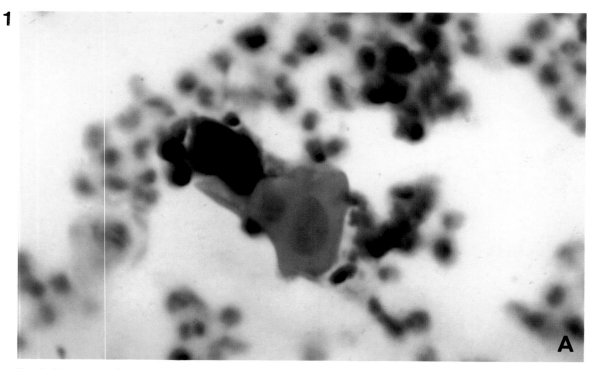

Fig. 1. Sputum cytology. **A,** Initial screening specimen shows markedly atypical squamous cells. **B** through **D,** Induced sputum reveals large squamous carcinoma cells, singly and in clumps. (Papanicolaou stain.)

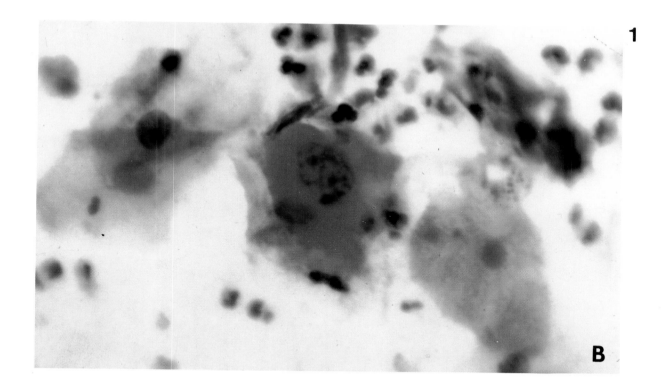

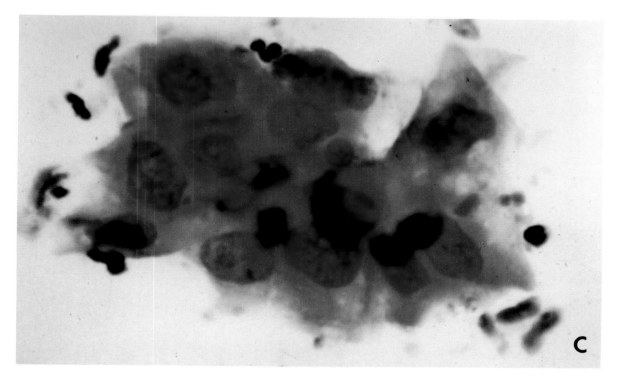

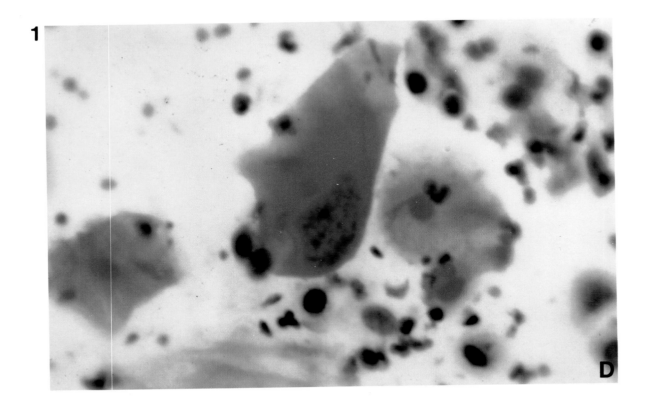

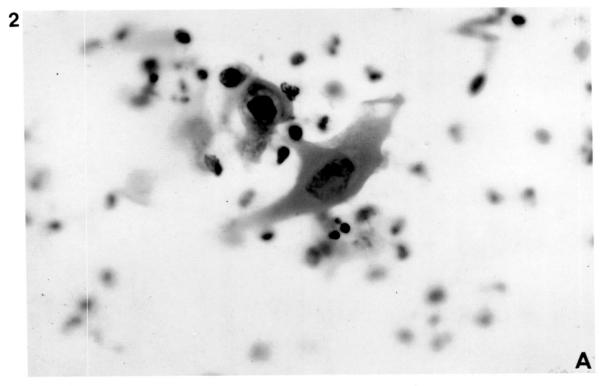

2

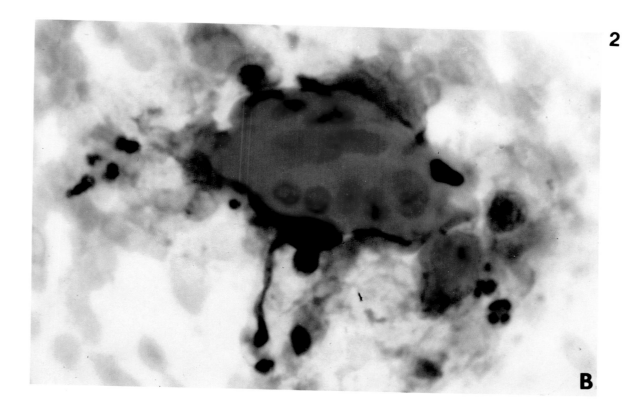

B

Localizing Bronchoscopy

A fiberoptic bronchoscopy was performed 3½ weeks after the first abnormal sputum and revealed a tiny tumor just inside the left upper-lobe bronchus along the inferior wall. There was also a suspicious area in the anterior segment of the right lower lobe, where the RB8 (a-b) bronchial spur was thickened.

Bronchial brushings of the left upper lobe (LB1,2,3) were positive for squamous cancer cells (Fig. 2A). Brushings from RB8 showed a few moderately atypical squamous cells (Fig. 2B). All others were negative.

Bronchial biopsy specimens from the left upper lobe and the RB8 (a-b) spur were positive for squamous cell cancer (Fig. 2C and D). Other areas showed only squamous metaplasia or normal mucosa.

Opposite Page

Fig. 2. A, Bronchial brushing from LB1,2 shows carcinoma cells, squamous type. **B**, Bronchial brushing from RB8 shows a clump of moderately atypical squamous cells. (Papanicolaou stain.) **C**, Biopsy specimen from left upper-lobe bronchus reveals squamous cell carcinoma. **D**, Biopsy specimen from RB8 shows squamous cell carcinoma. (Hematoxylin and eosin stain.) **E**, Fiberbronchoscopic view shows tumor (**arrow**) involving inferior wall of left upper-lobe bronchus. **F**, Fiberbronchoscopic view shows thickened RB8 (a-b) spur (**arrow**).

2

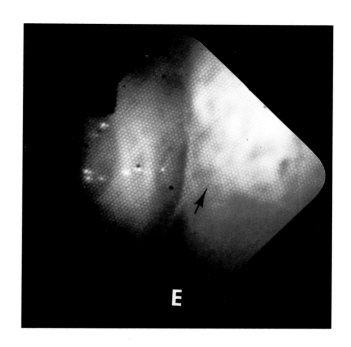

C

E

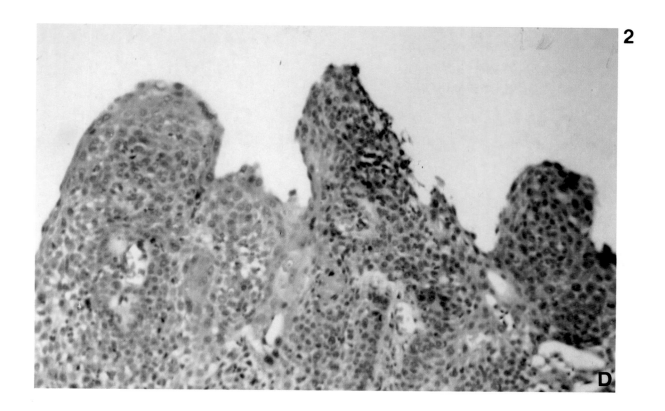

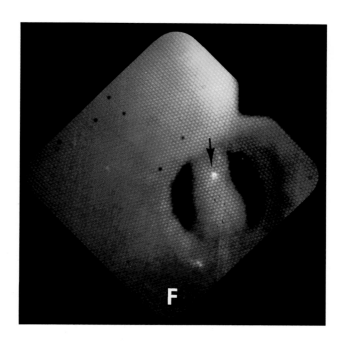

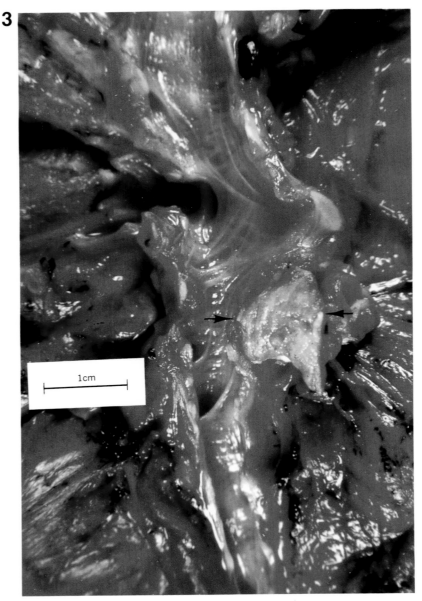

Fig. 3. Resected left upper lobe from first operation with triangular "window" from left upper-lobe bronchus removed as initial surgical procedure. Margin of this specimen was involved by tumor (**arrows**) (fresh frozen section). Left upper lobectomy was performed. Bronchial margin was free of tumor.

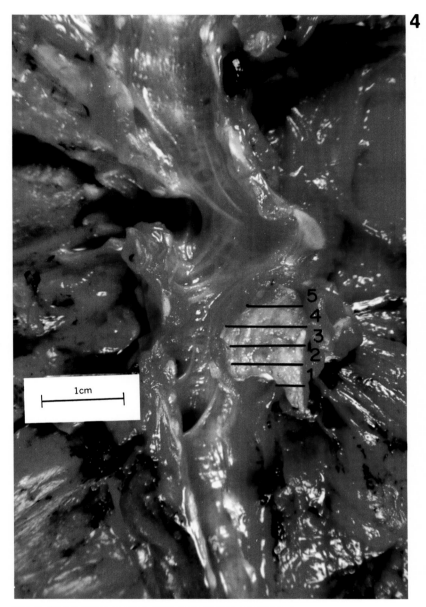

Fig. 4. Serial block section of "window" was carried out
as diagramed. Remainder of bronchial tree was blocked
and sectioned.

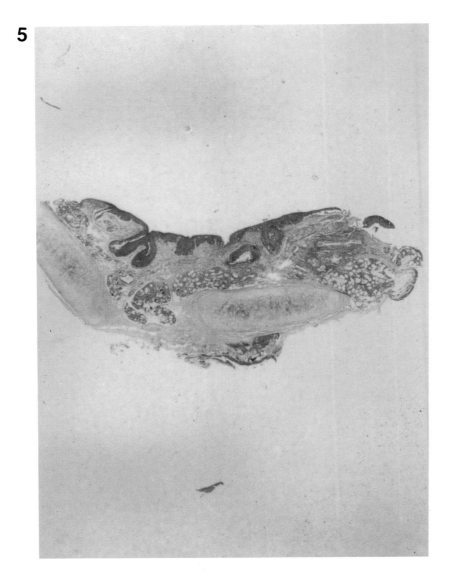

5

Fig. 5. First cross section of left upper-lobe "window" (see diagram). Entire surface epithelium is altered, with extension into ducts of mucous glands.

6

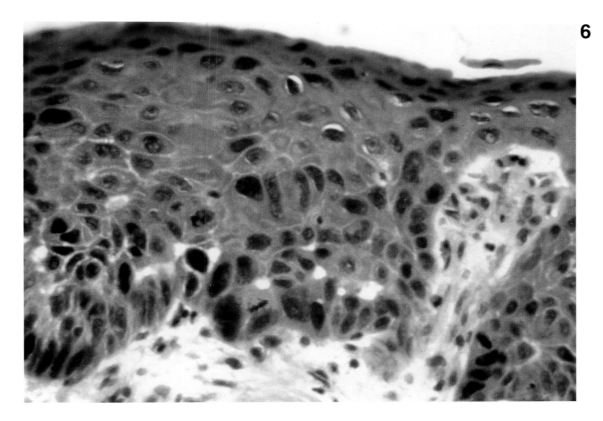

Fig. 6. Higher magnification demonstrates squamous cell carcinoma in situ, with considerable surface maturation.

7

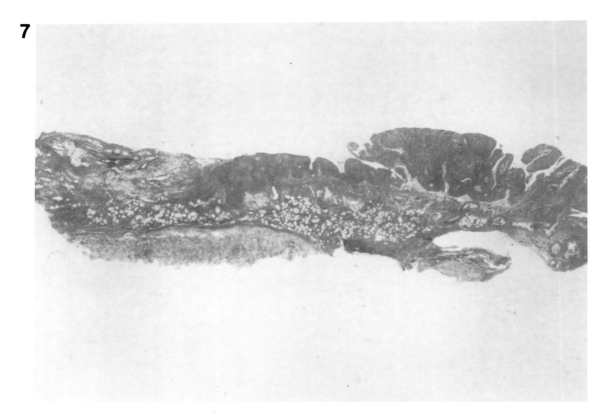

Fig. 7. Second cross section of left upper-lobe "window." Much of surface epithelium is replaced by warty tumor.

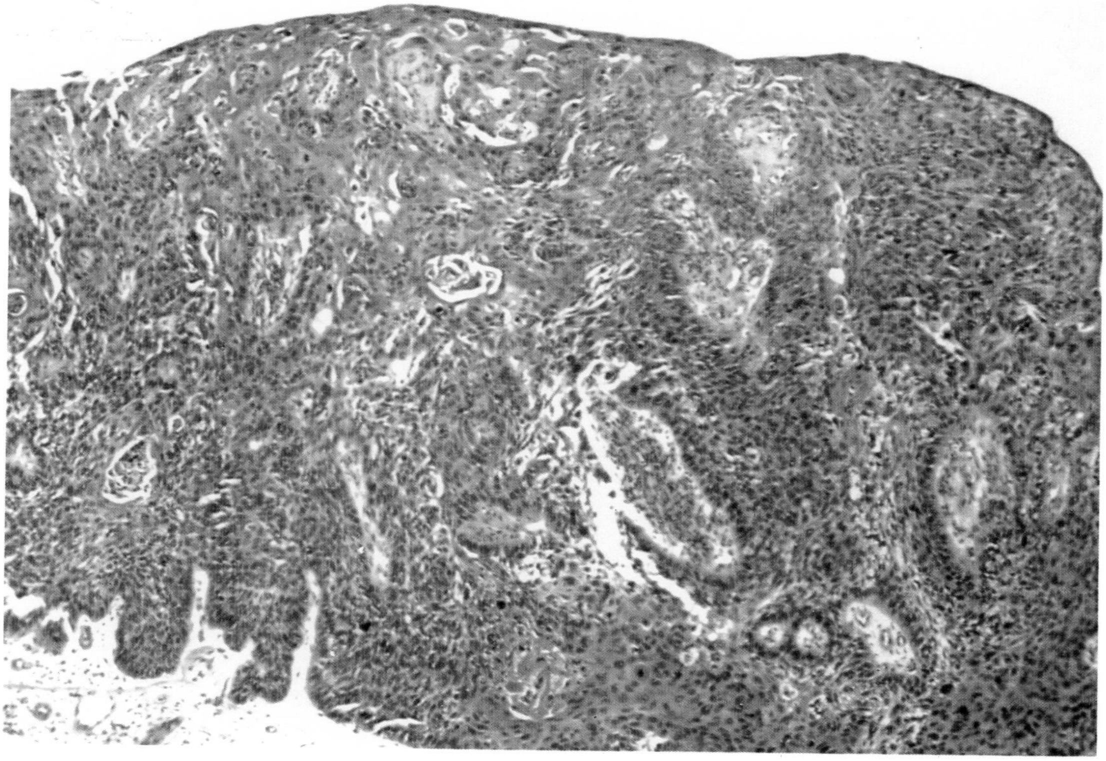

Fig. 8. Higher magnification demonstrates thickened plaque of squamous cell carcinoma.

9

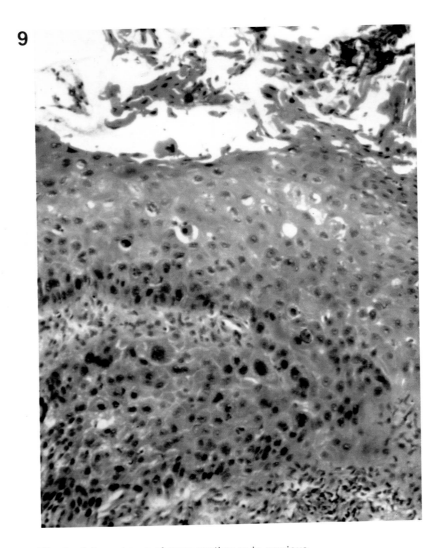

Fig. 9. Adjacent area of same section as in previous figure shows highly keratinized in situ carcinoma with focal mucosal invasion (0.1 cm in depth).

10

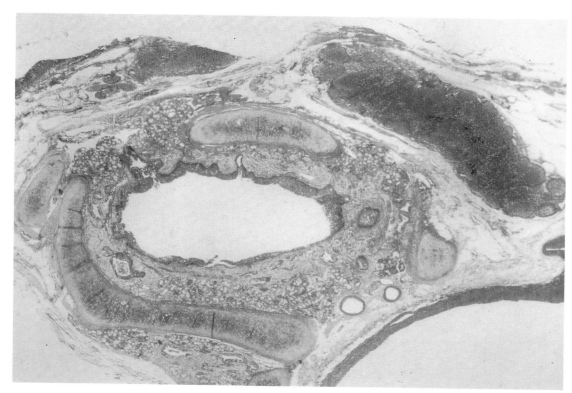

Fig. 10. First cross section of LB3 (unopened). There is obvious epithelial alteration of entire surface. (Five more distal blocks through LB3 were similarly involved.)

11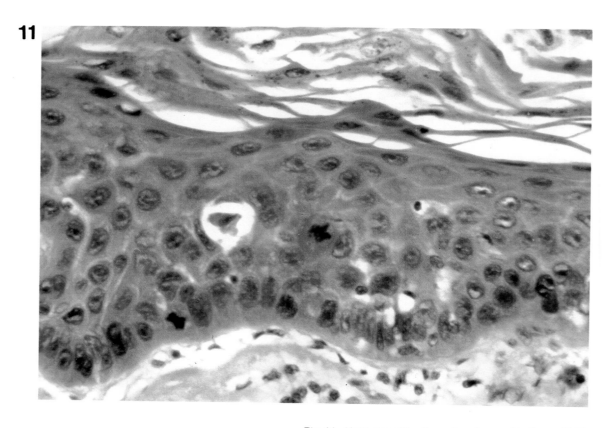

Fig. 11. High magnification of surface epithelium of LB3 shows well-differentiated squamous cell carcinoma in situ.

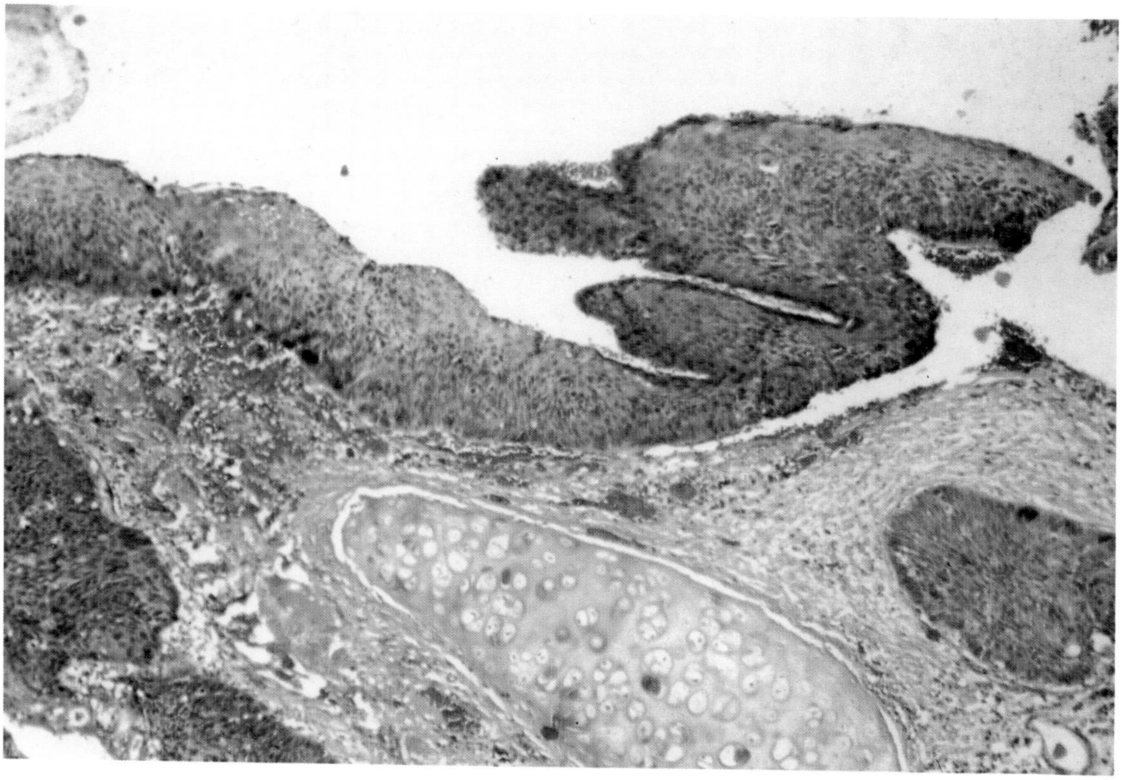

Fig. 12. Longitudinal section of peripheral 0.45 cm of LB1 (see Fig. 18). In situ squamous cell carcinoma is present, with extension into ducts of mucous glands.

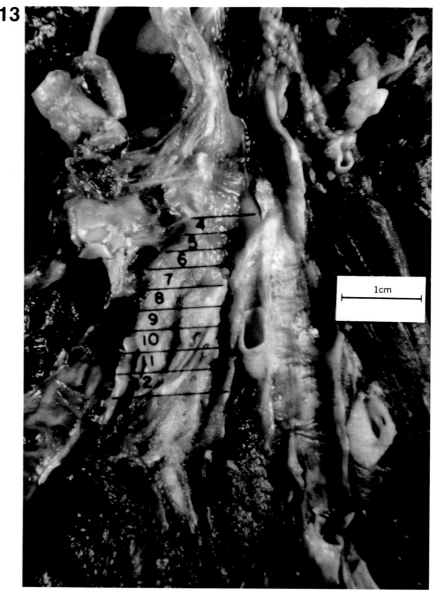

Fig. 13. Resected right lower lobe from second operation 1 month later. Warty tumor involved proximal RB8 and serial block sectioning of RB8 was carried out as diagramed. Tumor was demonstrated in nine consecutive blocks (3 cm in length).

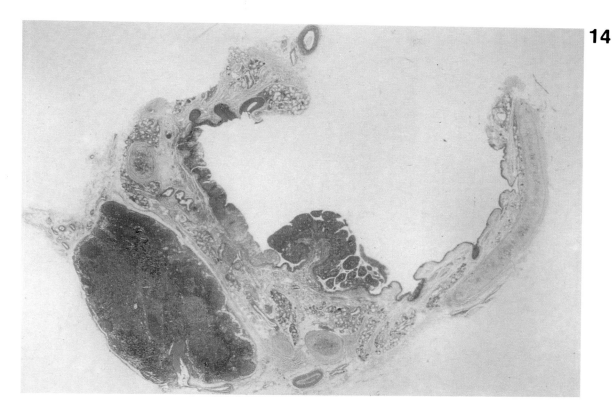

14

Fig. 14. First cross section through tumor (see diagram). In situ carcinoma with warty projection involves more than half of circumference of RB8.

15

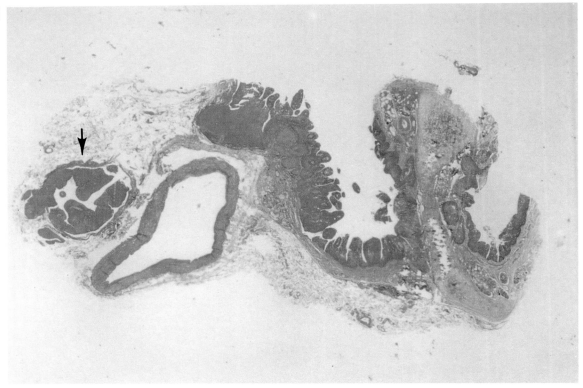

Fig. 15. Fifth cross section through tumor (RB8). In situ squamous cell carcinoma is present in RB8 and subsegmental branch. Focus of invasive squamous cell carcinoma appears within adjacent pulmonary parenchyma (**arrow**).

16

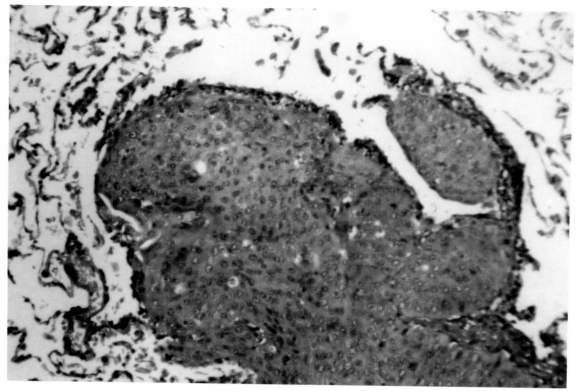

Fig. 16. High magnification shows intraparenchymal extension of carcinoma (0.3 cm in depth).

17

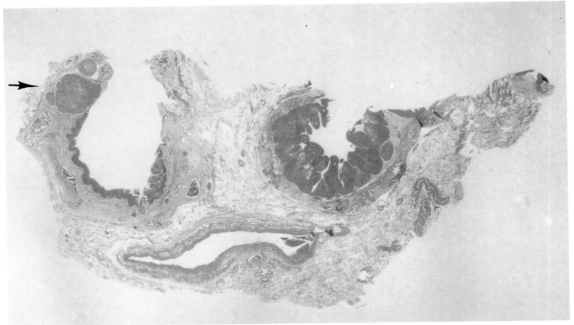

Fig. 17. Eleventh cross section of tumor (RB8). Both
subsegmental bronchi contain in situ carcinoma, with
slight focal invasion in one area (**arrow**).

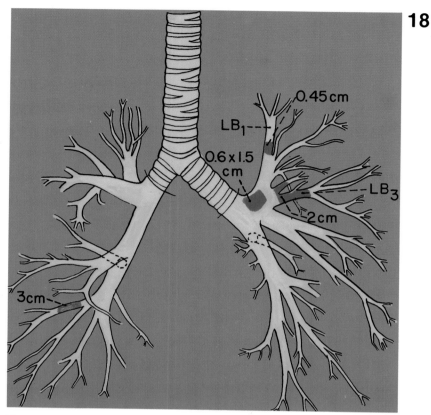

18

Fig. 18. Diagram of tracheobronchial tree showing locations of synchronous bilateral multicentric squamous cancers encountered in this case.

Summary

Diagram shows multicentric squamous cell carcinoma involving three separate foci of the left upper lobe and one basal segmental bronchus of the right lower lobe (see above). The lesions in the left upper-lobe bronchus and in RB8 were visible to the bronchoscopist and were also seen on pathologic examination. Lesions involving LB1 and LB3 were not visible to the bronchoscopist or to the pathologist. Histologically, the lesion is in situ squamous cell carcinoma in all sites with focal microinvasion, 0.1 cm in depth, in the left upper-lobe bronchus; there was also extension through the bronchial wall and into the adjacent pulmonary parenchyma in one block of RB8 (0.3 cm in depth). A small peribronchial lymph node was metastatically involved in the region of the tumor at this site.

Section 6

RADIOLOGY AND PATHOLOGIC CORRELATIONS

W. Eugene Miller, M.D.

John R. Muhm, M.D.

Frederick P. Stitik, M.D.

Lewis B. Woolner, M.D.

The cases in this chapter illustrate the early radiologic features of bronchogenic carcinoma. With one exception, all cases were detected by the prospective screening programs of the NCI Cooperative Early Lung Cancer Group. The exception in Case 5, in which a tumor that was inapparent on standard radiographic examination of the thorax was clearly localized by computed axial tomography. Two other radiologically oriented localizing techniques are also considered. They are percutaneous needle aspiration and tantalum bronchography.

Many of the cases demonstrate the well-documented (and humbling) observation that once a tumor has been detected radiographically, it can often be recognized retrospectively on earlier films. This occurred in the present group of cases despite the fact that every radiograph was independently interpreted by at least two qualified observers. Nevertheless, it is encouraging that most tumors were detected while they were still less than 3 cm in diameter. Thus, perodic radiologic screening of persons who have an increased susceptibility to lung cancer ("high-risk" groups) appears to be helpful in early detection of lung cancer.

Approximately half of all bronchogenic carcinomas arise **centrally,** in the area occupied by the main-stem, lobar, segmental, and subsegmental bronchi, all of which are within visual range of the bronchofiberscope. Early central cancers may either be radiographically inapparent ("occult") or present as hilar or perihilar densities.

The remaining bronchogenic cancers are located **peripherally,** beyond broncho-fiberscopic visibility. Their early radiologic manifestations are nodular or irregular densities, sometimes associated with areas of pneumonitis. It is in cases of peripheral tumors that percutaneous needle aspiration has its greatest applicability.

Prompt radiologic detection of lung cancer requires optimum equipment, strict quality control of the filming process, and lateral or stereoscopic projections of the thorax as well as the standard posteroanterior view. The importance of multiple radiologic interpretations by skilled observers should be emphasized. So too should the value of comparison with previous "reference" films. Finally, one must develop a high degree of alertness for any "indeterminate" nodular or fibrotic lesions that may occur in persons within the "high-risk" group.

Part I: Central Cancers

Case 1

63-year-old man

Tumor: Small ("oat") cell carcinoma.

Location: Medial portion of right upper lobe, right upper hilus, and adjacent mediastinum.

Treatment: Unresectable. Palliative radiotherapy and chemotherapy were administered.

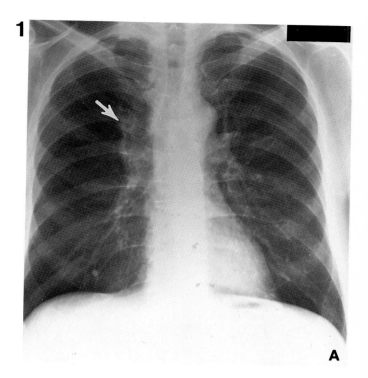

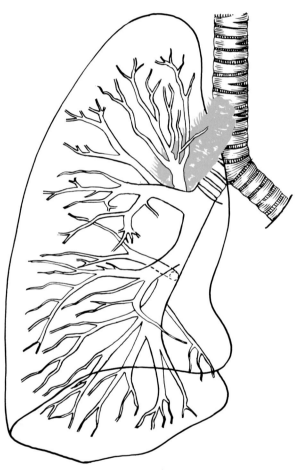

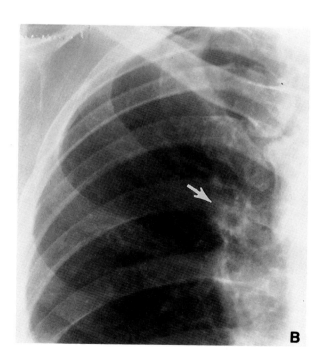

Radiology

Fig. 1. Initial screening x-ray was interpreted as showing no tumor, but in retrospect there appears to be some enlargement of right upper hilus and an irregular density extending into suprahilar area (**arrows**). **A,** Posteroanterior view of chest. **B,** Localized view of right upper hilus and upper lung.

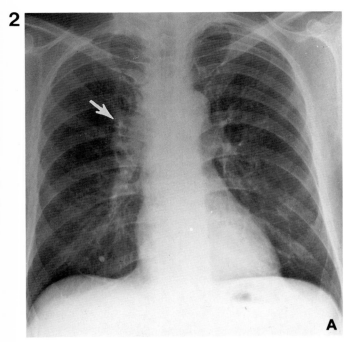

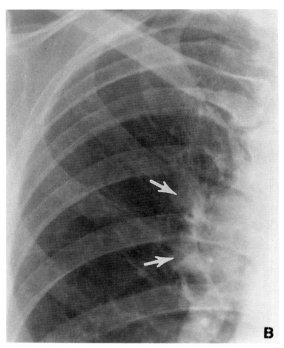

Fig. 2. X-ray 4 months later, when cancer was detected. There is definite enlargement of right middle and upper hilar regions. Irregular density extends into medial

aspect of right upper lung (**arrows**). **A,** Posteroanterior view of chest. **B,** Right upper hilus and upper lung.

Pathology

Fig. 3. Histologic section of biopsy specimen from mediastinoscopy shows small ("oat") cell undifferentiated bronchogenic carcinoma.

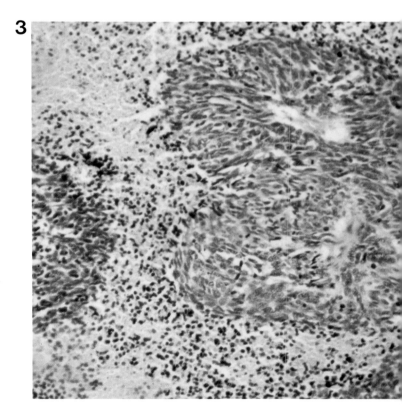

Comment

Small cell bronchogenic carcinoma is difficult to diagnose in its early stages. Radiologic detection is usually possible before cytologic detection. Most small cell cancers are hilar tumors that enlarge rapidly and soon spread to the surrounding lymph nodes, to the mediastinal structures, and to distant sites, especially brain, bone and liver. These tumors are rarely resectable, but they sometimes respond to chemotherapy or chemotherapy combined with radiotherapy.

Case 2

52-year-old man. Recurrent pneumonia, left upper lobe.

Tumor: Squamous cell carcinoma.

Location: Left upper-lobe bronchus centrally.

Treatment: Left pneumonectomy was necessary because of the proximity of the tumor to the left main bronchus.

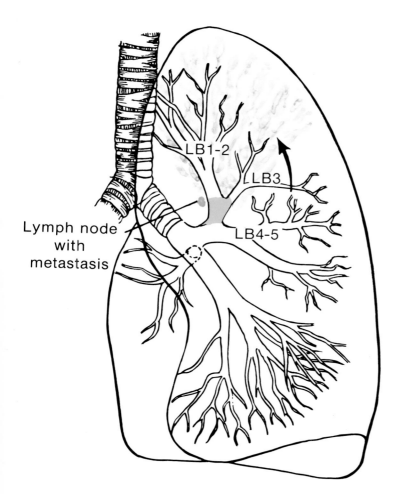

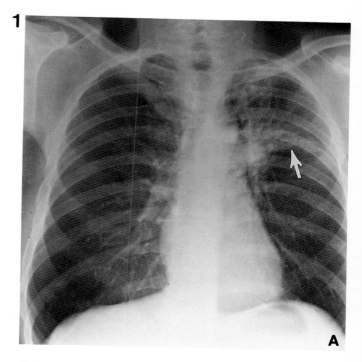

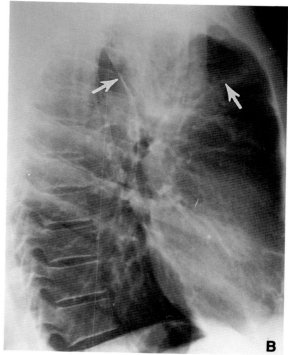

Radiology

Fig. 1. Initial screening x-ray shows pneumonitis and loss of volume in left upper lobe (**arrows**), with sparing of lingula. **A,** Posteroanterior view of chest. **B,** Lateral view.

Pathology

A small squamous cell carcinoma (1.5 by 1.0 by 0.4 cm) was present in the upper-lobe bronchus and caused obstructive pneumonitis, with abscess formation and loss of volume in the apical-posterior (LB1&2) and anterior (LB3) segments. In addition to involving the origins of these bronchi, the tumor extended proximally to the junction with the left main-stem bronchus. The lingula (LB4,5) was not involved. One peribronchial lymph node was metastatically involved.

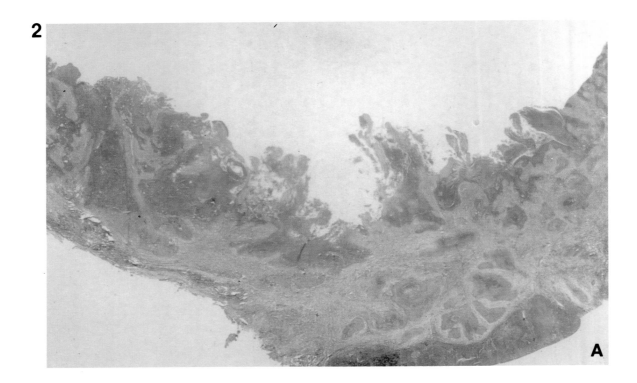

Comment

Symptoms of recurring pneumonia with radiographic evidence of lobar or segmental involvement are often associated with advanced lung cancer. However, occasionally, as in this case, a small, resectable central tumor may cause these findings.

This case is a good example of an "early" lung cancer requiring a pneumonectomy

Fig. 2. A, Low-power mounted microscopic section through left upper-lobe bronchus shows invasive squamous cell cancer. **B**, Higher magnification of section of tumor.

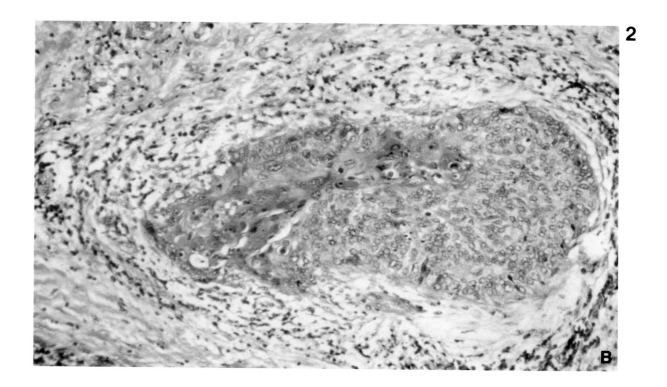

because of encroachment on the adjacent main-stem bronchus.

A radiologic clue to the small size of the tumor is provided by the sparing of the lingular segments (LB4,5). This has produced an obstructive pneumonitis configuration atypical for the left upper lobe but characteristic of the trisegmented right upper lobe.

Case 3

64-year-old man

Tumor: Small ("oat") cell carcinoma.

Location: Left upper lobe, perihilar location.

Treatment: Left upper lobectomy, plus chemotherapy.

Radiology

Fig. 1. Initial screening chest x-ray was interpreted as normal. **A,** Posteroanterior view of chest. **B,** Localized view of left upper lung.

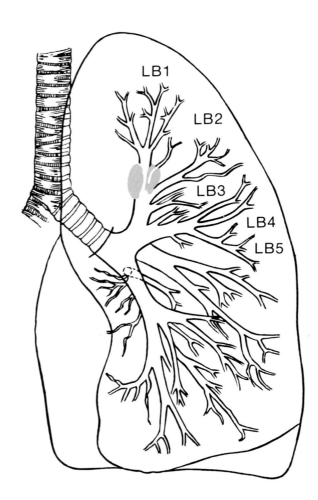

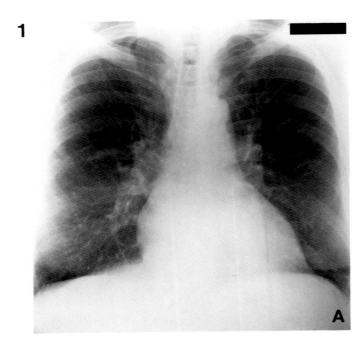

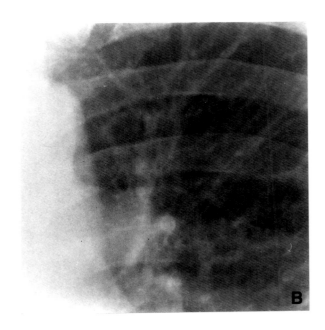

2

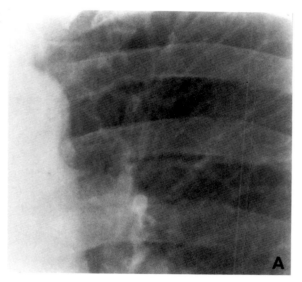

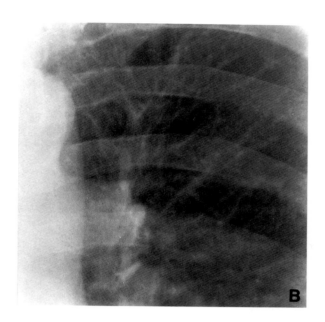

Fig. 2. Prospective sequential localized views of left upper lung show no change. **A,** Four months after initial x-ray. **B,** Twenty-eight months afterward. **C,** Thirty-two months afterward.

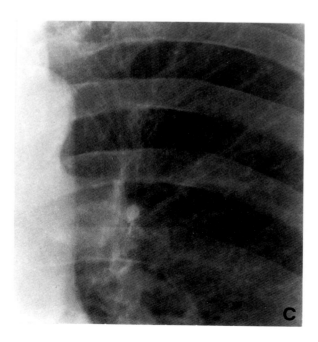

3

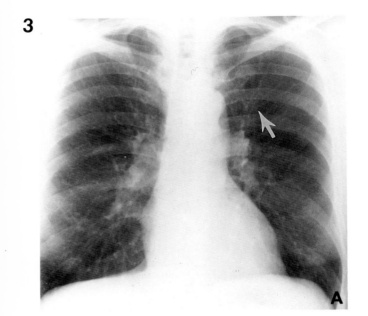

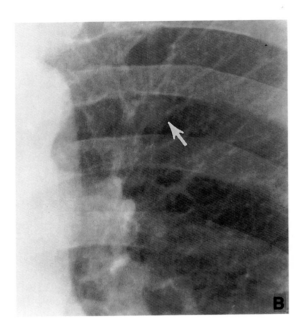

Fig. 3. X-ray 3 years after initial film. It was interpreted as representing no change, but in retrospect there may be a small, faint, irregular density (**arrow**) above left hilus. **A**, Posteroanterior view of chest. **B**, Left upper lung.

4

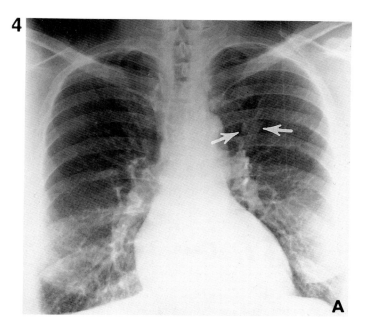

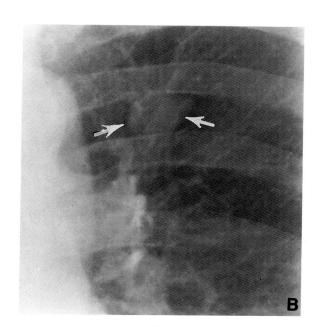

Fig. 4. X-rays 4 months later, when tumor was detected. There is now an irregular nodule (**arrows**) above left hilus. **A**, Posteroanterior view of chest. **B**, Left upper lung. **C**, Hilar tomogram shows relationship of tumor to LB1 bronchus.

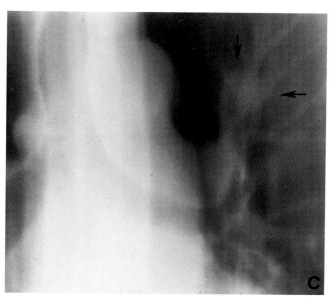

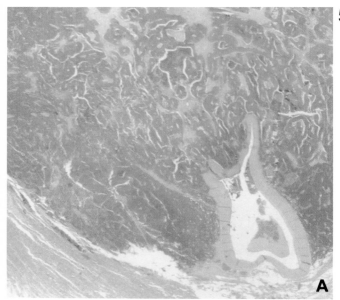

5   Pathology

This 2-cm ill-defined small cell carcinoma was located in the apical segment (LB1) of the left upper lobe. The tumor involved and constricted this bronchus and infiltrated the adjacent pulmonary parenchyma. Lymph nodes were not involved.

Fig. 5. A, Low-power mounted microscopic section of intraparenchymal tumor shows relatively smooth border. **B**, Low-power section of small ("oat") cell cancer. **C**, High-power magnification of same area.

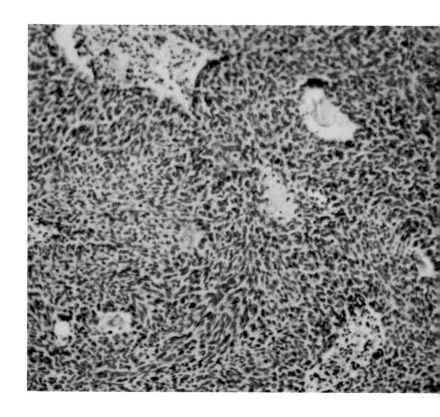

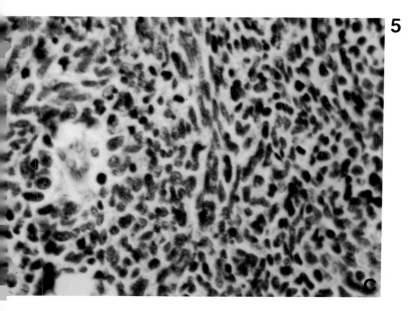

5

Comment

Although most small cell carcinomas are unresectable, some, such as this one, may be circumscribed and distal to the hilus when first discovered. If so, resection may be attempted, but adjuvant chemotherapy, with or without radiotherapy, should also be administered.

This is a case of carcinoma visible retrospectively on review of earlier films. Such an occurrence is not uncommon when chest x-rays are taken sequentially and each new set of films is compared with the previous ones.

Case 4

60-year-old man

Tumor: Squamous cell carcinoma.

Location: Perihilar, in apical-posterior segment of left upper lobe (LB1&2).

Treatment: Left upper lobectomy.

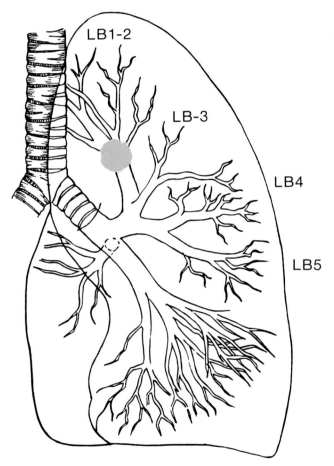

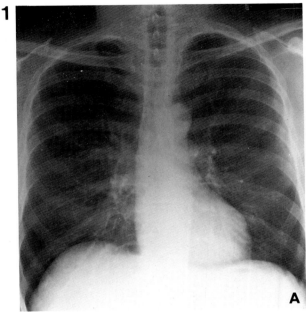

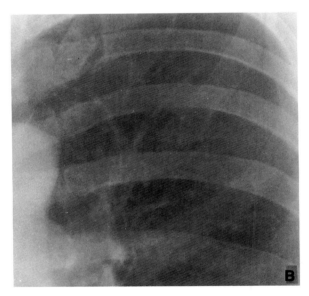

Radiology

Fig. 1. Initial screening chest x-ray was interpreted as normal. **A,** Posteroanterior view of chest. **B,** Localized view of left upper hilus and lung where tumor was later discovered.

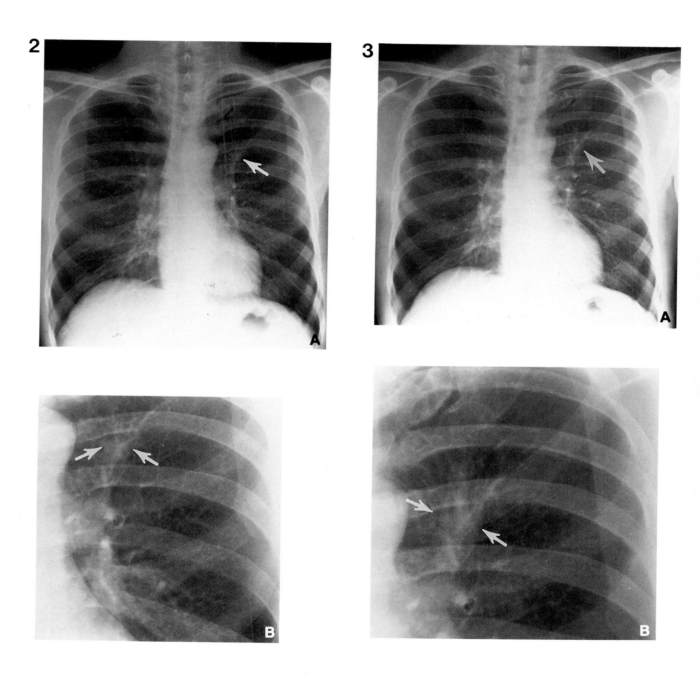

Fig. 2. Follow-up x-ray, obtained 20 months later, was interpreted as negative. In retrospect, there is an ill-defined density (**arrows**) in left suprahilar area, appearing to accentuate upper "horn" of hilus. **A,** Posteroanterior view of chest. **B,** Local view of left hilar and perihilar regions.

Fig. 3. X-ray 2 years after initial film, when cancer was detected. There is an ill-defined but definite ovoid density (**arrows**) above left hilus. **A,** Posteroanterior view of chest. **B,** Local view of left upper hilus and lung.

3

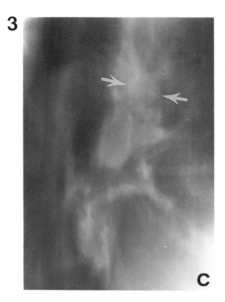

Fig. 3. C, Tomogram—55° left posterior oblique—best demonstrates tumor (**arrows**).

Pathology

Fig. 4. Resected left upper lobe shows sessile tumor, 2.4 by 1.5 by 0.6 cm, involving LB1 & 2 bronchus (**arrows**). Lymph nodes were not involved.

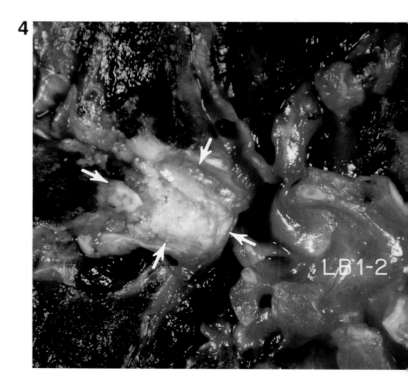

5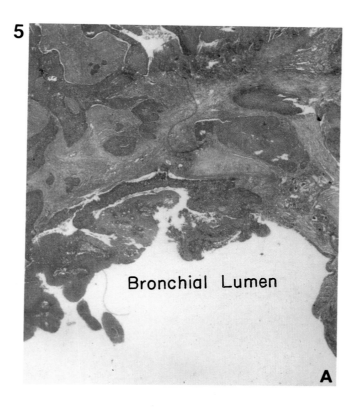

Bronchial Lumen

Comment

This is another example of a tumor that was visible in retrospect when sequential chest radiographs were reviewed. This case demonstrates the value of 55° posterior oblique tomography for enhancing visualization of the hilar and perihilar regions.

Fig. 5. A, Cross section of LB1 & 2 bronchus. Squamous cell carcinoma is present within lumen and extends through bronchial wall. **B**, Higher magnification of keratinizing squamous cell carcinoma adjacent to bronchial cartilage.

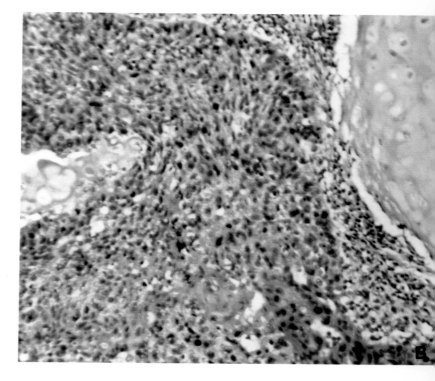

Case 5

51-year-old woman

(Not in early lung cancer screening program)

Tumor: Bronchogenic adenocarcinoma ("occult"; referred for localization).

Location: Perihilar region of left upper lobe.

Treatment: Trisegmentectomy: Apical-posterior (LB1&2) and anterior (LB3) segments of left upper lobe.

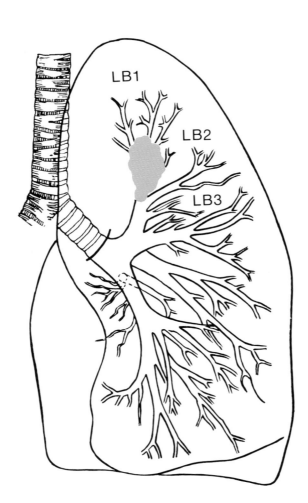

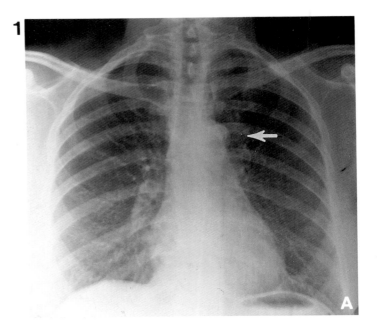

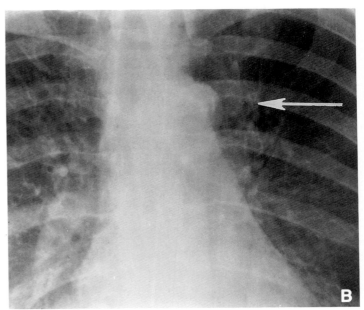

Radiology

Fig. 1. Initial x-rays of chest obtained because of episodic hemoptysis were interpreted as negative. In retrospect, there may be a very slight abnormality in left suprahilar area (**arrow**), but this is questionable at best. **A,** Posteroanterior view of chest. **B,** Localized view of left hilar and perihilar areas.

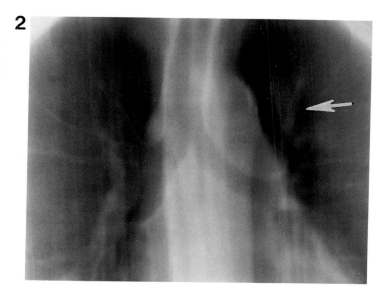

Fig. 2. Hilar tomograms were obtained because of finding of adenocarcinoma cells in sputum and negative posteroanterior chest x-ray. Ill-defined elongated density (**arrow**) above left hilus appears to impinge on "air bronchogram" of bronchus to apical segment of left upper lobe (LB1).

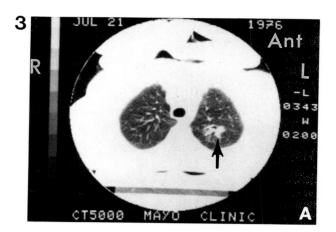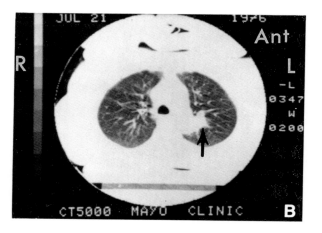

Fig. 3. Computed axial tomographic views of upper portion of thorax, emphasizing pulmonary and mediastinal structures (cross sections of thorax, viewed from below, with top of photograph representing anterior aspect of patient). Tumor appears as white lesion (**arrows**) in left lung, posteriorly. **A,** Cross section near apices of lungs. **B,** Cross section of suprahilar region.

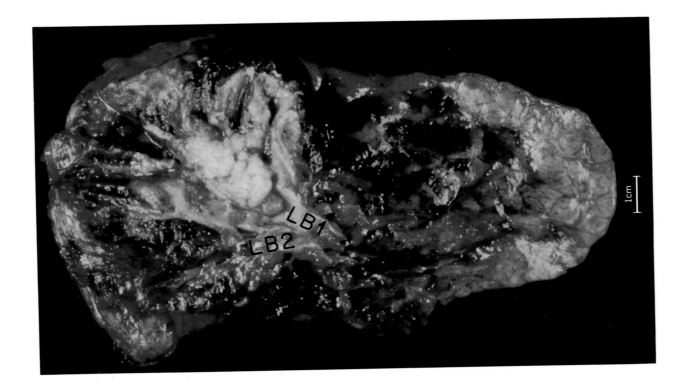

Pathology

Fig. 4. Gross specimen of tumor. Resected segments (LB1&2, LB3) of left upper lobe, showing polypoid tumor largely within LB1 bronchus.

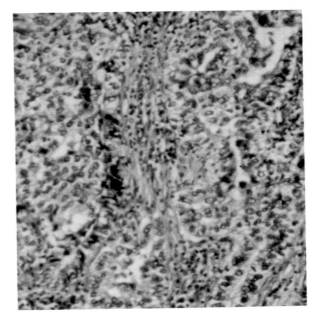

Fig. 5. Microscopic features. Histologic section of poorly differentiated bronchogenic adenocarcinoma.

Comment

If bronchoscopy fails to localize an "occult" tumor, computed axial tomography may be helpful. This technique appears to be more sensitive than whole-lung tomography, although the two procedures tend to complement each other. In this case the bulk of the "occult" tumor probably was a significant factor in its detection by computed tomography.

Part II: Peripheral Cancers

Case 6

80-year-old man

Tumor: Large cell undifferentiated carcinoma.

Location: Subpleural, in apical segment of right upper lobe (RB1).

Treatment: Right upper lobectomy.

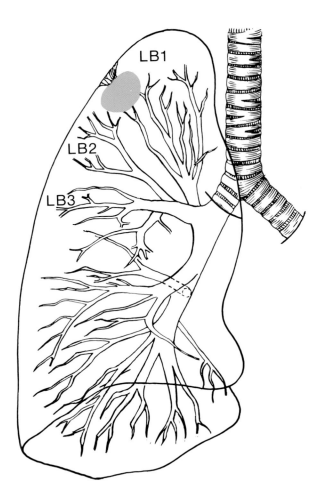

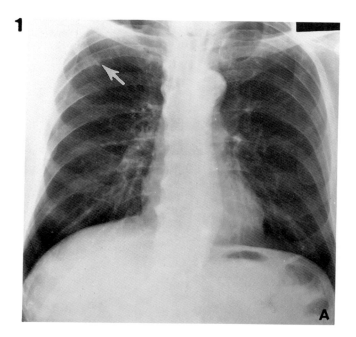

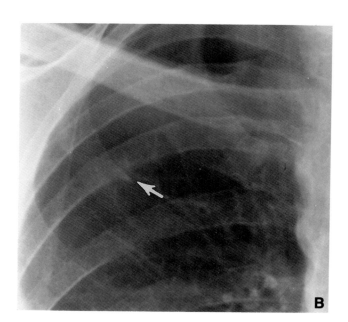

Radiology

Fig. 1. Initial x-ray shows small, localized, irregular peripheral nodule (**arrow**) in right upper lobe. X-ray was obtained 2 years before detection of tumor. Lesion was overlooked. **A,** Posteroanterior view of chest. **B,** Localized view of right upper lobe.

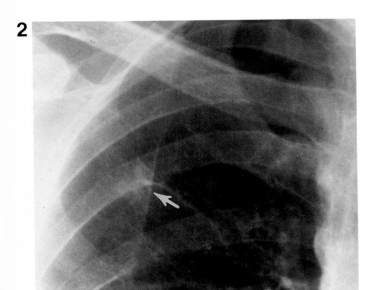

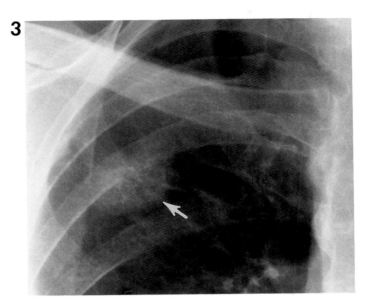

Fig. 2. Follow-up localized view of right upper lobe 1 year later. Lesion (**arrow**) is larger, but it was still not detected. It is partially obscured by overlying rib and scapula.

Fig. 3. Follow-up film of right upper lobe another year later, when tumor was finally detected. Lesion (**arrow**) was further enlarged, with linear strands extending toward thickened overlying pleura.

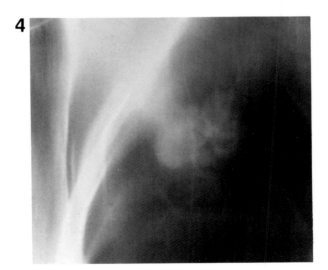

Fig. 4. Localized tomogram of tumor site. Tumor appears to contain area of radiolucency, and therefore bronchioloalveolar carcinoma was suspected. Adjacent pleura is thickened by what seemed to be tumor extension but proved to be only fibrous reaction.

Pathology

Fig. 5. Microscopic features of tumor, which was 2 cm in diameter and did not involve either pleura or lymph nodes. **A**, Low-power mounted microscopic section of tumor shows subpleural location and some fibrous septa extending from tumor to pleura (**arrow**). **B**, High-power section of large cell undifferentiated bronchogenic carcinoma.

5

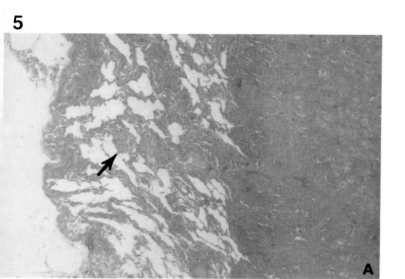

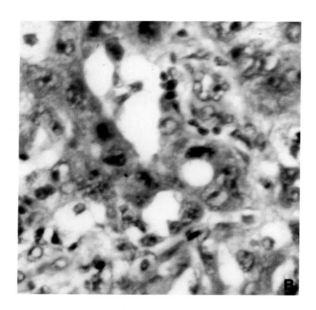

Comment

In this case the tumor seemed more advanced than it actually was. There appeared to be extension to the pleura, but fibrotic changes accounted for this. The case is also another example of retrospective visibility of an early lung cancer on review of serial x-rays.

Although 80 years old at the time of surgery, the patient was alive and well 6 years later. Age alone is not a contraindication to surgical treatment for lung cancer.

Case 7

61-year-old man

Tumor: Squamous cell carcinoma.

Location: Periphery of superior segment, right lower lobe (RB6).

Treatment: Right lower lobectomy.

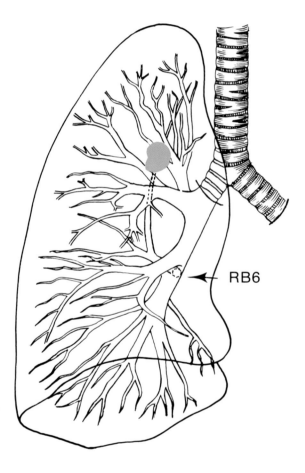

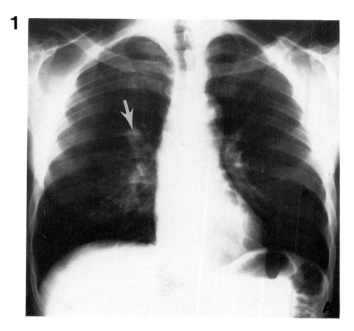

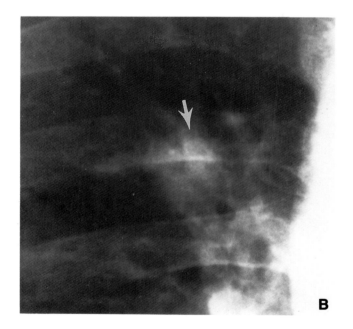

Radiology

Fig. 1. Initial chest x-ray shows rounded density (**arrow**) at level of upper right hilus. **A,** Posteroanterior view of chest. **B,** Localized view.

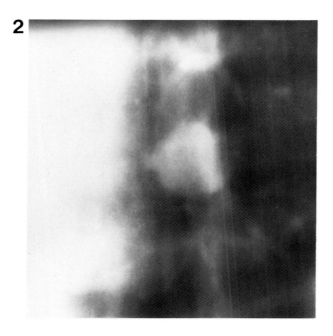

Fig. 2. Localized tomogram of lesion. Cut was obtained 3.5 cm from posterior chest; this places lesion in periphery of superior segment of right lower lobe (RB6). The tumor is round and has a smooth border. There is no evidence of calcification.

Pathology

Induced sputum was negative for cancer cells. Percutaneous needle aspiration biopsy was performed.

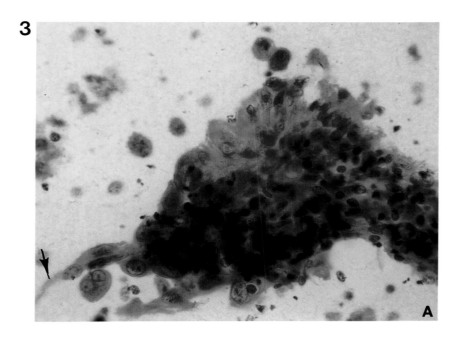

Fig. 3. Fragment of poorly differentiated carcinoma aspirated by needle. **A,** Low-power view shows tailing of cytoplasm (**arrows**), suggesting squamous differentiation.

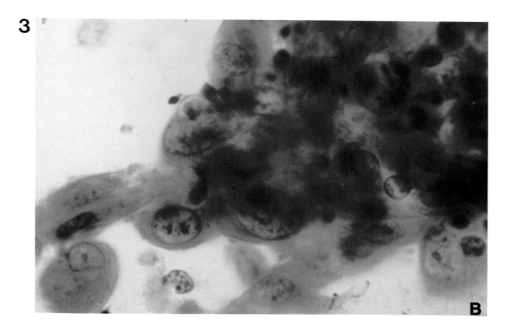

Fig. 3. B, High-power view shows dense, glassy cytoplasm and suggestion of intercellular bridging.

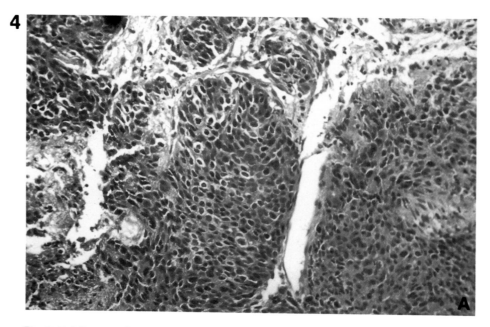

Fig. 4. A, Microscopic sections from resected cancer, which was 2 cm in diameter and situated in the apical subsegment (B6[2]) of the superior segment. No lymph nodes were involved. Although no keratin was present, identification of intercellular bridges supports diagnosis of squamous cell carcinoma. **A**, Low-power view. **B**, High-power view.

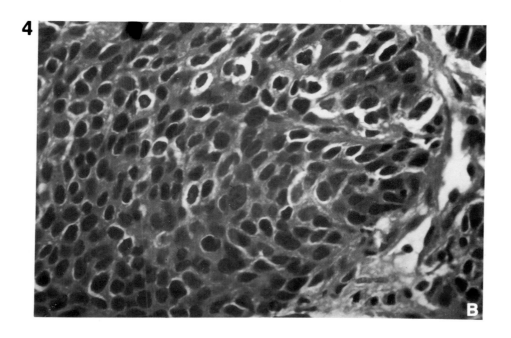

Comment

This cancer, like others to follow, had a smooth, round configuration that might suggest benign disease. However, malignant tumors may display similar contours. In a population with a high risk of developing lung cancer, any newly appearing lesion, regardless of shape, must be viewed with a high degree of suspicion.

Percuta. eous needle aspiration is an important diagnostic procedure in evaluating patients with localized indeterminate pulmonary disease. Intensified fluoroscopic images, biplane capabilities, improvements in needles, and increased accuracy of cytologic diagnosis have combined to make the procedure more accurate and safe. The range of indications for needle aspiration varies considerably. However, there is unanimity regarding its value in preoperative assessment of patients with pulmonary insufficiency or whenever the surgeon or the patient has misgivings about thoracotomy. Needle aspiration tends to complement fiberoptic bronchoscopy and it is especially applicable to small peripheral tumors, which are often exceedingly difficult to sample endoscopically. This is particularly true of tumors, like the present one, that are situated in the apical subsegment (B6 [a]) of the superior segment of the lower lobe.

Case 8

52-year-old man

Tumor: Squamous cell carcinoma.

Location: Peripheral portion of lateral basal segment, left lower lobe.

Treatment: Left lower lobectomy.

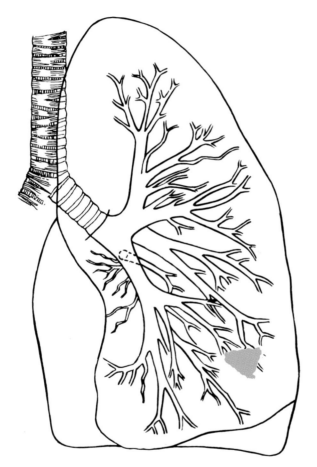

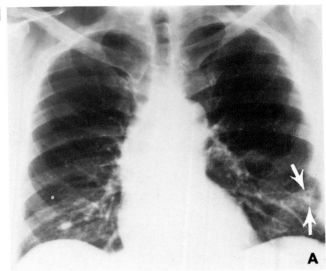

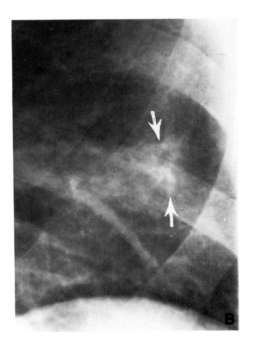

Radiology

Fig. 1. Initial screening chest x-ray shows small, ill-defined density in left lower lung field (**arrows**). **A,** Posteroanterior view of chest. **B,** Localized view of left lower lung.

2

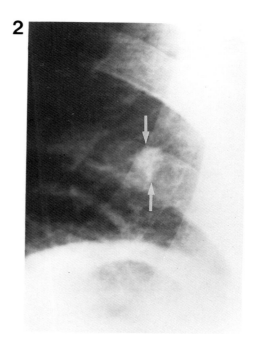

Fig. 2. Localized view of left lower lung on film taken 8 months earlier. In retrospect, lesion can be seen (**arrows**), but it is obscured by crossing ribs.

3

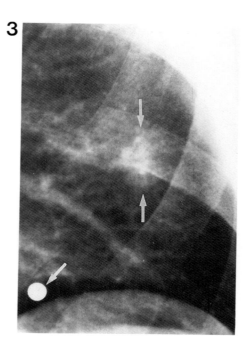

Fig. 3. Localized view of left lower lung. Film was taken shortly after initial screening x-ray. Nipple marker is in place (**lower arrow**). Nipple was obviously not responsible for radiographic abnormality (**upper arrows**).

4

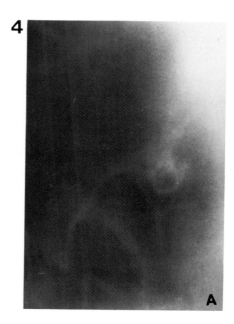

A

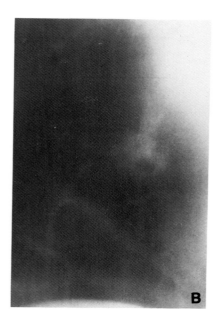

B

Fig. 4. Localized tomograms obtained 4 months after initial screening x-ray demonstrate ill-defined cavitary mass or infiltrate. **A,** Cut obtained 16 cm from posterior chest. **B,** Cut obtained 16.5 cm from posterior chest.

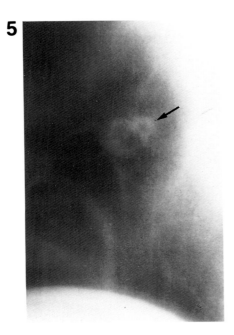

Fig. 5. Second tomogram 4 months later (8 months after initial screening x-ray). Cavitation has increased, but total size of lesion has decreased, and there is now a smaller nodular cavity projecting from superior-lateral aspect (**arrow**).

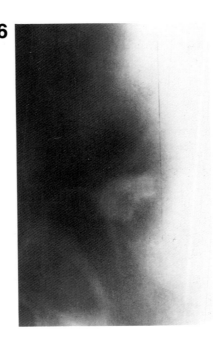

Fig. 6. Third tomogram 2 months later shows increase in size of lesion and little cavitation. Needle aspiration was positive for cancer cells at this time.

Pathology

Small, necrotic peripheral squamous cell carcinoma was associated with surrounding pneumonitis. Lymph nodes were not involved.

Fig. 7. Low-power view of tumor with central cavitation (**arrows**) and surrounding pneumonitis.

Fig. 8. High-power photograph shows squamous cell cancer and associated inflammatory reaction.

Comment

At first, the tumor appeared to decrease in size, presumably because of a decrease in the surrounding inflammation. Even small bronchogenic carcinomas may be associated with peripheral pneumonitis. In this case, needle aspiration confirmed that an indeterminate lesion of fluctuating size and configuration was, in fact, a cancer.

7

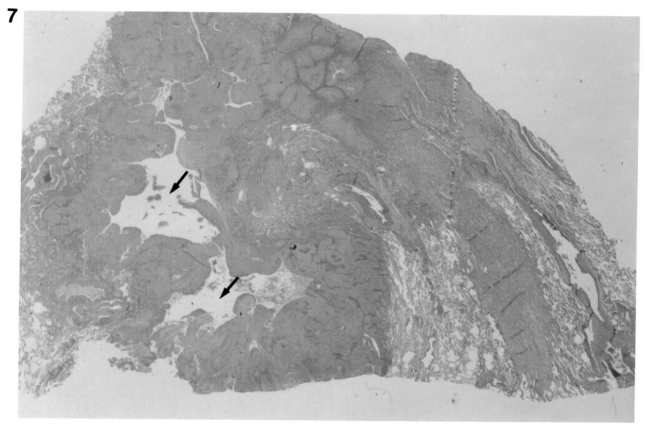

8

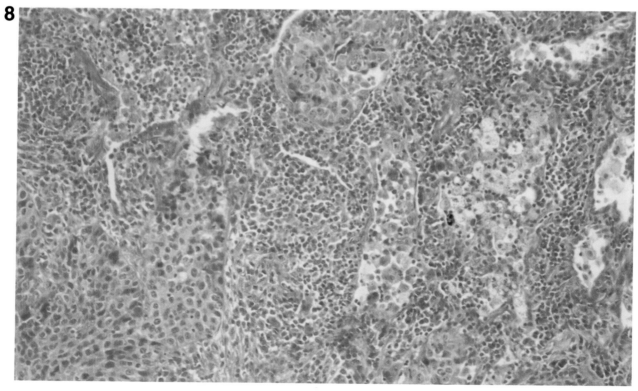

Case 9

59-year-old man

Tumor: Bronchogenic adenocarcinoma.

Location: Peripheral, in fissure between right upper and middle lobes.

Treatment: Bilobectomy, right upper and middle lobes.

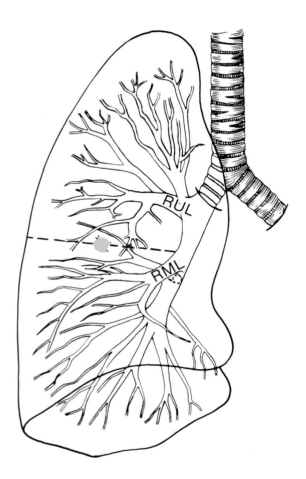

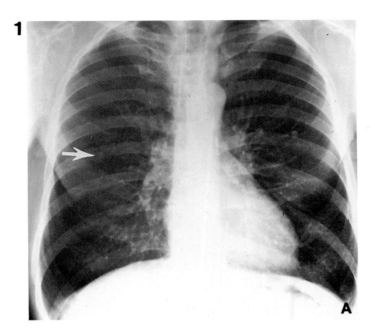

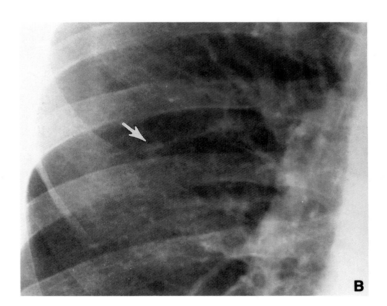

Radiology

Fig. 1. Initial screening film, interpreted as negative by three trained observers. In retrospect, there is a very faint irregular density (**arrow**) in right mid lung. **A,** Posteroanterior view of chest. **B,** Enlarged view of right mid lung.

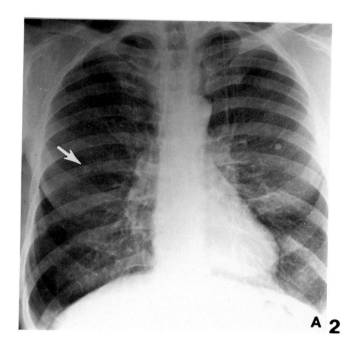

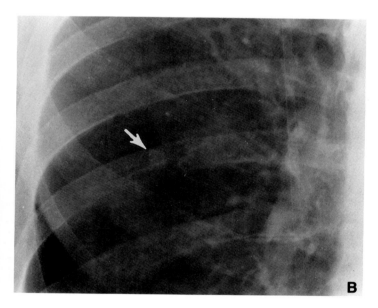

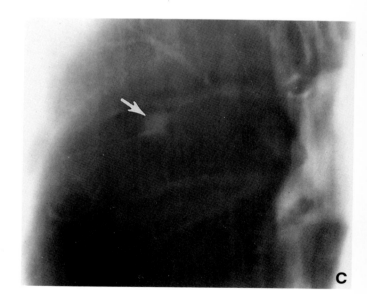

Fig. 2. Films obtained 8 months later, when lesion (**arrow**) was first detected. Lesion is now more dense and discrete but is only questionably larger. **A,** Posteroanterior view of chest. **B,** Local view of right mid lung. **C,** Tomogram of tumor.

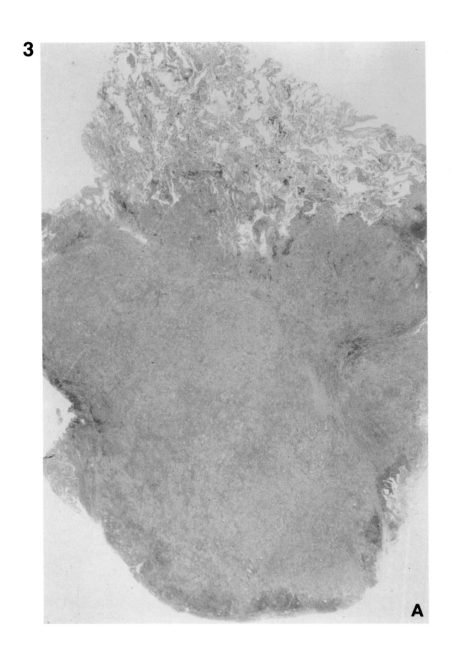

3

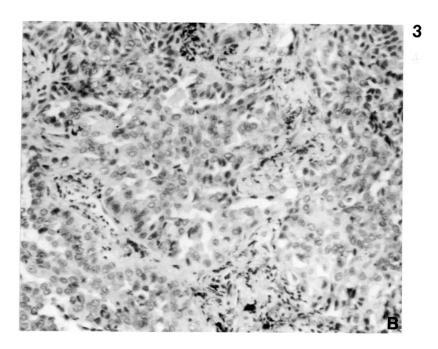

B

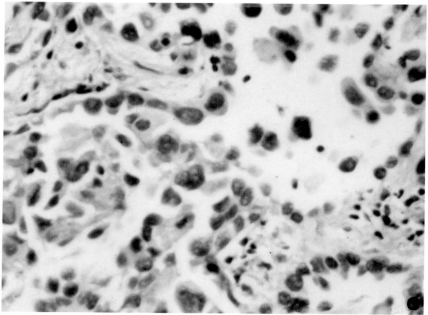

Pathology

Fig. 3. Microscopic pathologic features (no lymph nodes were involved). **A,** Low-power mounted microscopic section through entire tumor (1 cm in diameter). Margin of tumor is irregular. **B,** Section through center of tumor shows poorly differentiated bronchogenic adenocarcinoma. **C,** Higher power section of margin of tumor.

Comment

Like case 2, this is a small tumor that required extensive resection because of its location. Again it was an early tumor, visible retrospectively even on the initial screening film.

Case 10

61-year-old man

Tumor: Squamous cell carcinoma.

Location: Periphery of posterior segment of right upper lobe (RB2).

Treatment: Right upper lobectomy.

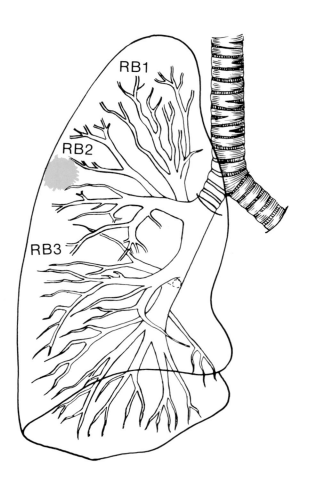

Radiology

Fig. 1. Initial screening chest x-ray shows irregular nodule in right mid-lung field laterally (**arrow**). It was overlooked at that time and was later regarded as an area of fibrosis. **A,** Posteroanterior view of chest. **B,** Local view of right mid lung.

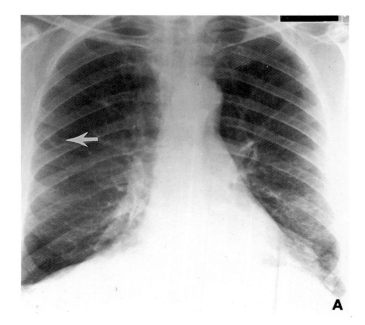

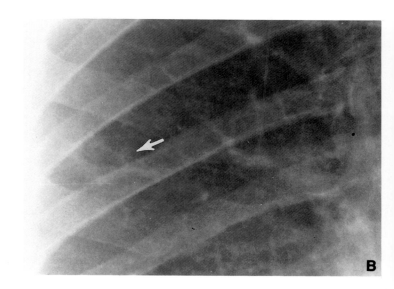

Fig. 2. Eight months later. X-ray was interpreted as unchanged. In retrospect, density in periphery of right lung (**arrow**) was slightly more consolidated. **A,** Posteroanterior view of chest. **B,** Local view, right mid lung.

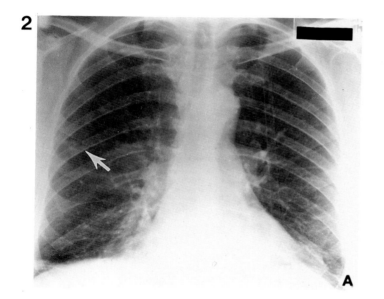

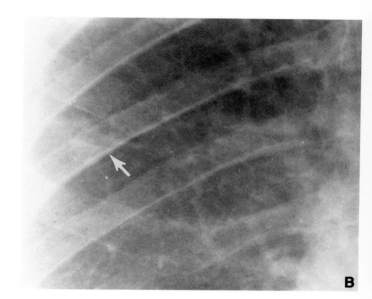

3

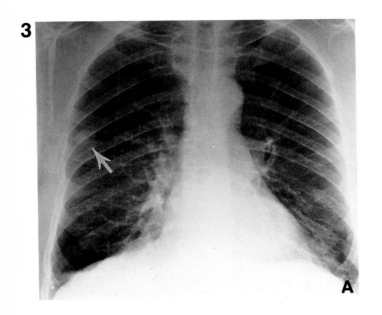

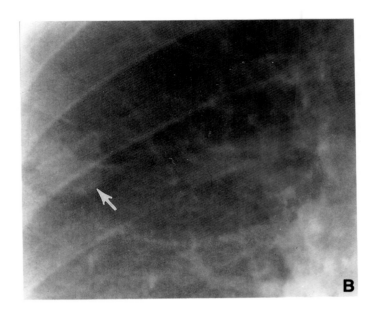

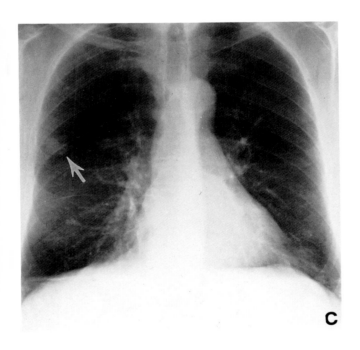

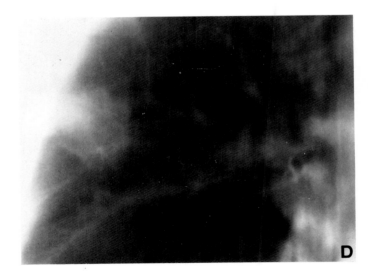

Fig. 3. One year later, when tumor was detected. Lesion (**arrows**) is now larger, although margin remains somewhat irregular. **A,** Posteroanterior view of chest. **B,** Local view of right mid lung. **C,** Films taken at 350 kV. Peripheral lesion is more obvious with rib shadows suppressed. **D,** Tomogram demonstrates that lesion has irregular margin and abuts against pleura.

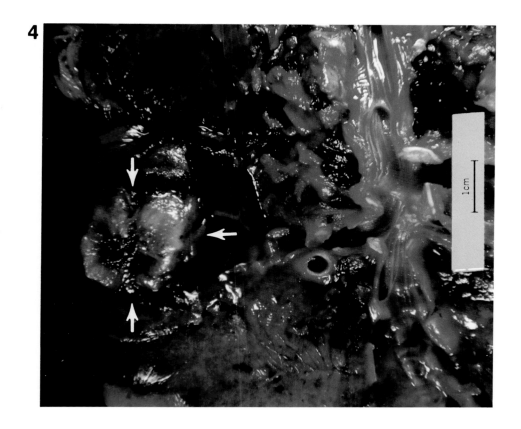

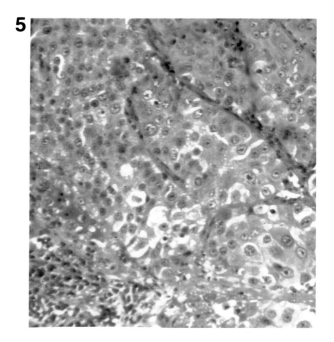

Pathology

Fig. 4. Resected right upper lobe shows subpleural carcinoma (**arrows**), 2.5 cm in diameter. Tumor involved and puckered overlying visceral pleura. Lymph nodes contained only noncaseating granulomas.

Fig. 5. Histologic section reveals poorly differentiated squamous cell carcinoma.

Comment

This and the two previous tumors are rather typical of the many early peripheral carcinomas that present as small, subtle, ill-defined, solitary densities that may be overlooked or considered benign. Only close observation and a high degree of alertness will succeed in revealing their cancerous nature at an early stage. Radiographs obtained at high kilovoltage (such as 350 kV) may aid in identification of tumors located in the extreme periphery of the lungs, where they might otherwise be obscured by the ribs, mediastinum, or diaphragm.

Case 11

69-year-old man

Tumor: Large cell undifferentiated carcinoma.

Location: Subpleural parenchyma, posterior segment of right upper lobe.

Treatment: Bisegmentectomy, posterior segment of right upper lobe and superior segment of right lower lobe (limited resection because of reduced respiratory reserve).

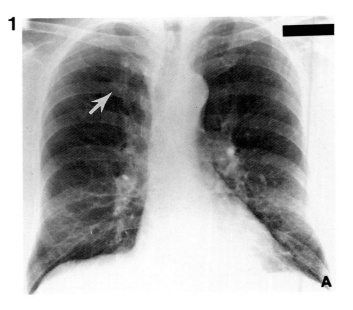

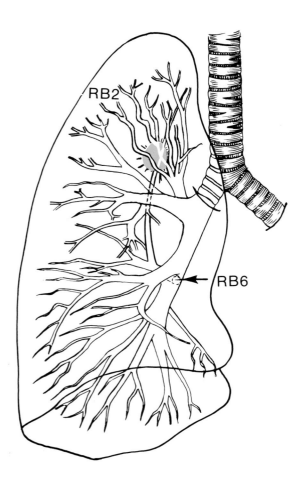

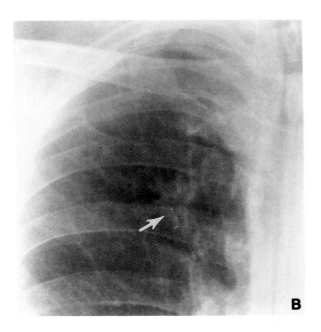

Radiology

Fig. 1. Initial screening film shows poorly defined nodular density in medial portion of right upper-lung field (**arrow**) which was not considered significant until retrospective review. **A,** Posteroanterior view of chest. **B,** Localized view of right upper lung.

2

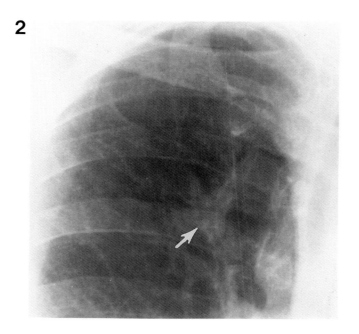

Fig. 2. Right upper lung 1 year later. Although considered stable at this time, lesion has, in retrospect, enlarged and become more nodular (**arrow**).

3

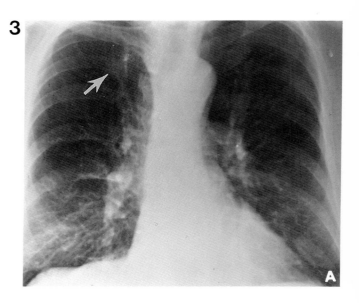

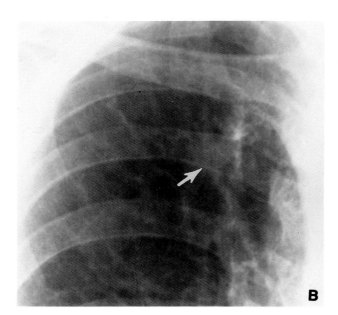

Fig. 3. Film taken 4 months later. Interpretation is of stable lesion, except in retrospect. It is still ill-defined (**arrows**) and is partially obscured by rib shadow. **A,** Posteroanterior view of chest. **B,** Local view of right upper lung.

4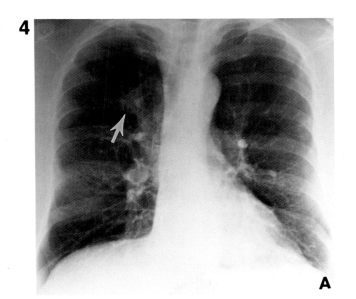

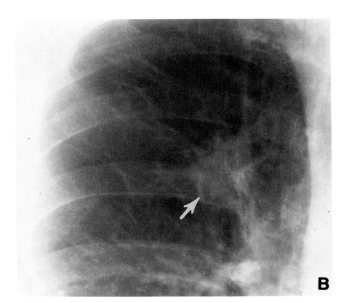

A

B

Fig. 4. Chest x-ray 20 months after initial film, when tumor was first detected. Lesion is now definitely larger, rounder, and more discrete (**arrow**). **A**, Posteroanterior view of chest. **B**, Local view of right upper lung. **C**, Tomogram of tumor shows "corona radiata," or spiculated linear densities (**arrow**) extending outward from tumor, with intervening lucent areas. This phenomenon has been well described* as a sign that is often, but not invariably, indicative of cancer.

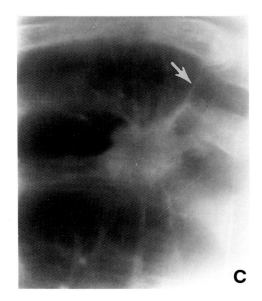

C

*Heitzman ER, Naeye RL, Markarian B: Roentgen pathological correlations in coal workers' pneumoconiosis. Ann NY Acad Sci 200:510-526, 1972.

5

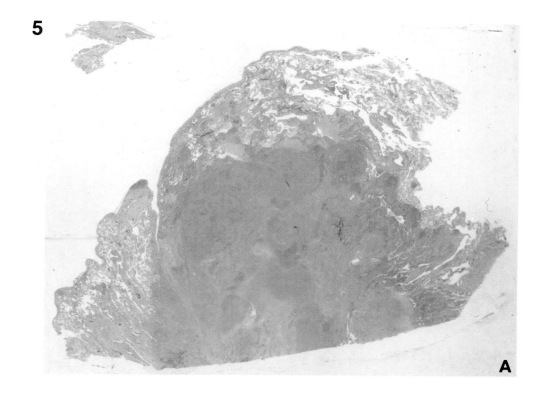

A

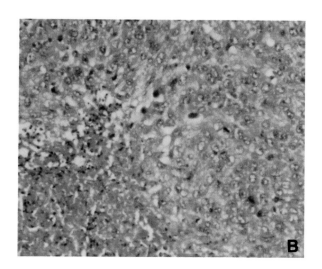

B

Pathology

Fig. 5. Microscopic features of tumor, which was 2 cm in diameter. Interlobar visceral pleura was involved, but lymph nodes were not. **A**, Low-power view of tumor shows subpleural location and irregular tumor margin. **B**, Partially necrotic large cell undifferentiated bronchogenic carcinoma.

Comment

This is another case emphasizing that ill-defined densities, especially in older heavy smokers, need to be regarded as carcinoma until proven otherwise. It is all too easy to consider, erroneously, that the lesion represents "nodular fibrosis," a diagnosis that should not be entertained unless serial films are available and show the abnormality unchanged for 2 years or more.

Tumors such as this one and those in cases 8-10 are extremely difficult to discern at an early stage because their borders gradually fade into a background of normal pulmonary parenchyma.

Case 12

60-year-old man

Tumor: Large cell undifferentiated carcinoma.

Location: Peripheral, in superior segment of right lower lobe (RB6).

Treatment: Right lower lobectomy.

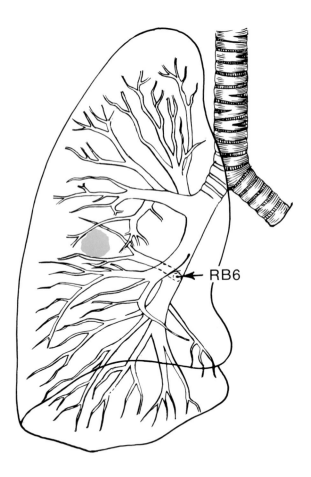

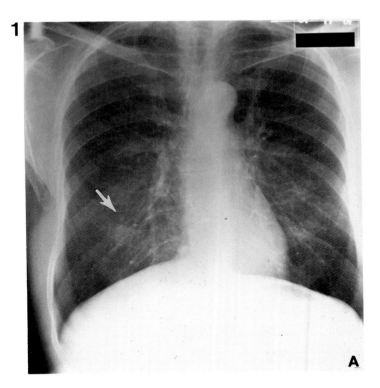

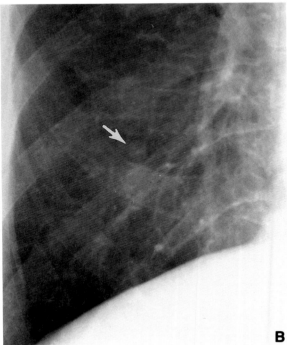

Radiology

Fig. 1. Initial screening chest x-ray. This was originally interpreted as normal, but in retrospect a subtle nodule (**arrow**) is visible in right lower lung. **A,** Posteroanterior view of chest. **B,** Enlarged view of right lower chest.

2

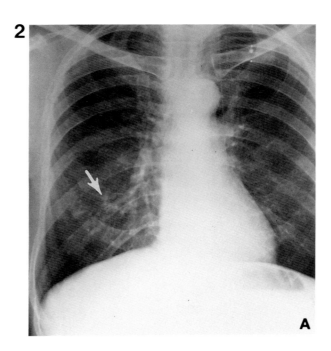

A

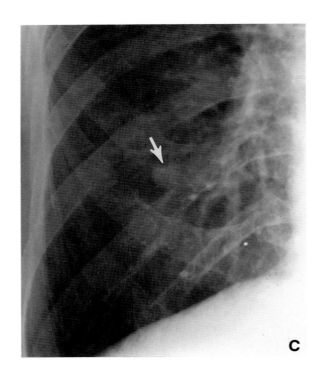

C

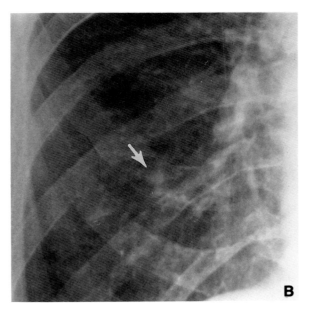

B

Fig. 2. X-rays 4 and 8 months later show nodule (**arrow**) gradually enlarging. On single posteroanterior films, it was erroneously interpreted by some observers as a nipple shadow. **A,** Posteroanterior view of chest 4 months later. **B,** Localized view of right lower chest, same film. **C,** Right lower chest, 8 months later.

3

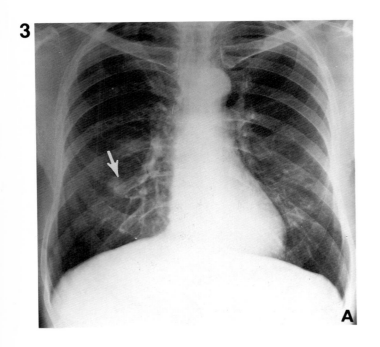

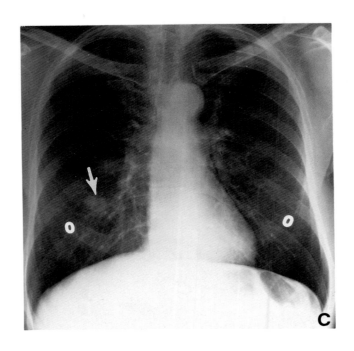

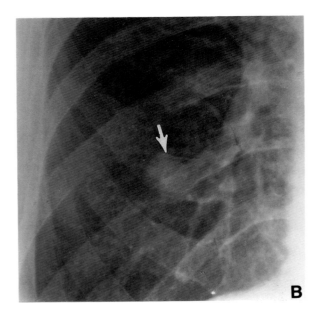

Fig. 3. Chest x-ray 1 year after initial screening film. Nodule (**arrow**) was now correctly interpreted as tumor. It has enlarged considerably. Like the tumors in cases 7 and 13, it has a spherical configuration and a smooth margin not typical of primary bronchogenic carcinoma. **A**, Posteroanterior view of chest. **B**, Enlarged view of right lower chest. **C**, Posteroanterior view of chest,

3

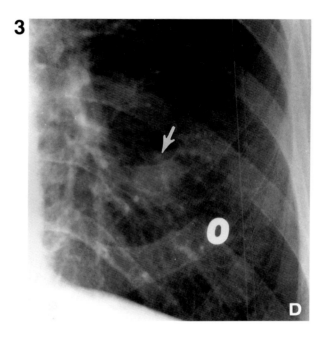

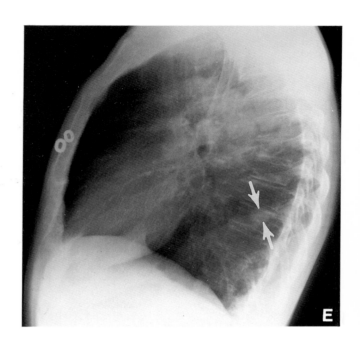

showing relative position of nipple markers and nodule.
D, Right lower chest with nipple marker. **E**, Lateral
projection with nipple markers on anterior chest wall
and tumor far posteriorly. **F**, Lateral projection,
localized view of posterior portion. Note smooth
rounded margin of tumor.

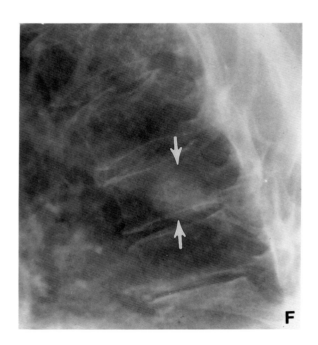

4

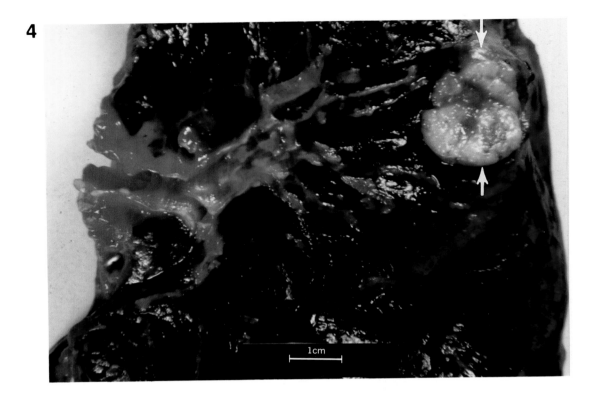

Pathology

Fig. 4. Resected right lower lobe shows peripheral carcinoma, 2.5 cm in diameter (**arrows**), with slight central necrosis. Tumor was located 1.5 cm beneath pleura. Lymph nodes were not involved.

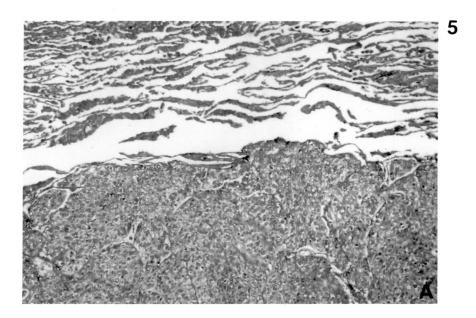

5

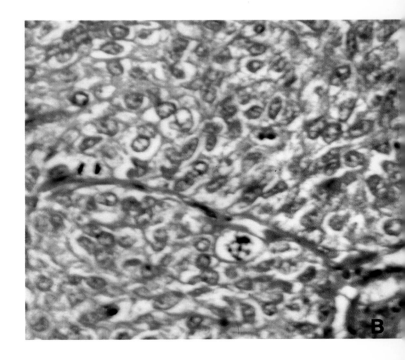

Fig. 5. A, Low-power histologic view demonstrates smooth tumor margin. **B,** Histologic section showing large cell undifferentiated bronchogenic carcinoma.

Comment

There were two aspects of this case that impeded diagnosis. First, during its early stages, the location of the tumor on the posterior anterior view of the chest was suggestive of a nipple shadow. This problem was resolved by application of nipple markers. In addition, the smooth rounded contour of the lesion gave the appearance of a granuloma, but, as already demonstrated, cancers may exhibit similar features.

Case 13

56-year-old man

Tumor: Bronchogenic adenocarcinoma.

Location: Apex of left upper lobe.

Treatment: Left upper lobectomy with intrapericardial resection (radical). Dissection of involved mediastinal nodes from branch of pulmonary artery.

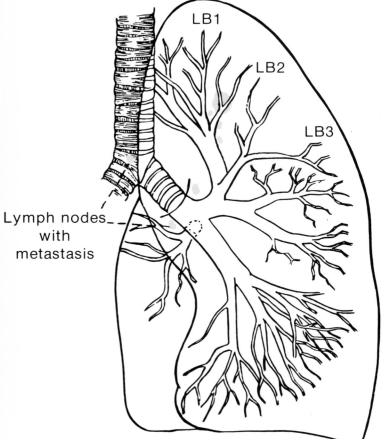

Lymph nodes with metastasis

LB1
LB2
LB3

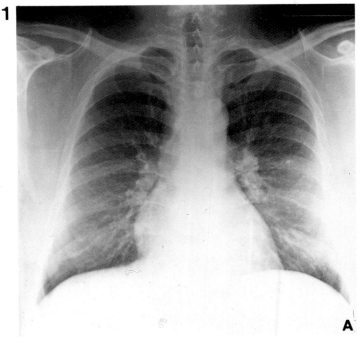

A

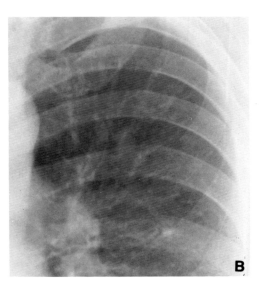

B

Radiology

Fig. 1. Initial chest x-ray was negative, even in retrospect. **A,** Posteroanterior view of chest. **B,** Localized view of left upper lobe.

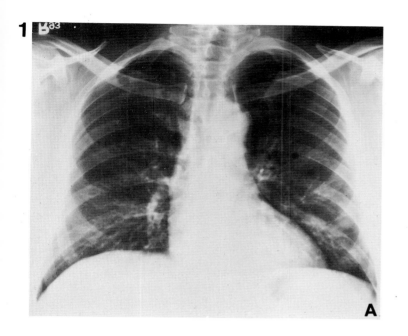

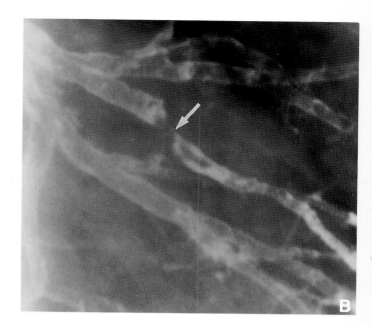

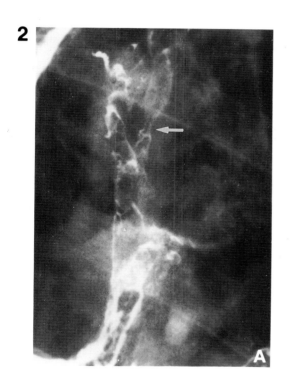

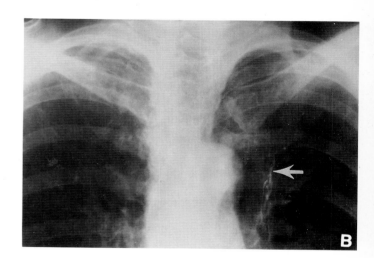

Section 7

CASE PRESENTATIONS

Robert S. Fontana, M.D.

Wilmot C. Ball, Jr., M.D.

In this section case studies are presented to illustrate early manifestations of the various cell types of bronchogenic carcinoma included in the classifications of the American Joint Committee and World Health Organization. Each case has been selected to demonstrate certain clinical features considered to be important. Emphasis has been given to management of the medical problem. Details concerning radiography, cytology, bronchoscopy, and pathology have been described in other sections.

CASE 1

A 57-year-old livestock auction worker had a cigarette-smoking history of 35 pack-years. He sought medical advice after experiencing a transient syncopal episode. Physical examination, chest x-ray, and sputum cytology test were negative (Fig. 1).

Four months later, the chest x-ray and the sputum cytology test were repeated as screening tests for lung cancer. The radiograph was again negative, but squamous cancer cells were detected in the sputum (Fig. 2).

Otolaryngologic examination and bronchoscopy using a rigid, open-tip bronchoscope were negative. "Pooled" bronchial secretions and washings were positive for squamous cancer cells.

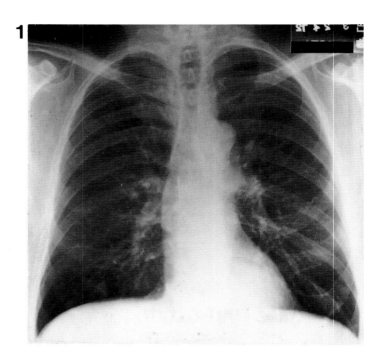

Fig. 1. Chest x-ray film shows no abnormality

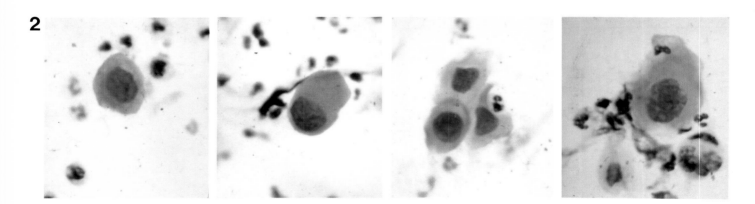

Fig. 2. Four microscopic views of squamous cancer cells observed in sputum.

3

Detailed fiberbronchoscopy was carried out under general anesthesia. No tumor was visualized, but bronchial brushings from the anterior segment of the right upper lobe (RB3) contained squamous cancer cells (Fig. 3 and 4).

Since no tumor was observed by direct vision, fiberbronchoscopy was repeated 3 days later, with identical results.

4

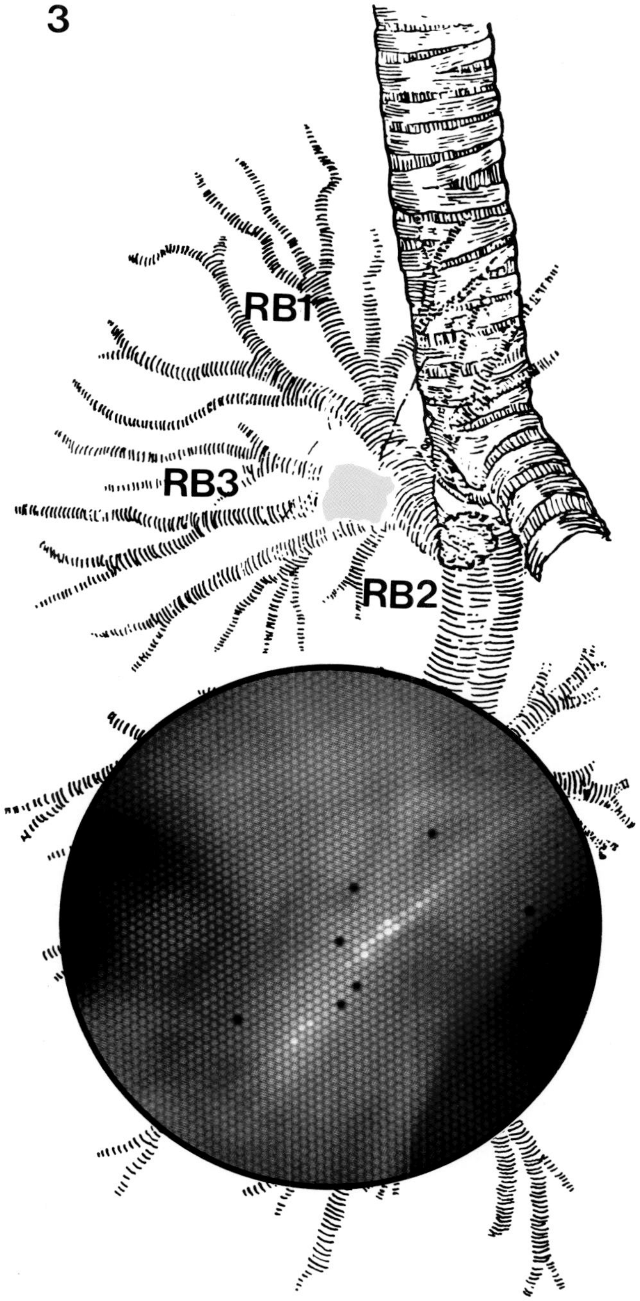

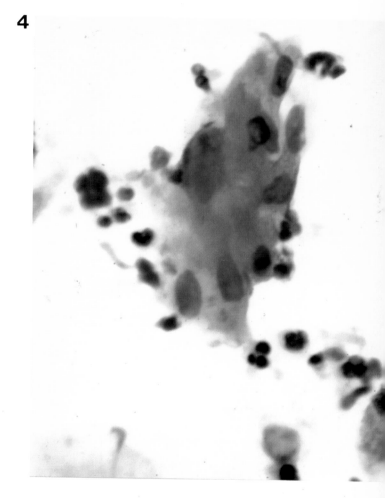

Fig. 3. Encircled photograph of anterior segment of right upper lobe bronchus (RB3) as seen through fiberbronchoscope. No tumor is visible. Photograph is superimposed on diagram of right side of tracheobronchial tree, with the area of positive brushing shown in blue.

Fig. 4. Clump of squamous carcinoma cells from bronchial brushing from RB3.

One week later, right thoracotomy was performed. No tumor was palpated, but right upper lobectomy was carried out. Examination of the specimen of lung revealed a nodular mucosal tumor involving a subsegment of RB3 (Fig. 5 through 9).

The patient made an uneventful recovery from surgery. He was alive and fully active without evidence of recurrent tumor 6 years later.

5

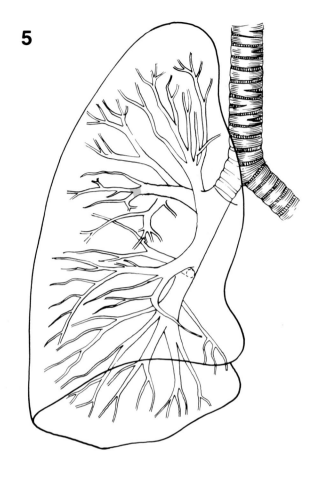

Fig. 5. Right upper lobe bronchi with area of mucosal tumor colored blue.

Fig. 6. Gross specimen of tumor in subsegment of RB3.

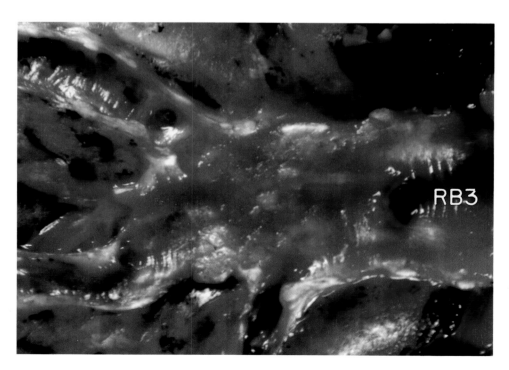

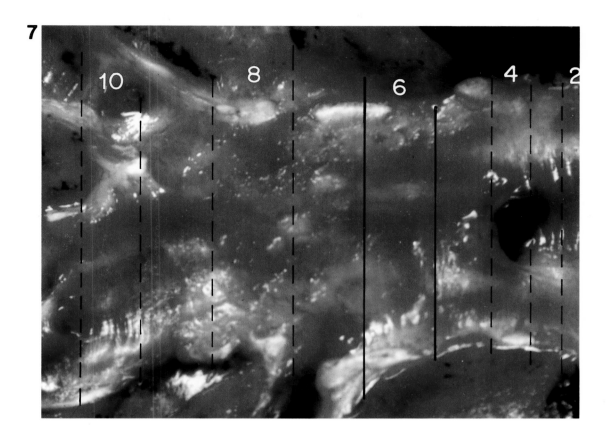

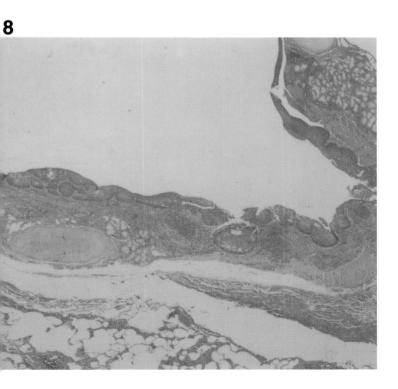

Fig. 7. Enlarged view of gross specimen indicates sites of serial block sectioning.

Fig. 8. Low-power microscopic view of bronchial wall (section 6) shows in situ squamous cell carcinoma limited to surface epithelium and ducts of mucosal glands.

Comment

1. This case demonstrates the value of meticulous, detailed bronchoscopic examination with careful sampling of individual bronchial segments when cancer cells are present in sputum and bronchial secretions but no tumor is visible radiographically or endoscopically.

2. Under these circumstances, sampling from the same bronchus (in this case RB3) should be positive on at least two separate occasions before one can regard the tumor as localized and contemplate performing thoracotomy.

3. Pathologically, the tumor in this case was a squamous cell carcinoma in situ limited entirely to the surface epithelium and the ducts of the mucosal glands.

4. Most radiographically "occult" bronchogenic carcinomas are of the squamous cell type.

9

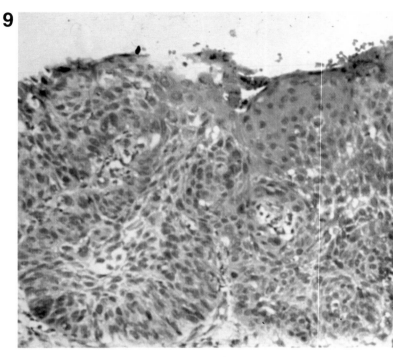

Fig. 9. Higher-power microscopic view of tumor.

CASE 2

A 54-year-old heavy smoker was hospitalized with acute gout. Despite a normal chest x-ray, a sputum cytology test was obtained because he was a smoker and because of a history of weight loss. The test was positive for squamous carcinoma cells (Fig. 1). Bronchoscopy showed roughening of the spur between the anterior and lateral basal segmental bronchi in the right lower lobe (RB8-9). There was also narrowing of the orifice of the anterior basal segmental bronchus (RB8). Washings and brushings from the right lower lobe were positive for cancer cells, and biopsy of the RB8-9 spur disclosed in situ squamous cell carcinoma.

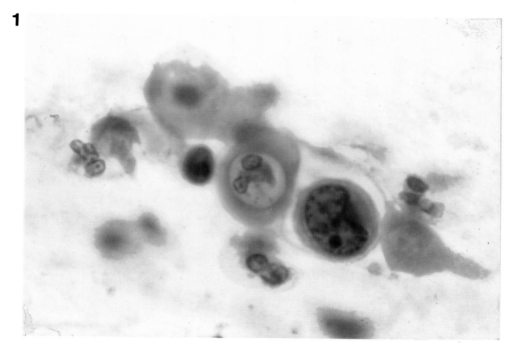

1

Fig. 1. Squamous carcinoma cells in sputum.

Thoracotomy was performed. After resection of the right lower lobe, the proximal bronchial margin was positive for squamous cell carcinoma in situ, and therefore the right middle lobe also was resected. The specimen (Fig. 2) showed invasive squamous cell cancer involving the right lower lobe bronchus in the region of the origins of the anterior, lateral, and posterior basal segmental bronchi. In addition, there was widespread in situ carcinoma involving the right lower lobe bronchus and all of its segmental bronchi, including the bronchus to the superior segment.

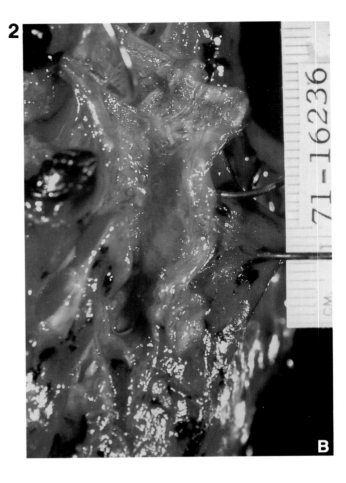

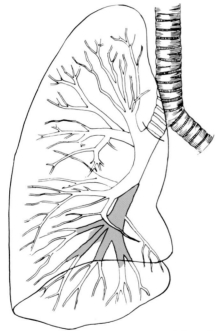

A

Fig. 2. Resected right middle and lower lobes. **A,** Diagram shows a 6-mm invasive squamous cell carcinoma (in red) and extensive contiguous in situ carcinoma (in blue). **B,** Mucosal surface of invasive cancer is rough and irregular, whereas in situ carcinoma of the more proximal bronchus (top of picture) retains its longitudinal ridges.

Postoperatively, the patient remained well; he had repeatedly negative sputum cytology tests for 2 years. Then a single sputum specimen showed metaplastic squamous cells with moderate atypia (Fig. 3). Six months later another specimen showed markedly atypical metaplastic squamous cells (Fig. 4). The patient declined further investigation and was lost to follow-up for the next 18 months. At this point he experienced hemoptysis and returned for evaluation. Chest radiographs revealed the interval development of a right hilar mass, and the sputum was again positive for squamous cancer cells. Bronchoscopy showed the presence of recurrent tumor, for which the patient received radiation therapy. He died of metastatic lung cancer 5 years after his resectional surgery.

3

4

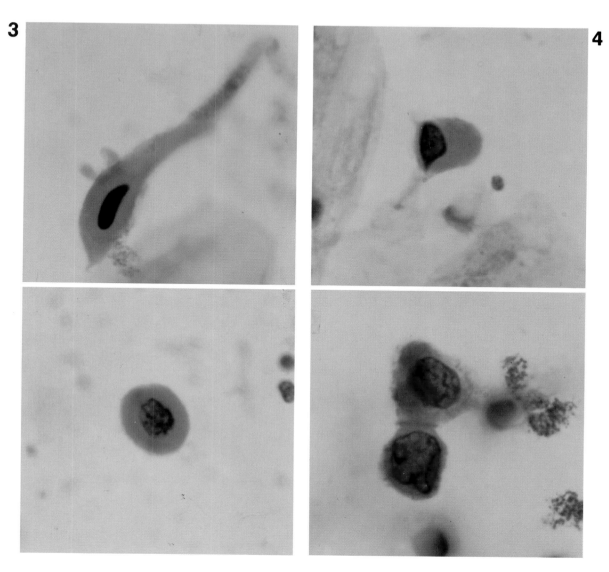

Fig. 3. Follow-up sputum preparation shows metaplastic squamous cells with moderate atypia.

Fig. 4. Sputum specimen 6 months later shows markedly atypical squamous cells.

Comment

1. The operative specimen in this patient showed extensive in situ squamous cell carcinoma, despite the limited extent of the invasive cancer. Because of uncertainty concerning the ultimate consequences of leaving in situ cancer at the margin of resection, a more extensive resection should be performed if the patient's pulmonary status permits.

2. This case also illustrates a progressive increase in degree of cellular atypia in serial sputum specimens obtained postoperatively, a finding that often precedes the development of either recurrent tumor or a second primary cancer.

CASE 3

A 52-year-old trucker had a cigarette-smoking history of 53 pack-years, a chronic productive cough, and two recent episodes of tussive syncope. For these reasons, a chest x-ray and a sputum cytology test were obtained. The x-ray showed a healed fracture of the right fifth rib, scattered metallic fragments posteriorly, and a bullet lodged near the spine—the results of an old hunting accident (Fig. 1).

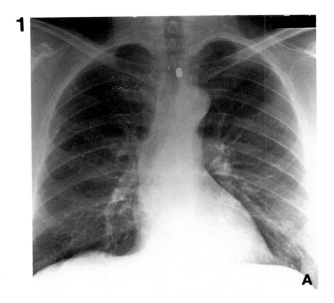

Fig. 1. A, Chest x-ray with old fracture of right fifth rib, metallic fragments posteriorly, and a bullet adjacent to spine. Both lungs appear normal.

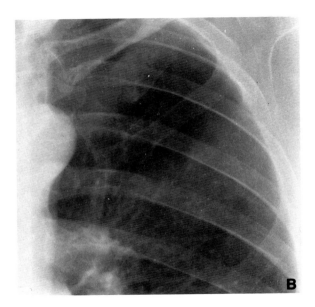

Fig. 1. B, Localized view of upper lobe of left lung, where an "occult" cancer was ultimately found.

The sputum cytology study revealed markedly atypical squamous cells. Because of this, additional sputum specimens were examined. Five such specimens showed persistence of marked atypia and a sixth, unequivocal cancer cells (Fig. 2). A specimen of induced sputum was also positive.

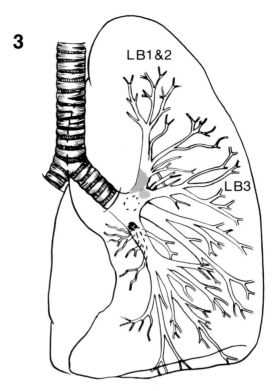

Fig. 3. Bronchial diagram with location of tumor colored blue (in situ portion) and red (microinvasion).

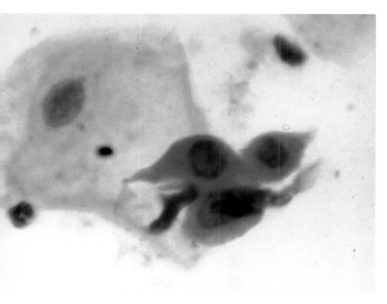

Fig. 2. Squamous cancer cells in sputum.

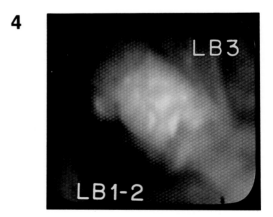

Fig. 4. Fiberbronchoscopic view of nodular tumor involving spur between LB1 and 2 **(lower left)** and LB3 **(upper right)**.

Otolaryngologic examination showed only polypoid changes of the vocal cords. Fiberoptic bronchoscopy under general anesthesia revealed diffuse bronchitis and a small verrucous tumor involving the spur between the apical-posterior and anterior segmental bronchi of the left upper lobe (LB1 & 2-3) (Fig. 3 and 4). Biopsy of the tumor disclosed squamous cancer (Fig. 5).

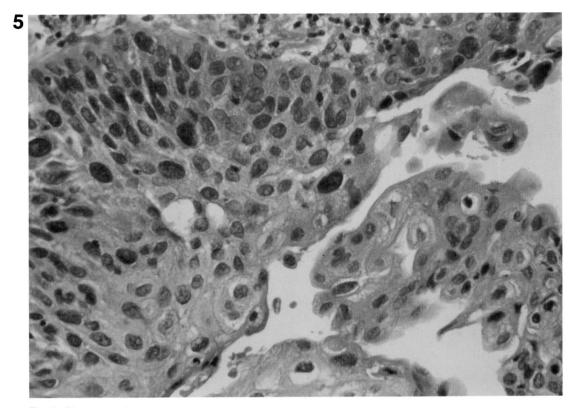

Fig. 5. Biopsy specimen shows squamous cancer.

Left thoracotomy was performed. No tumor could be palpated, but the left upper lobe was resected together with adjacent hilar lymph nodes.

Pathologic examination showed in situ squamous cell cancer with foci of superficial microinvasion along the common bronchus of LB1 and 2 and the adjacent spur between this bronchus and LB3 (Fig. 6 and 7). The total mucosal surface involved was 0.84 cm². The line of resection and the lymph nodes were free of tumor.

6

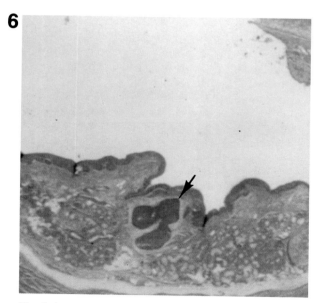

Fig. 6. Low-power magnification of cross section of bronchus at site of cancer, with localized area of superficial microinvasion indicated by **arrow**.

Comment

1. This case demonstrates the importance of close and continuing observation of persons with negative chest x-rays but with sputum containing markedly atypical squamous cells.

2. Repeated findings of squamous cells with marked atypia strongly suggest the presence of cancer, and would warrant otolaryngologic examination and bronchoscopy.

3. The cancer in this case was small, and its location was beyond the range of the rigid, open-tube bronchoscope, as most early lung cancers are. Yet it was easily visualized with the fiberbronchoscope— which demonstrates the value of this instrument.

4. Despite its small size, the tumor exhibited all the characteristics of a typical squamous cell bronchogenic carcinoma, including microinvasion. Although the procedure is at times difficult from a technical standpoint, it is now possible to localize such tumors with regularity and, in most instances, to accomplish resection.

7

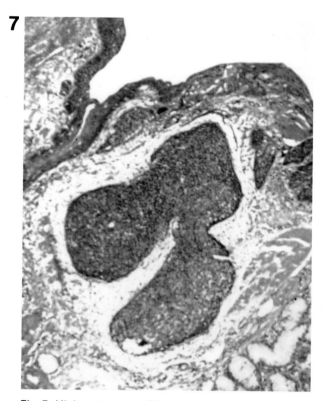

Fig. 7. High-power magnification of area of superficial microinvasion of squamous cancer between bronchial glands.

CASE 4

A 64-year-old smoker had been treated for a bronchogenic carcinoma by resection of the apical-posterior and anterior segments (LB1&2, LB3) of the left upper lobe 4 years before his first screening. Review of his records and the pathologic material showed a moderately well-differentiated squamous cell carcinoma (Fig. 1) with carcinoma in situ at the proximal margin of the bronchial resection (Fig. 2). At the time of screening for lung cancer, the man was essentially asymptomatic. The x-ray showed typical postoperative changes (Fig. 3), but the sputum test was positive for squamous cancer cells (Fig. 4).

1

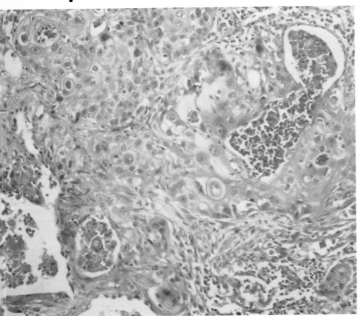

Fig. 1. Microscopic section of tumor resected 4 years earlier shows moderately well-differentiated squamous cell carcinoma.

2

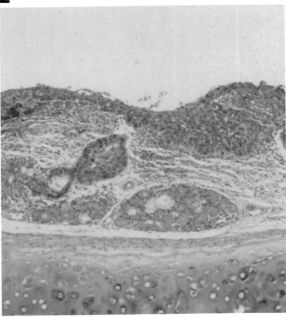

Fig. 2. Microscopic section of resected bronchial margin shows carcinoma in situ on the surface and within glands.

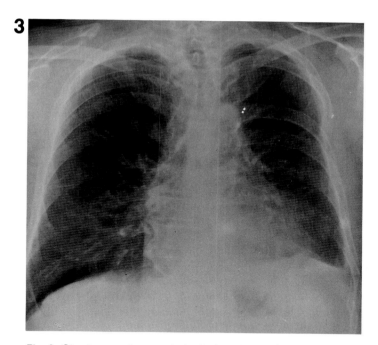

Fig. 3. Chest x-ray shows only typical postoperative changes.

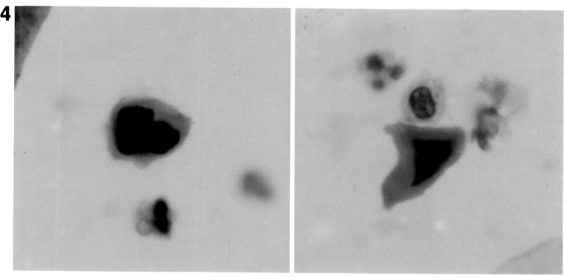

Fig. 4. Cells shed from squamous cell carcinoma into sputum (4 years after surgery).

Fiberoptic bronchoscopy was performed which showed thickening and roughening of the mucosa of the stump of the left upper lobe bronchus. In the lingular area there was a friable mass (Fig. 5). Biopsies and brushings from the left upper lobe stump, the lingular mass, and the left lower lobe bronchus were all positive for squamous cell carcinoma.

A completion pneumonectomy was performed, and the specimen of lung showed extensive squamous cell carcinoma in situ involving the lower lobe, lingula, and left main bronchus (Fig. 6). No area of invasive carcinoma was present. The patient died on the 14th postoperative day with massive consolidation of the right lung. Autopsy revealed multiple small pulmonary emboli and a "shock lung," but detailed examination of the right bronchial tree showed no evidence of in situ or invasive carcinoma.

5

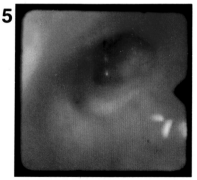

Fig. 5. Appearance of lingular area at fiberoptic bronchoscopy.

Comment

1. In situ squamous cell carcinoma remaining in the bronchial stump persisted for 4 years in this case without the development of invasive tumor. Because the right lung at autopsy was completely free of tumor, it is presumed that the in situ cancer had spread gradually within the mucosa of the left bronchial tree.

2. In situ squamous cell carcinoma is often inapparent endoscopically. Endoscopically inapparent cancer is invariably in situ. However, this case demonstrates that carcinoma in situ may also present as an exophytic lesion, and invasiveness cannot be determined from an endoscopic view of the surface of such a tumor.

6

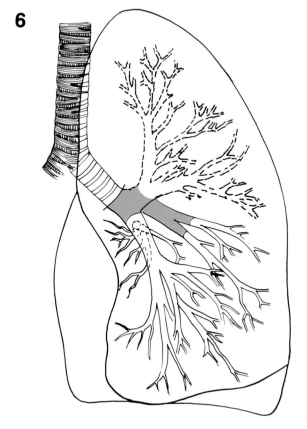

Fig. 6. Diagram of resected specimen, with extent of in situ carcinoma shown in blue.

CASE 5

A 55-year-old construction foreman had smoked four packs of cigarettes daily for many years. He was asymptomatic when he underwent screening by chest radiography and sputum cytology testing. The sputum

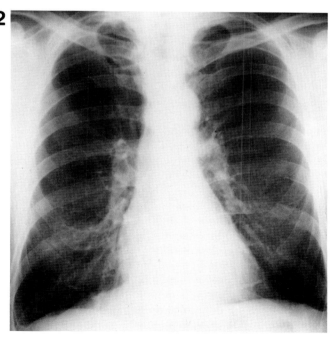

Fig. 1. Sputum specimen contains squamous carcinoma cells.

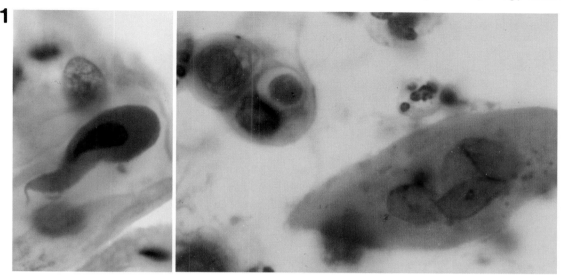

Fig. 2. Chest x-ray shows no abnormality.

test was positive for squamous carcinoma cells (Fig. 1). Chest radiographs (Fig. 2), including oblique films and whole-lung tomograms, were negative. A tantalum dust bronchogram showed only changes of chronic bronchitis.

Fiberoptic bronchoscopy revealed no evidence of a tumor, but there were subtle mucosal changes in the bronchi to the lateral and posterior basal segments of the right lower lobe (RB9 and 10). Washings from the right lower lobe showed squamous carcinoma cells.

A second bronchoscopy was performed 2 weeks later, with biopsy of an area of mucosal pallor at the RB9-10 spur (Fig. 3). The biopsy specimen showed squamous cell carcinoma (Fig. 4).

A right lower lobectomy was performed. The resected lobe contained an infiltrating carcinoma in the posterior basal segment (RB10) and large areas of carcinoma in situ involving the lateral basal, posterior basal, and superior segmental bronchi (RB9, RB10, RB6) (Fig. 5). The bronchial margin and the hilar nodes were free of tumor.

For a year after surgery he did well; sputum repeatedly showed only slightly to moderately atypical metaplastic squamous cells. He resumed smoking 10 months after surgery.

3 **4**

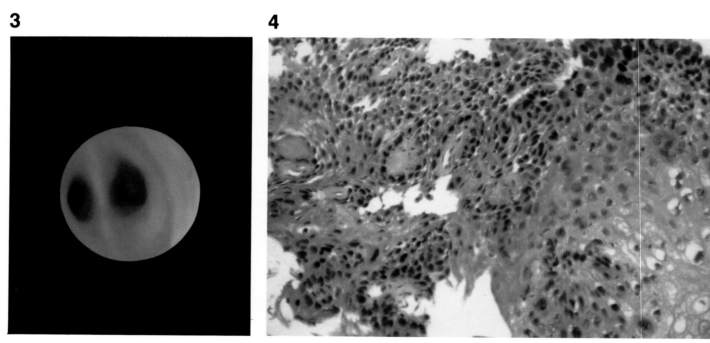

Fig. 3. View of RB9-10 through fiberoptic bronchoscope shows mucosal pallor.

Fig. 4. Biopsy from RB9-10 spur shows invasive squamous cell carcinoma.

During the second and third years following lobectomy, metaplastic squamous cells with marked atypia (Fig. 6) were repeatedly observed in the sputum, and 3 years postoperatively, squamous cancer cells were again detected (Fig. 7). His chest x-ray had been stable, with no suggestion of recurrence. However, a repeat tantalum dust bronchogram (Fig. 8) showed delayed clearance from the anterior segment of the left upper lobe.

5

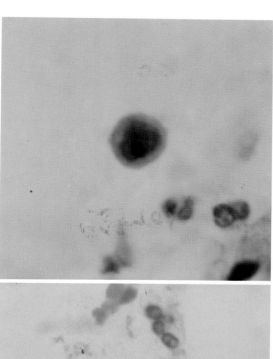

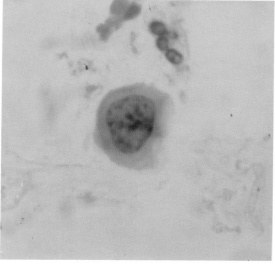

Fig. 5. Diagram of right lung shows area of invasive carcinoma (in red) and areas of in situ carcinoma (in blue).

Fig. 6. Postoperative sputum preparation contains cells that exhibit squamous metaplasia with marked atypia.

Fiberoptic bronchoscopy showed friability of the mucosa of the bronchus leading to this segment (LB3), and biopsy of the area disclosed squamous cell carcinoma. At thoracotomy, the tumor was densely adherent to the undersurface of the left pulmonary artery and was unresectable. Radiotherapy was administered to the area of the left upper lobe and adjacent mediastinum, but the patient died of metastasis 17 months after the second operation and 5 years after resection of the right lower lobe.

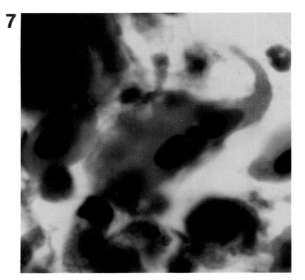

Fig. 7. Sputum specimen contains squamous carcinoma cells.

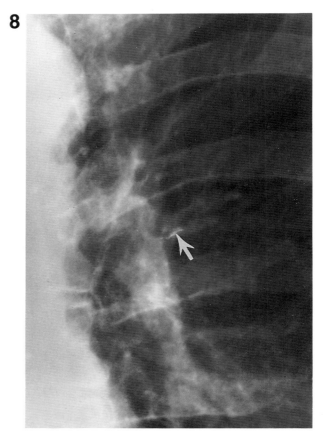

Fig. 8. Delayed clearance of tantalum (**arrow**) from anterior segment of left upper lobe (LB3). Chest radiograph was taken 48 hours after bronchography.

Comment

1. In this chronic heavy smoker, two presumably separate radiographically occult squamous cell carcinomas developed 3 years apart. The first was a tiny localized lesion that was resected by lobectomy; the second was unresectable at the time of exploration.

2. Although the extent of invasive cancer in the right lower lobe was very small, there was a large contiguous area of carcinoma in situ and a separate area of in situ cancer which had not been visible at bronchoscopy. Relatively large areas of in situ carcinoma may be encountered in association with small areas of invasion.

3. Serial cytopathologic examinations of sputum after resection of the first cancer showed a gradual progression of metaplastic squamous cells with increasingly pronounced degrees of cellular atypia before obvious cancer cells were again detected. Such changes may be predictive of the later development of squamous cell cancer.

4. Not all radiographically occult squamous cancers are resectable. Some, such as the one in Case 7 that follows, cannot be completely removed because of their proximal location. Others, as in the present case, have already undergone metastasis by the time the tumor is first detected.

CASE 6

A 60-year-old retired banker was seen for a general medical examination. He had smoked an average of 30 cigarettes daily for 45 years. He had a chronic cough that was productive of mucoid sputum. A chest x-ray was interpreted as showing bilateral pulmonary fibrosis and bullous changes, most prominent in the basilar regions (Fig. 1). A sputum cytology test was negative.

Four and eight months later, chest x-rays obtained for lung cancer screening purposes

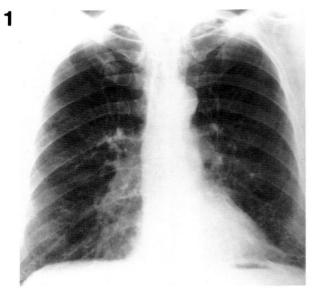

Fig. 1. Initial chest x-ray shows diffuse bilateral pulmonary fibrosis.

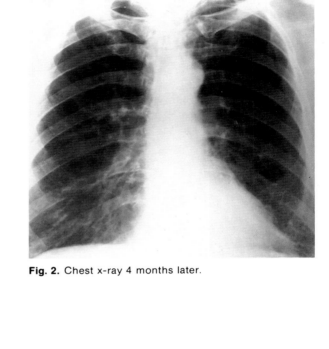

Fig. 2. Chest x-ray 4 months later.

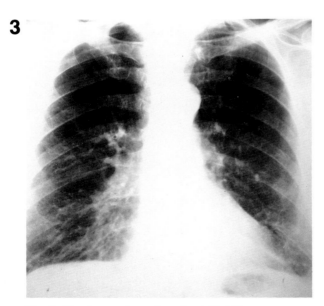

Fig. 3. Chest x-ray 8 months after initial film.

were interpreted as showing no change. Sputum cytology tests continued to be negative (Fig. 2 and 3).

Four months afterward (1 full year after the initial chest x-ray), a tumor was detected radiographically (Fig. 4).

4

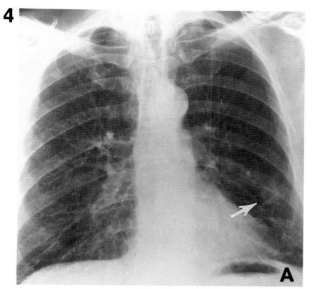

Fig. 4. **A,** Chest x-ray 1 year after initial film. Tumor is clearly visible in left lower lung (**arrow**).

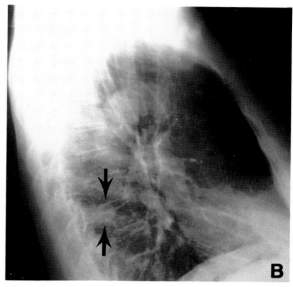

Fig. 4. **B,** Lateral chest x-ray shows posterior location of tumor (**arrows**).

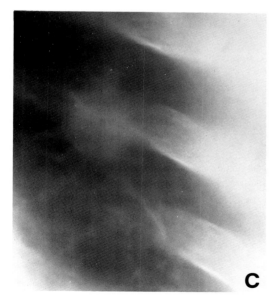

Fig. 4. **C,** Tomogram of tumor, which is surrounded by radiolucent halo interspersed with linear radiating densities ("corona radiata"). (See reference: Heitzman, et al., Case 11, Section 6: Radiology.)

5

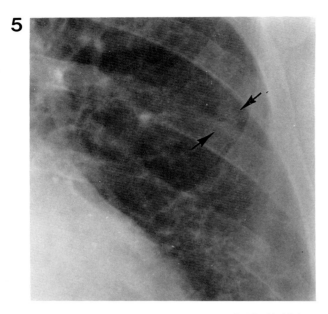

Fig. 5. Localized view of left lower lung field of initial chest x-ray. Small tumor (**arrows**) was overlooked because of surrounding diffuse pulmonary fibrosis.

6

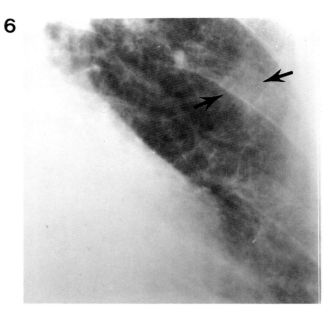

Fig. 6. Localized view of left lower lung 4 months after initial x-ray, with enlarging tumor (**arrows**), which was again overlooked.

7

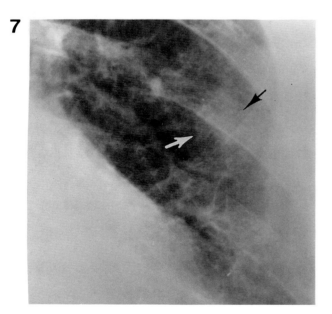

Fig. 7. Localized view of left lower lung 4 months later. Tumor (**arrows**) had enlarged further but still remained undetected.

8

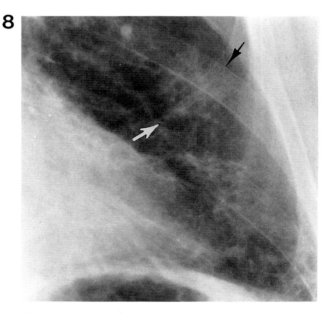

Fig. 8. Localized view of left lower lung field of film on which tumor (**arrows**) was ultimately detected, 1 full year after original x-ray.

9

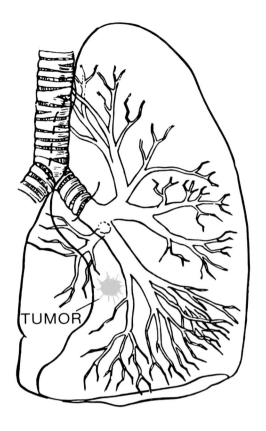

In retrospect, a small tumor could be observed on the original chest x-ray but was overlooked because of the background of pulmonary fibrosis (Fig. 5). The tumor was more obvious on the x-rays taken 4 and 8 months later (Fig. 6 and 7). It had enlarged considerably before it was finally detected (Fig. 8).

Repeated sputum cytologic examinations were negative. Fiberbronchoscopic examination disclosed only chronic bronchitis.

Left thoracotomy was performed. This revealed diffuse anthracosis and disseminated microbullous disease. In addition, there was a circumscribed tumor, 1.5 cm in diameter, situated in the periphery of the lower lobe. There was puckering of the pleura with infiltration of its visceral layer by tumor. Lymph nodes were not involved. The tumor was excised by left lower lobe lobectomy (Fig. 9 through 11).

Fig. 9. Diagram of tumor in periphery of left lower lobe.

Fig. 10. Low-power microscopic view of tumor shows peripheral location and associated scarring.

10

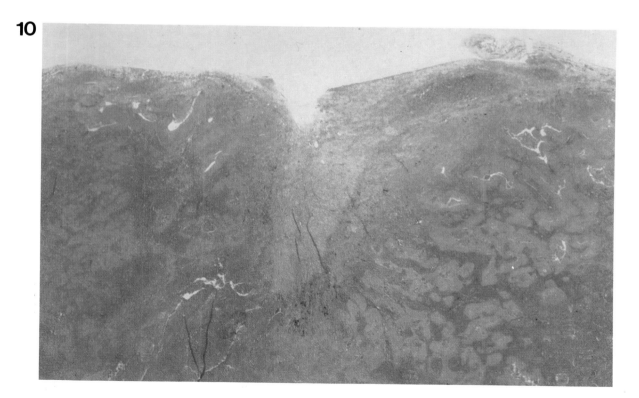

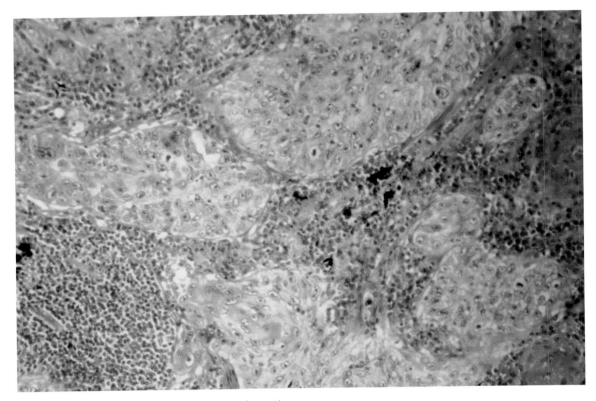

Fig. 11. Higher magnification reveals keratin formation characteristic of squamous cell carcinoma.

Comment

1. In this case the background of diffuse pulmonary fibrosis and bullous disease obscured a slowly enlarging tumor.

2. This case demonstrates the importance of careful scrutiny and comparison of sequential chest x-rays in the radiographic detection of early lung cancer.

3. The "corona radiata" surrounding the tumor on the tomographic view is often seen in association with peripheral lung cancers but is not diagnostic.

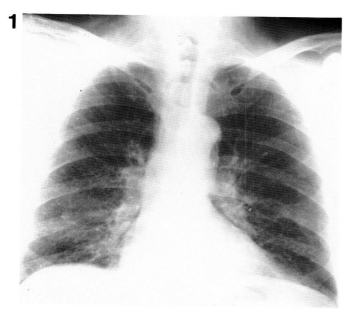

Fig. 1. Chest x-ray, interpreted as negative.

CASE 7

A 64-year-old retired pipefitter had smoked an average of 30 cigarettes a day for 30 years. He had arteriosclerosis obliterans and chronic obstructive pulmonary disease with limited respiratory reserve. He had recently undergone right hemicolectomy as treatment for a localized colonic carcinoma. During a postoperative checkup, a chest x-ray was obtained which was unremarkable (Fig. 1). However, a sputum cytology test at that time revealed markedly atypical squamous cells. Repetition of the cytology test disclosed squamous cancer cells (Fig. 2).

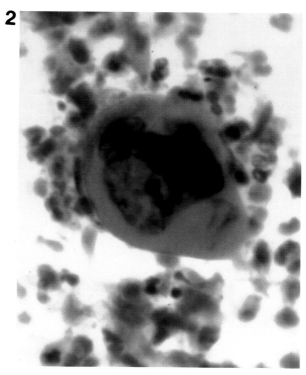

Fig. 2. Squamous carcinoma cell from specimen of sputum.

3

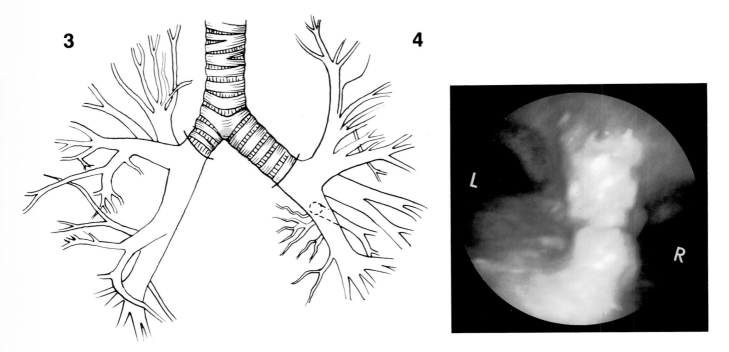

4

Fig. 3. Diagram shows site and extent of squamous cell cancer at tracheal bifurcation. In situ cancer is colored blue and invasive tumor, red.

Fig. 4. Endoscopic view of squamous cell cancer involving tracheal bifurcation.

5

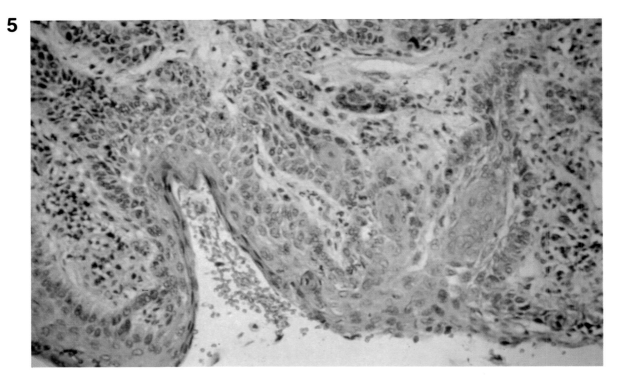

Fig. 5. Microscopic section of biopsy specimen from lower trachea shows in situ and infiltrative squamous cell carcinoma. (From Sanderson DR, Neel HB III,

Payne WS, Woolner LB: Cryotherapy for bronchogenic carcinoma: report of a case. Mayo Clinic Proc 50:435-437, 1975.)

Otolaryngologic examination was negative, but bronchoscopy revealed an indurated nodular tumor involving the distal posterior trachea, the tracheal bifurcation, and the proximal portions of both main bronchi (Fig. 3 and 4). Biopsy showed in situ and infiltrative squamous cell carcinoma (Fig. 5).

Because of the location of the tumor and the patient's other significant medical problems, radiation was selected as the primary treatment. Follow-up examinations, including sputum cytology tests, were negative until 13 months later, when repeat bronchoscopy again disclosed tumor at the tracheal bifurcation (Fig. 6). Biopsy revealed residual infiltrative squamous cancer (Fig. 7).

6

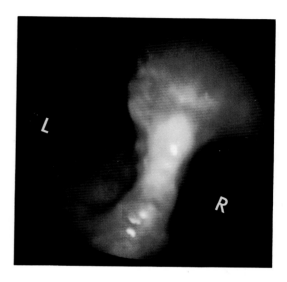

Fig. 6. Distal trachea and bifurcation, showing persistent or recurrent tumor.

7

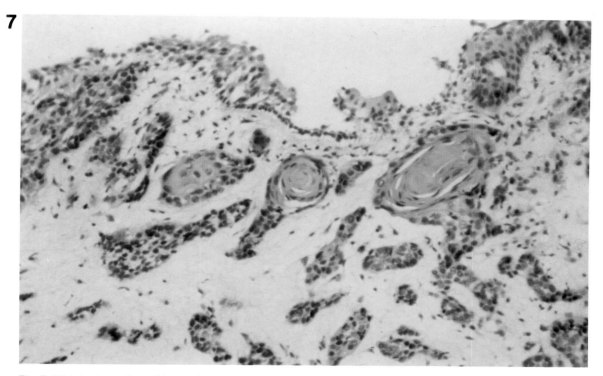

Fig. 7. Histologic section of tumor demonstrates postirradiation changes and residual infiltrative squamous cell carcinoma. (From Sanderson DR, Neel HB III, Payne WS, Woolner LB: Cryotherapy for bronchogenic carcinoma: report of a case. Mayo Clin Proc 50:435-437, 1975.)

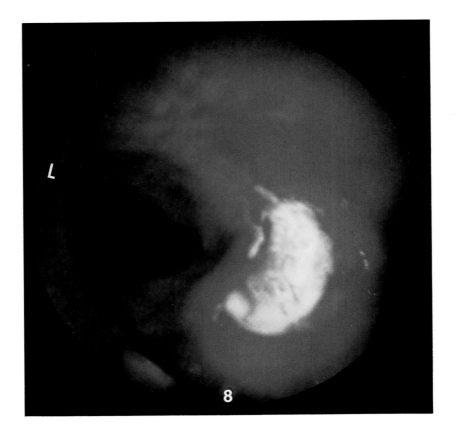

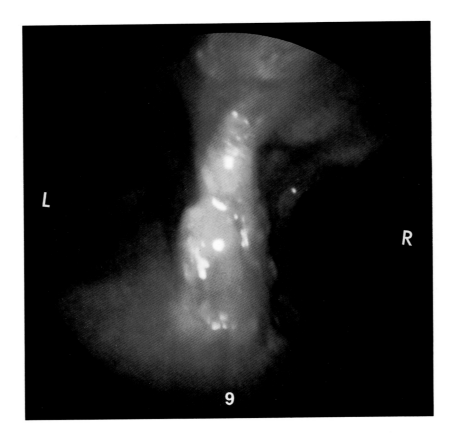

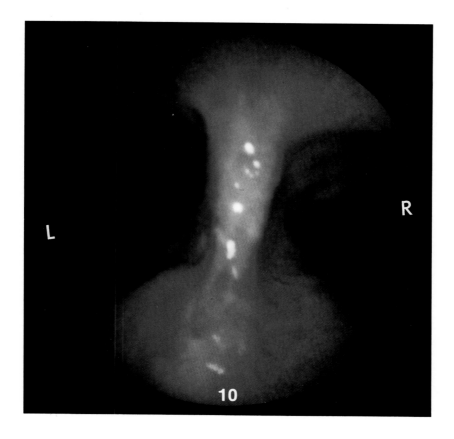

Fig. 8. Left side of tracheal bifurcation during cryotherapy treatment, demonstrating characteristic localized "ice ball" of frozen tissue, with surrounding erythema.

Fig. 9. Distal trachea and bifurcation after three cryotherapy treatments, showing regression of tumor.

Fig. 10. Tracheal bifurcation after fourth treatment. There has been further regression of tumor.

Of the various forms of palliative treatment available, cryotherapy was selected because of the accessibility and localized nature of the tumor, and because of the availability of an effective therapeutic cryoprobe adapted for use through a rigid open-tube bronchoscope. Cryotherapy was administered on five occasions during the ensuing 7 months. Each time, the procedure was well tolerated and definite regression of the local tumor was observed (Fig. 8 through 11).

About 1 month after the last cryotherapy treatment, the patient died suddenly of myocardial infarction sustained while mowing his lawn on a warm day. Postmortem examination, performed elsewhere, disclosed no gross abnormality of the tracheobronchial tree, and no evidence of recurrent or metastatic cancer was reported. However, serial histologic sections of the distal trachea and its bifurcation were not obtained.

11

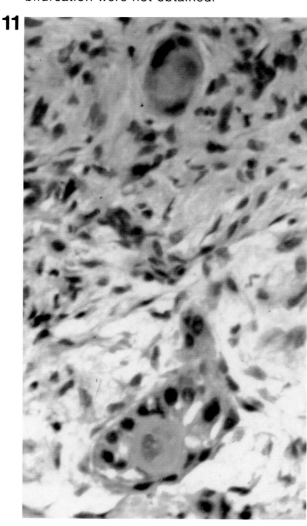

Fig. 11. Microscopic focus of residual squamous cancer in biopsy specimen obtained after fourth treatment. (From Sanderson DR, Neel HB III, Payne WS, Woolner LB: Cryotherapy for bronchogenic carcinoma: report of a case. Mayo Clin Proc 50:435-437, 1975.)

Comment

1. This case illustrates how a bronchogenic carcinoma, despite being limited in extent and of favorable cell type, may still be unresectable because of its location (see Case 5 in this section for further comment).

2. In this instance a small, localized squamous cell cancer was situated at the tracheal bifurcation. Extensive surgery would have been necessary, and this was precluded by the patient's pulmonary insufficiency and other medical problems.

3. A combination of vigorous local treatment, using radiation and cryotherapy, controlled the tumor, and the patient eventually died of other causes.

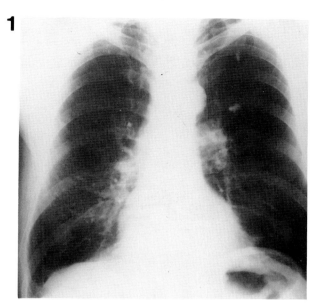

1

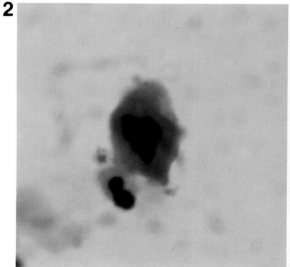

Fig. 1. Chest x-ray shows no abnormality.

CASE 8

A 53-year-old man was a chronic heavy cigarette smoker. He had no medical complaints at the time of his initial screening for lung cancer. The chest x-ray (Fig. 1) was normal, but the sputum cytology examination showed markedly atypical squamous cells (Fig. 2), a finding confirmed by repeated examination.

Although a definite diagnosis of cancer could not be made from the sputum cytology tests, bronchoscopy was considered indicated. A detailed examination was performed using the fiberbronchoscope. On the left side, tumor was seen (Fig. 3) extending upward from the orifice of the lingular division of the upper lobe (LB4, 5)

2

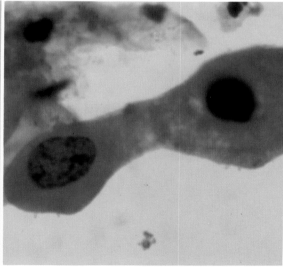

Fig. 2. Sputum cytology specimen shows markedly atypical squamous cells.

to the spur between the anterior and the apical-posterior segmental bronchi (LB1 & 2-3).

Biopsy of this area showed squamous cell carcinoma in situ. Although no definite abnormality was seen on the right side, brushings from the right upper lobe bronchus were also positive for squamous cancer cells.

The patient's general physical condition and pulmonary function were good, and it was believed that resection of the obvious lesion involving the left upper lobe could be followed by a limited contralateral resection if this was later required. At thoracotomy, the left upper lobe was removed. The specimen showed in situ squamous cell carcinoma at the LB1 & 2-3 spur and a separate focus in LB4 (Fig. 4).

Postoperatively, the sputum was positive for squamous carcinoma cells. Bronchoscopy 8 weeks after surgery was normal except for a 2.5-mm area of suspicious mucosal change in the right upper lobe bronchus (Fig. 5). Excisional biopsy of this area was carried out utilizing a cup forceps. Although no tumor was identified in the fragments of tissue obtained, the patient's sputum cytology test has been negative for the 18 months that have elapsed since the excisional biopsy, the chest x-ray has shown no change, and the patient has remained clinically well.

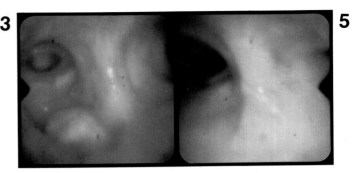

Fig. 3. View of lingular and upper-division bronchi of left upper lobe through fiberbronchoscope shows presence of tumor.

Fig. 5. View of right upper lobe spur shows small area of mucosal change thought to represent tumor.

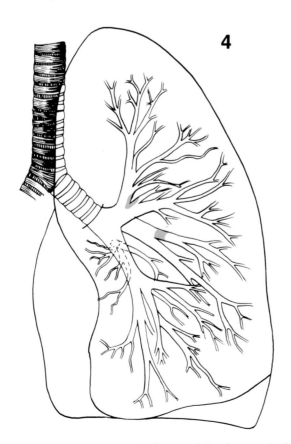

Fig. 4. Diagram of resected left upper lobe shows extent of two areas of carcinoma in situ (in blue).

Comment

1. The evidence of bilateral independent primary squamous cancers in this patient was obtained only by routine brushing of bronchi that appeared normal on visual examination, even though an obvious tumor had already been observed elsewhere. This approach has proven important for precise and complete diagnosis in cases of "occult" cancer, which exhibit a tendency to be multicentric.

2. Despite the absence of cancerous tissue in the excisional biopsy material, it seems likely that this patient's second primary tumor was in fact located in the right upper lobe and that it was successfully removed endoscopically. In selected cases of squamous carcinoma in situ, this is a therapeutic approach that might be considered, particularly in patients for whom surgical resection is contraindicated.

3. Once again, the presence of markedly atypical squamous cells in repeated specimens of sputum indicated the presence of cancer.

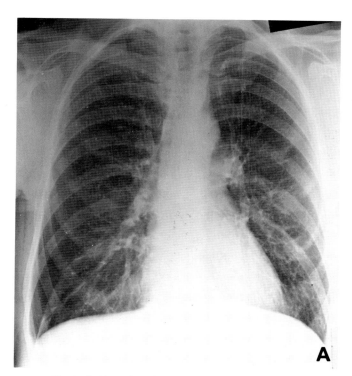

Fig. 1. **A**, Negative chest x-ray 3 years before discovery of tumor. **B**, Localized view, left mid-lung.

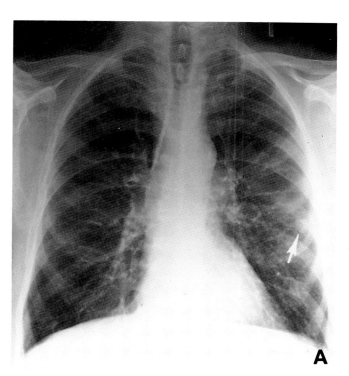

Fig. 2. **A**, Chest x-ray at time of detection of peripheral nodule (**arrow**). **B**, Localized view of left mid-lung. Nodule is identified by **arrow**.

CASE 9

A 64-year-old man with a cigarette-smoking history of 75 pack-years experienced symptoms suggesting intermittent partial obstruction of the small intestine. Results of the abdominal investigation were negative, and his symptoms of obstruction subsided. He had a history of chronic pancreatitis, and 3 years previously he had undergone subtotal pancreatectomy and

1

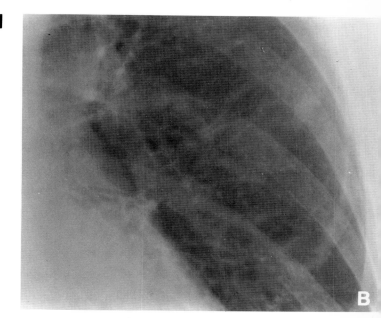

2

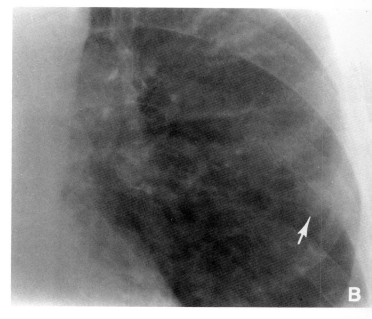

pancreaticojejunostomy. At that time a chest x-ray was negative (Fig. 1).

A chest x-ray taken during evaluation of his possible bowel obstruction disclosed a rounded density in the periphery of the left mid-lung (Fig. 2).

A cytologic examination of his sputum revealed moderately atypical squamous cells. An induced-sputum specimen was obtained, and this disclosed markedly atypical squamous cells suggesting possible cancer (Fig. 3).

Bronchoscopy revealed no obvious endobronchial tumor, but random mucosal biopsies indicated squamous cell cancer at the junction of the upper and lower lobe bronchi on the left side (Fig. 4).

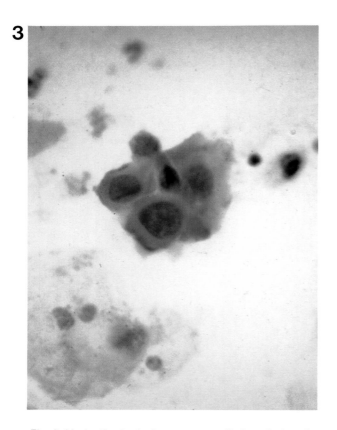

Fig. 3. Markedly atypical squamous cells from induced sputum.

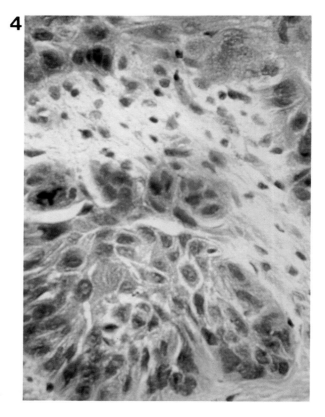

Fig. 4. Squamous cell cancer in situ from biopsy of mucosa at junction of left upper and left lower lobe bronchi.

Left thoracotomy was performed. A circumscribed squamous cell cancer, 1.8 cm in diameter, was present in the periphery of the lingular division of the left upper lobe. A second, centrally located or "hilar type" in situ squamous cell cancer was found in the left lower lobe bronchus just below the take-off of the left upper lobe bronchus. This tumor measured 4 by 7 mm. Pneumonectomy was required in order to remove both tumors (Fig. 5 through 10).

5

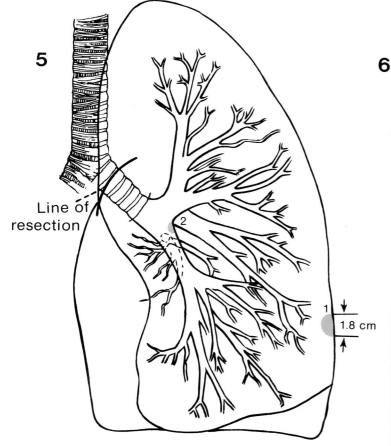

Fig. 5. Diagram of left lung shows locations of peripheral circumscribed invasive (red) squamous cell cancer and central in situ (blue) squamous cell cancer (simultaneous, or synchronous, primary tumors).

Fig. 6. Gross specimen of peripheral cancer located in extreme left lower corner of photograph and identified by **arrows**.

6

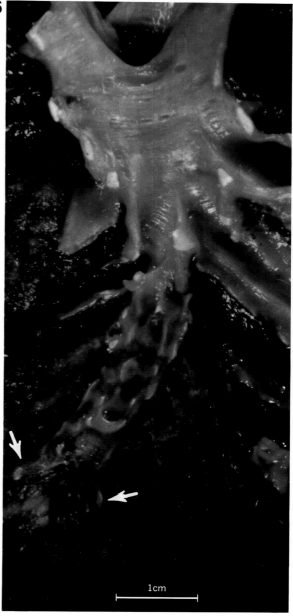

1cm

7

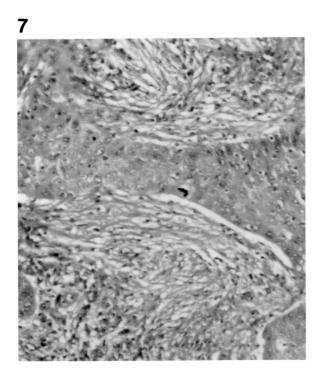

Fig. 7. Microscopic section of peripheral squamous cell cancer.

8

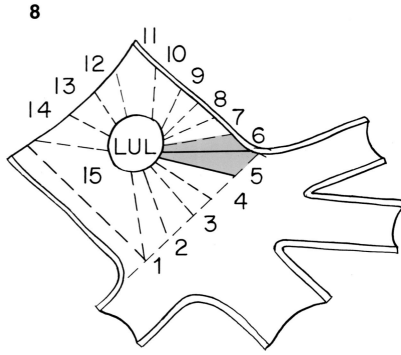

Fig. 8. Diagram of junction between upper lobe of left lung (LUL) and lower lobe shows sites of serial block sections obtained for microscopic study; 5-6 block best demonstrated in situ squamous cell cancer discovered at junction of the two lobes.

9

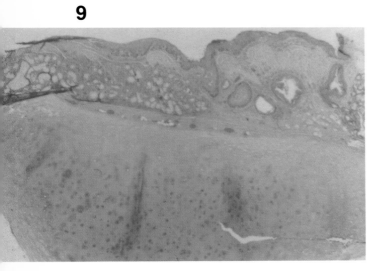

Fig. 9. Low-power view of microscopic section of in situ squamous cell cancer situated between upper and lower lobes.

Comment

1. Both the sputum cytology and the chest x-ray were abnormal in this case. However, the radiographic abnormality was both small and peripheral; this raised suspicion, later confirmed, that it was not the source of the abnormal cells.

2. This combination of observations should suggest multicentric cancers, at least one of which is "occult."

3. Multicentric lung cancers, whether occurring simultaneously (synchronous) or at different times (metachronous) are most often of the squamous cell type.

4. In this case, no tumor was visualized bronchoscopically, but the in situ squamous cell cancer was localized by systematic, sequential sampling of individual bronchi and their spurs. The great importance of this technique is thus evident.

5. Because the bronchial mucosal cancer was both radiographically and endoscopically "occult," it could have been presumed to be, and in fact was, entirely in situ.

10

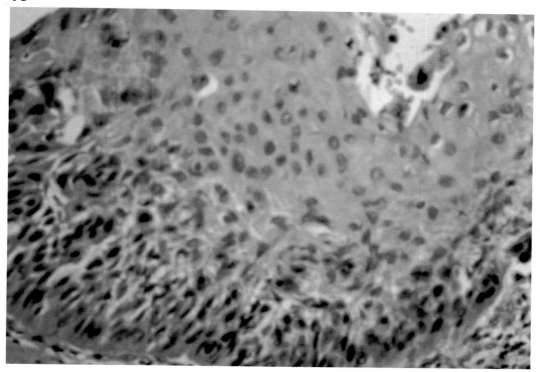

Fig. 10. High-power view of mucosal surface of in situ cancer. Tumor involved surface epithelium and ducts of mucous glands but did not penetrate bronchial wall beyond this level.

CASE 10

A 60-year-old copper mine foreman had a cigarette-smoking history of 45 pack-years. He also had inhaled considerable amounts of pipe tobacco smoke. He had a chronic cough that was productive of mucoid sputum. The cough had become worse, and dyspnea and wheezing had commenced after exposure to smoke during a fire 6 years previously; this eventually led him to seek medical attention. His chest x-ray was negative (Fig. 1).

Pulmonary function studies disclosed moderately severe but partially reversible obstructive changes. Cytologic examination of a specimen of sputum showed metaplastic squamous cells with marked atypia. The test was repeated, with the same results (Fig. 2).

Carcinoma of the respiratory tract was suspected because of the repeated finding of marked cellular atypia, even though frankly cancerous squamous cells were not observed. Rigid, open-tube bronchoscopic examination performed under topical anesthesia was unremarkable except for diffuse bronchitis. Differential bronchial washings from each lung revealed markedly atypical squamous cells on the right side and a few metaplastic squamous cells on the left but again no obviously cancerous cells.

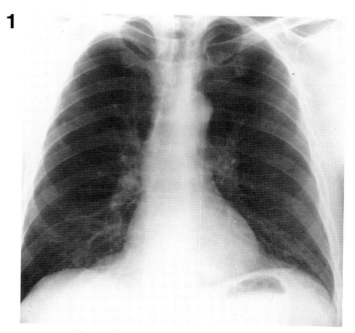

Fig. 1. Chest x-ray, interpreted as negative.

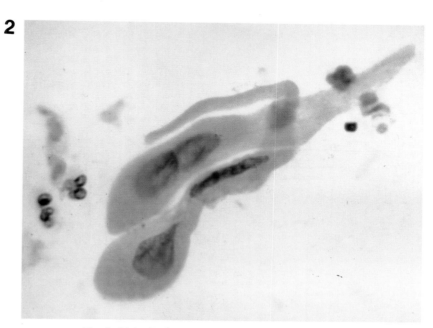

Fig. 2. Metaplastic squamous cells with marked atypia which were observed on two consecutive sputum cytologic examinations.

3

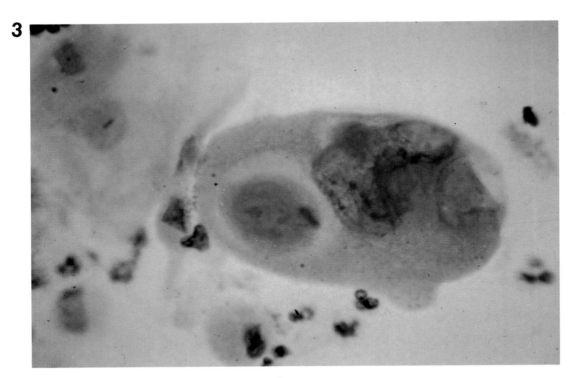

Fig. 3. Squamous carcinoma cell in sputum specimen collected 4 months after initial one.

A sputum cytology test obtained 1 month later showed only moderately atypical cells, but 3 months after this another test disclosed squamous cancer cells (Fig. 3), a finding confirmed by induced-sputum study. The chest x-ray remained negative (Fig. 4).

Bronchoscopy was repeated, with the use of general anesthesia and a fiberbronchoscope. Detailed inspection again showed only bronchitis, but brushings from the lingular bronchi (LB4, 5) were positive for squamous cancer cells (Fig. 5).

Because no tumor was actually visualized, fiberbronchoscopy was repeated. This time brushings from LB4 and LB5 contained a few cells that were regarded as "probably cancerous." However, the evidence was not considered strong enough to justify thoracotomy.

4

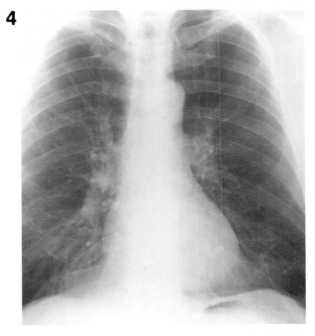

Fig. 4. Negative chest x-ray taken 4 months after initial film.

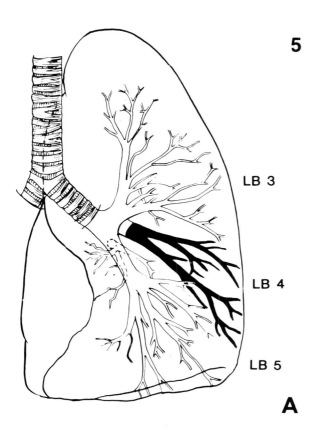

5

LB 3

LB 4

LB 5

A

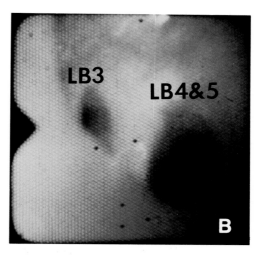

LB3 LB4&5

B

Fig. 5. A, Bronchial diagram with lingular bronchi emphasized in black. **B**, Fiberbronchoscopic view of orifice of left upper lobe. Anterior segment (LB3) on left, next to pointer. Lingular bronchi (LB4 & 5) on right. **C**, Squamous cancer cells from bronchial brushings of LB4 and 5.

A fourth bronchoscopic examination was performed with almost identical results, except that this time a few definitely cancerous cells were observed on the brushings from LB4 and 5 (Fig. 6).

Left thoracotomy was carried out. Because no tumor had actually been seen, the surgeon had determined preoperatively that he would resect the lingula. If he found no tumor, he would then complete removal of the left upper lobe. If this failed to disclose any grossly visible tumor, the procedure would be terminated, because of uncertainties regarding the location of the tumor and the patient's respiratory reserve. Further action would then depend on the results of microscopic pathologic studies.

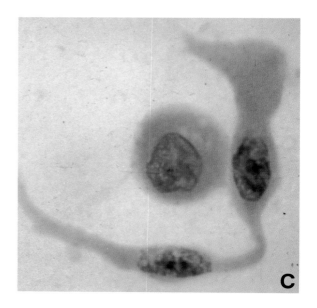

C

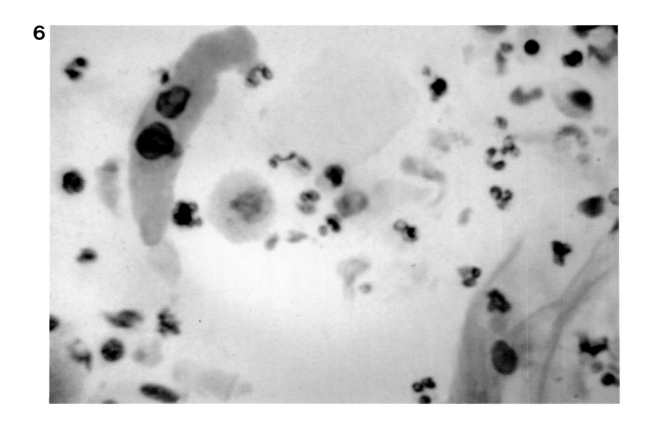

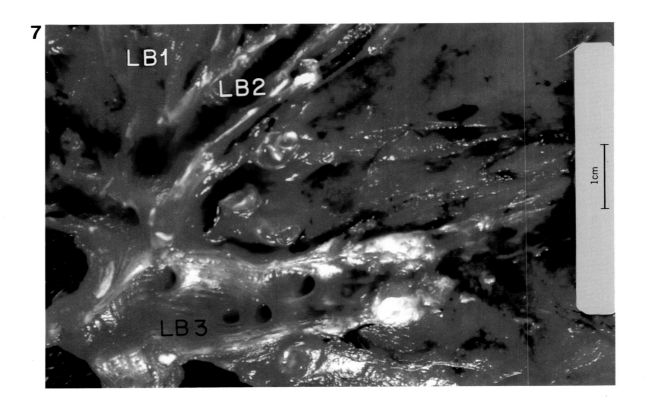

At operation, no tumor could be palpated. The lingula was resected, but on gross inspection of LB4 and LB5 no tumor was evident.

The remainder of the left upper lobe was then resected. Examination of its anterior segment bronchus (LB3) revealed an in situ and superficially invasive squamous cell carcinoma 1.5 cm in length, arising 2.5 cm from the origin of the bronchus.

Fig. 6. Squamous cancer cells from brushings of LB4 and 5 at fourth bronchoscopy.

Fig. 7. Gross specimen of tumor involving LB3. Bronchus has been opened longitudinally to demonstrate "napkin ring" configuration of well-localized squamous cell carcinoma. LB1 and 2 are shown for orientation.

Fig. 8. Diagram shows actual location of cancer, 2.5 cm from orifice of LB3.

Fig. 9. Enlarged view of tumor. Note abrupt transition from normal-appearing bronchus to tumor.

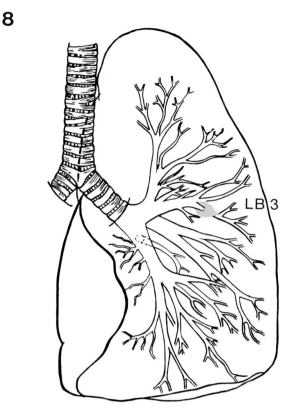

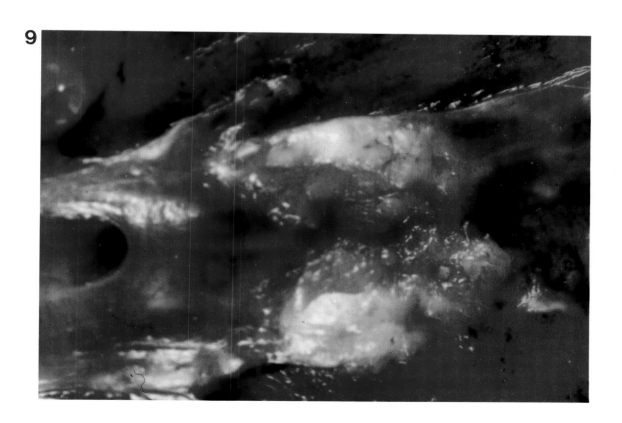

Convalescence from surgery was uneventful. A chest x-ray film 3 weeks afterward showed only the expected postoperative changes on the left side (Fig. 13).

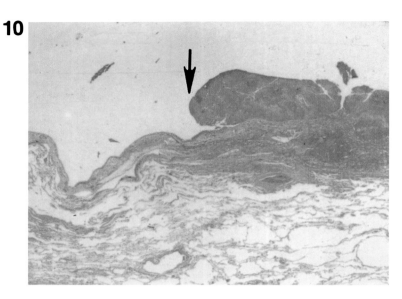

Fig. 10. Microscopic view of tumor demonstrates sharp demarcation (**arrow**) between normal bronchial mucosa and tumor.

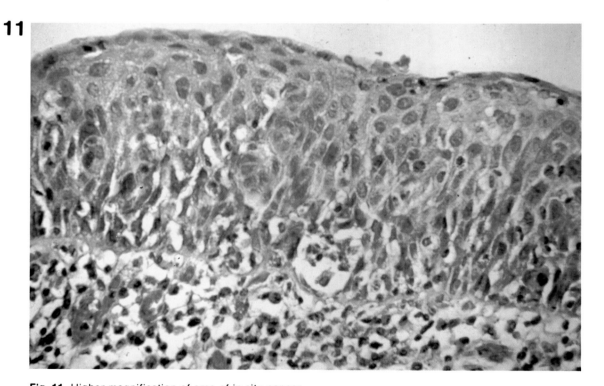

Fig. 11. Higher magnification of area of in situ cancer.

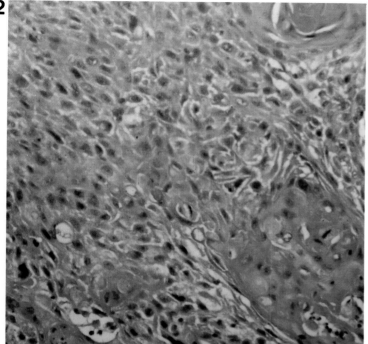

Fig. 12. High-power magnification shows zone of infiltrating, keratinized cancer. Focal infiltration extended 2 mm into bronchial wall.

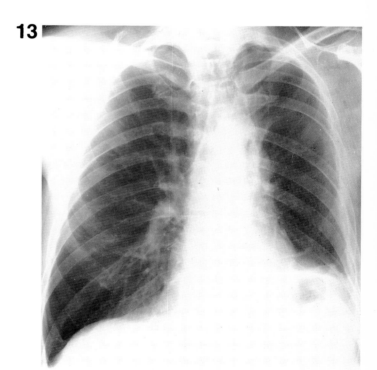

Fig. 13. Chest x-ray 3 weeks after surgery shows postoperative changes on left.

Six months later, the patient noted increasing dyspnea. He contacted his primary physician, who obtained another chest x-ray. This revealed a definite increase in the size of the right hilar shadow, suggesting new or recurrent carcinoma and possible hilar adenopathy (Fig. 14).

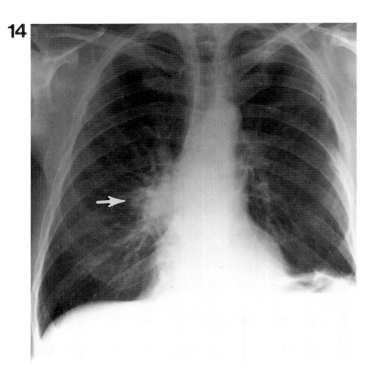

Fig. 14. Chest x-ray 7 months postoperatively. There is definite enlargement of right hilar density (**arrow**).

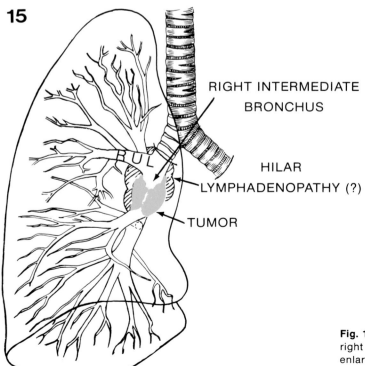

Fig. 15. Diagram of invasive squamous cell cancer in right intermediate bronchus. Degree of hilar enlargement radiographically suggests associated lymphadenopathy.

Another bronchoscopic examination was performed. This disclosed a polypoid tumor almost completely obstructing the intermediate bronchus on the right side just below the level of the upper lobe bronchus (Fig. 15). Biopsy revealed squamous cell carcinoma (Fig. 16).

The patient's ventilatory reserve was considerably reduced. Removal of the right-sided tumor, if possible at all, would have required resection of at least the middle and lower lobes. For these reasons, further surgery was not advised and radiation therapy was administered. This was followed by regression of the right hilar enlargement and amelioration of the dyspnea (Fig. 17).

16

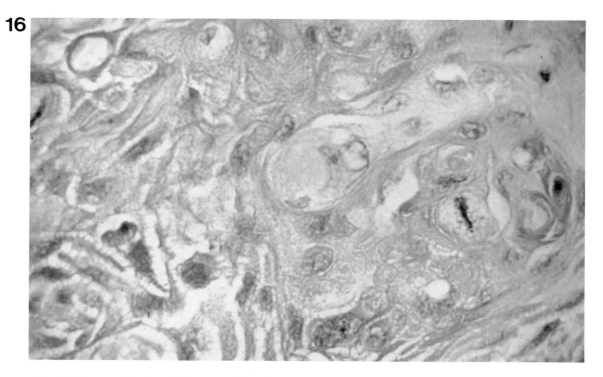

Fig. 16. Microscopic view of biopsy specimen from intermediate bronchus confirms diagnosis of squamous cell carcinoma.

During the ensuing 5 years, there was no evidence of recurrent or metastatic lung cancer. Repeated sputum cytologic examinations were negative for carcinoma cells. Radiation fibrosis of the right lower lung developed, as did progressive obstructive lung disease and episodes of congestive cardiac failure. Recurrent pericardial effusion twice necessitated drainage procedures, but the aspirate was negative for cancer cells on each occasion. A chest x-ray 5 years after completion of radiotherapy showed cardiomegaly, postoperative changes on the left, and fibrosis of the right lung medially and inferiorly (Fig. 18).

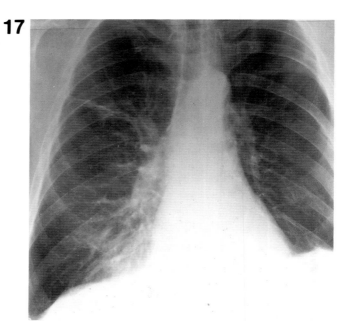

Fig. 17. Chest x-ray 4 months after completion of radiation therapy and 1 year after surgery. Right hilar density is much reduced in size. Residual postoperative changes persist on left.

Comment

1. There were two presumably separate primary squamous cell carcinomas in this case. The first was detected by sputum cytology testing and the second by chest radiography.

2. As previously noted, multiple primary cancers of the respiratory tract are usually squamous cell cancers.

3. The interval between detection of the two cancers was quite short (only 8 months), yet even in retrospect the initial chest x-ray was negative.

4. The first (radiographically "occult") cancer stresses the need for careful assessment of patients with cancer cells in the sputum but with negative chest x-rays and negative otolaryngologic and fiberbronchoscopic examinations. The presence of cancer cells in sputum cannot be ignored; nor can positive bronchial brushings. However, caution is advised whenever positive brushings are not confirmed by direct observation of a tumor or by bronchial biopsy.

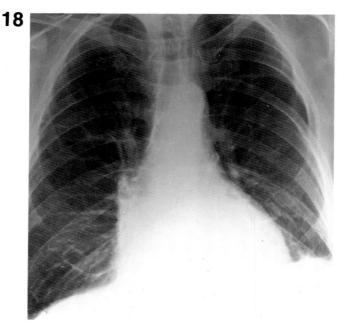

Fig. 18. Chest x-ray 5 years after radiation therapy.

5. Positive bronchial brushings collected from the same bronchus on two or more occasions are usually, but not invariably, sufficient to establish the location of an endoscopically inapparent cancer. In the present case the tumor was located in a bronchus adjacent to the one from which the positive brushings were obtained. Whether this was the result of mistaken bronchial identification or of cell "spillover" is moot.

6. In cases of suspected but radiologically and endoscopically "occult" lung cancer, the bronchoscopist and the cytopathologist must satisfy themselves and their surgical colleagues "beyond reasonable doubt" that a cancer is indeed both present and localized. The surgeon should then proceed with operation on this basis, realizing that no abnormality may be palpable or even visible but having a predetermined plan of action, as in the present case.

7. As a rule, radiation therapy for lung cancer is only palliative. However, it is recognized that radiation may at times eradicate the intrathoracic component of a bronchogenic carcinoma. This appears to have occurred in the second cancer encountered in this case. No evidence of recurrence or metastasis was noted 5 years after completion of treatment for the second tumor.

CASE 11

A 66-year-old retired sheet-metal worker with a cigarette-smoking history of 68 pack-years was seen for a medical checkup. He had moderate nerve deafness and a chronic morning cough productive of mucoid sputum.

A chest x-ray revealed diffuse, finely nodular densities scattered throughout both lungs (Fig. 1). When compared with previous films, the condition appeared stable. During his working years, he had done considerable soldering and welding, and it was presumed that the radiographic changes represented occupational pneumoconiosis. A sputum cytology test was negative.

During the next 2 years, screening chest x-rays and sputum cytology tests were obtained every 4 months. Both tests were consistently negative (Fig. 2).

Four months later, the chest x-ray was again reported as exhibiting no change. In retrospect, there was a faint, irregular new density in the peripheral portion of the right upper lobe (Fig. 3). Sputum cytologic examination remained negative.

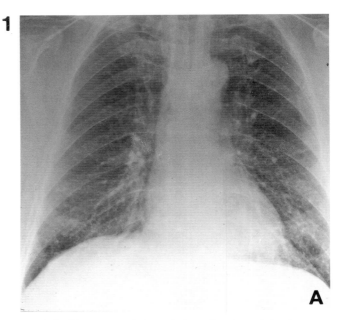

Fig. 1. A, Chest x-ray, interpreted as showing minimal diffuse nodular densities bilaterally and probably representing occupational pneumoconiosis.

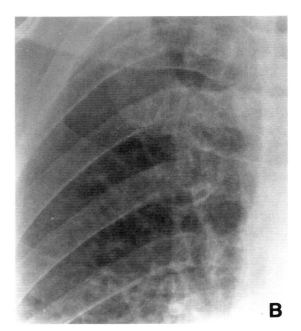

Fig. 1. B, Enlarged view of right upper lung.

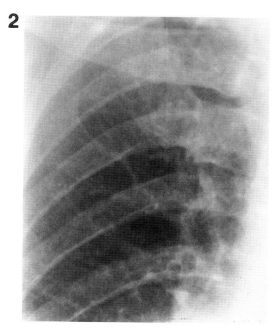

Fig. 2. Localized x-ray of right upper lung 2 years after first film. No significant change was noted.

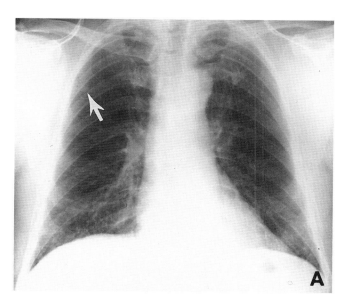

Fig. 3. A, Chest x-ray 28 months after first film, interpreted as showing no change. Note small, ill-defined density in periphery of right upper lobe, indicated by **arrow**.

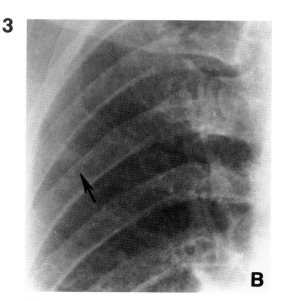

Fig. 3. B, Localized view of right upper lung and small, ill-defined density (**arrow**).

Four months after this, his chest x-ray revealed an obvious circumscribed density, 2 cm in diameter, in the periphery of the right upper lung. Tomograms showed partial cavitation but no calcification of the lesion (Fig. 4). Examination of spontaneous and induced-sputum specimens disclosed no cancer cells.

Fiberoptic bronchoscopy was negative. Bronchial brushings were obtained with the use of fluoroscopic guidance. Brushings and bronchial secretions were negative for cancer cells and for acid-fast bacilli.

Fig. 4. A, Chest x-ray 32 months after initial film shows noncalcified cavitary density in right upper lung (**arrow**). **B,** Localized view of right upper lung. Lesion (**arrow**) has a rounded contour and indistinct border. **C,** Whole-lung tomogram shows lesion in right upper lung and evidence of cavitation. **D,** Localized tomogram shows peripheral cavitary lesion without calcification.

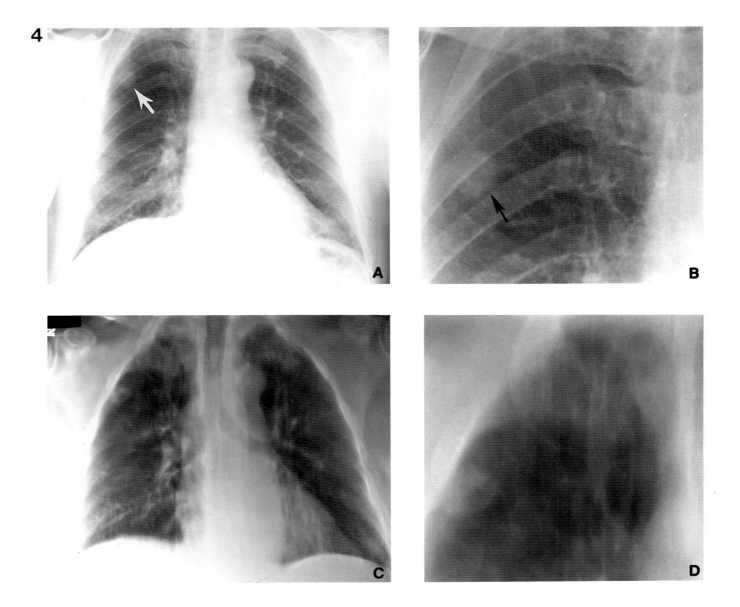

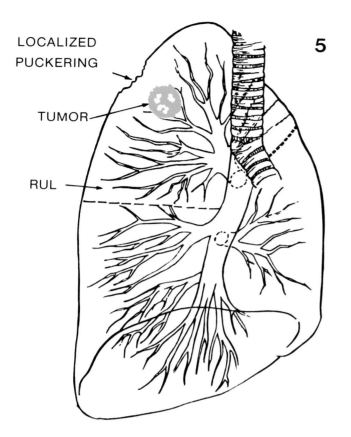

LOCALIZED PUCKERING

TUMOR

RUL

5

Right thoracotomy was recommended. At surgery, a 2-cm mass was palpated in the apical segment of the right upper lobe. Lobectomy was performed.

Pathologic examination revealed a peripheral, cavitating, bronchogenic type of adenocarcinoma. There was puckering of the overlying pleura, but neither the pleura not the transected bronchial stump was involved by tumor. Hilar and peribronchial lymph nodes were also negative (Fig. 5 and 6).

Fig. 5. Diagram of tumor shows cavitation plus puckering of overlying pleura.

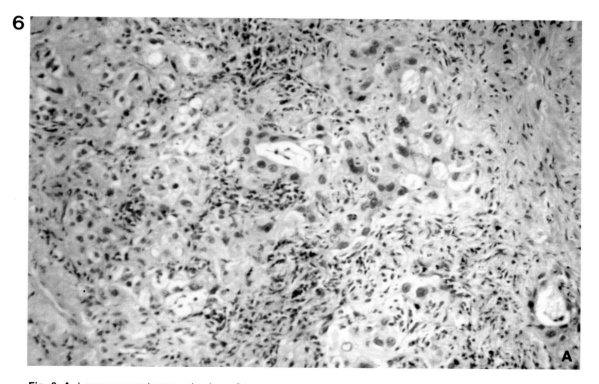

Fig. 6. A, Low-power microscopic view of tumor, a bronchogenic adenocarcinoma.

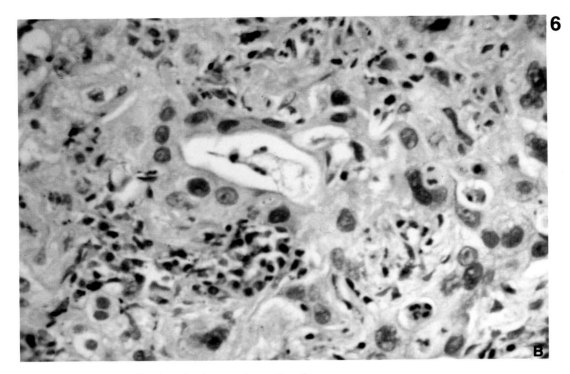

Fig. 6. B, Higher magnification of microscopic section of tumor.

The patient's postoperative course was satisfactory. Three years later he was alive and well, without evidence of recurrent or metastatic disease.

Comment

1. In this case there was rapid growth of the cancer. It grew from a lesion that was barely visible radiographically, even in retrospect, to one that was 2 cm in diameter in 125 days.

2. This case demonstrates the value of frequent repetition of chest x-rays in screening programs designed to detect early lung cancer.

3. The case also illustrates the complementary roles of chest radiography and sputum cytology in programs of lung cancer detection. All pulmonary cytology tests were negative, including tests of spontaneous and induced sputum and bronchial secretions and brushings.

4. Rapidly growing tumors cause concern over prognosis. However, in this instance the tumor was still small and localized at the time of surgery, and resected nodes were negative for cancer.

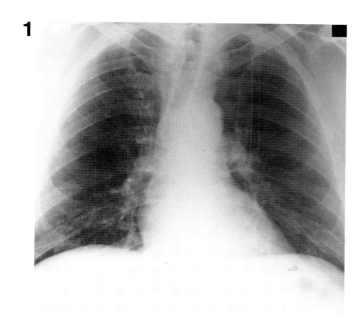

Fig. 1. Chest x-ray, interpreted as normal.

CASE 12

A 66-year-old retired businessman had a cigarette-smoking history of 125 pack-years. He sought medical advice because of a long-standing, productive cough and symptomatic ischemic peripheral vascular disease. A chest x-ray was normal (Fig. 1). A 3-day "pooled" spontaneous sputum specimen revealed metaplastic squamous cells but no atypia.

Lung cancer screening by chest radiography and sputum cytology testing was repeated every 4 months. The two tests were negative during the subsequent year. A chest x-ray taken 16 months after the first film was also interpreted as negative, although in retrospect a vague ill-defined semicircular density was present above the dome of the right diaphragm (Fig. 2). The sputum cytology test remained negative.

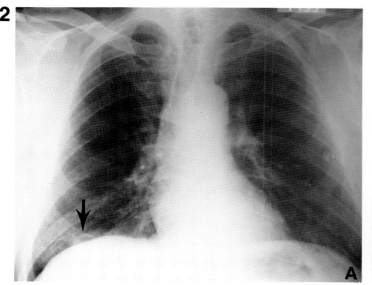

Fig. 2. A, Chest x-ray 16 months after initial film. Faint density is present above right diaphragm (**arrow**).

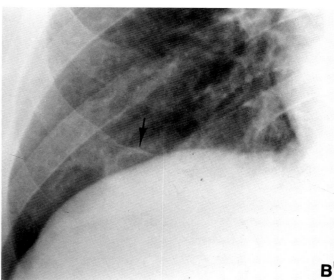

Fig. 2. B, Localized view of right lower lung and diaphragm shows vagueness of abnormality (**arrow**).

Four months later, the radiographic abnormality was clearly visible as an ovoid density visible above and below the dome of the right diaphragm (Fig. 3 **A** and **B**). On lateral view, there was an obvious triangular density in the posterior costophrenic angle (Fig. 3 **C**).

Simultaneously, adenocarcinoma cells were observed in the sputum (Fig. 4). Scattered rales and rhonchi were audible over the base of the right lung posteriorly.

Bronchoscopy revealed no tumor, but secretions from the lower lobe bronchus of the right lung were positive for adenocarcinoma cells.

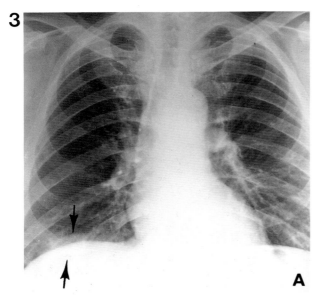

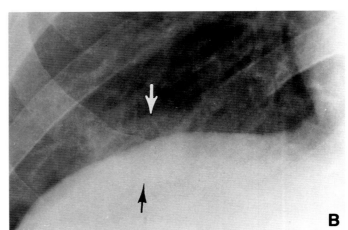

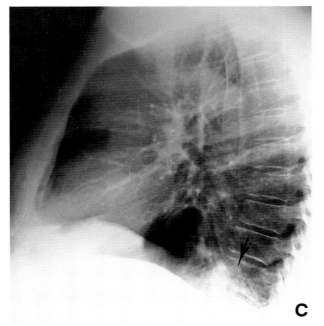

Fig. 3. A, Chest x-ray 20 months after first film. **Arrows** delineate upper and lower margins of tumor. **B,** Enlarged view of right lower lung field and tumor (**arrows**). **C,** Lateral chest x-ray demonstrates triangular density posteriorly, just above diaphragm (**arrow**).

Right thoracotomy was performed. In the center of the lower lobe was a tumor, 6 cm in diameter, having the consolidated, pneumonic characteristics of a bronchiolo-alveolar type of adenocarcinoma (Fig. 5).

Right lower lobectomy was carried out, and the diagnosis of bronchiolo-alveolar

carcinoma was verified histologically (Fig. 6). The lung-tumor interface was ill defined, with tumor gradually blending into normal lung. However, the line of bronchial transection, the peribronchial and hilar lymph nodes, and the pleura were all free of disease.

4

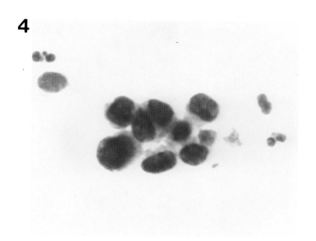

Fig. 4. Sputum cytologic preparation shows adenocarcinoma cells.

5

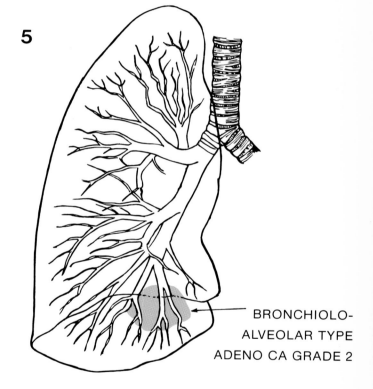

BRONCHIOLO-
ALVEOLAR TYPE
ADENO CA GRADE 2

Fig. 5. Diagram of tumor in right lower lobe.

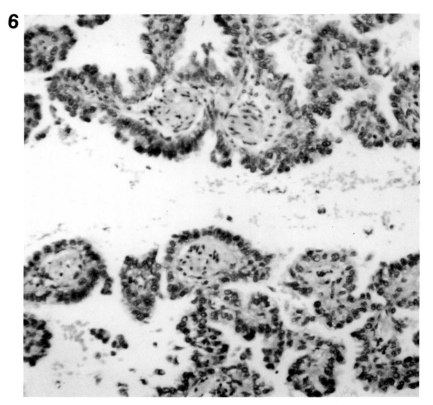

Fig. 6. Microscopic view of tumor shows well-differentiated adenocarcinoma of bronchiolo-alveolar type.

Comment

1. In this case the tumor was simultaneously detected by chest x-ray and by sputum cytology testing, an uncommon observation among cases of lung cancer discovered by screening with both tests every 4 months.

2. As a rule, the chest x-ray is more sensitive than the sputum cytology test in detecting peripheral lung cancers, whereas the sputum cytology test is superior for more centrally located ("hilar type") cancers.

3. However, in the present case the cancer was a low-grade, well-differentiated peripheral one. Its location permitted it to achieve considerable size before it was noted radiographically. As a consequence, when it was finally detected, its bronchial communications were sufficiently extensive to produce a positive cytology test.

4. The case also demonstrates the value of the lateral chest x-ray. In retrospect, the radiographic abnormality was present at least 4 months before the sputum cytology became abnormal. Unfortunately, only a posteroanterior chest x-ray was obtained at that time. Had a lateral view been taken, the tumor probably would have been obvious. It is situated in the posterior costophrenic angle, which is clearly visible on a lateral projection but relatively obscured on a posteroanterior film.

5. The radiographic appearance of the tumor was reminiscent of pneumonitis. The bronchiolo-alveolar type of adenocarcinoma may at times be misinterpreted as an inflammatory pneumonic process.

CASE 13

A 39-year-old asymptomatic machine repairman had a routine employment medical examination. At that time, a chest x-ray revealed scoliosis, an azygos lobe, and a localized density in the right upper lung field (Fig. 1).

He had a cigarette-smoking history of 10 pack-years but had not smoked in 7 years. His tuberculin skin test was negative. A chest x-ray taken 30 months previously had been negative. Tomograms of the right upper lung field disclosed that the lesion had an irregular border and contained multiple small radiolucent areas, presumably cavities (Fig. 2).

1
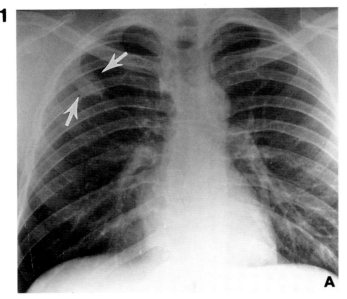 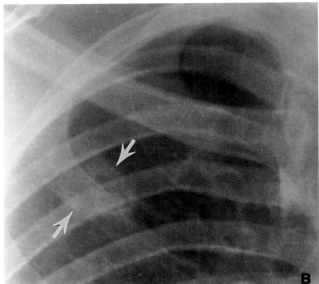

Fig. 1. A, Chest x-ray taken during routine medical examination. Localized density in right upper lung field (**arrows**). **B,** Enlarged view of lesion (**arrows**) shows suggestion of cavitation.

2
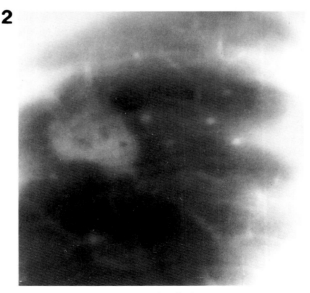

Fig. 2. Tomogram of cavitating lesion.

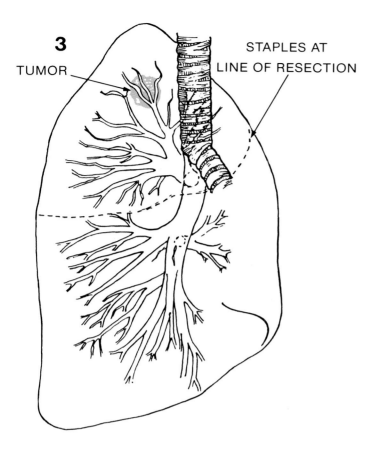

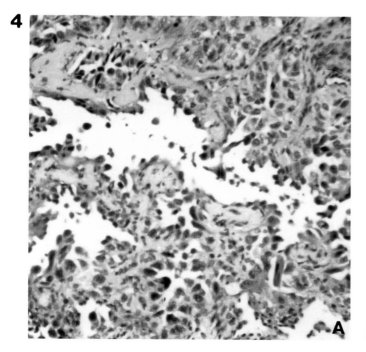

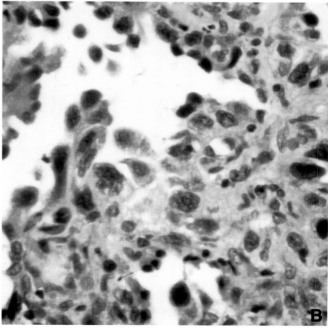

Bronchoscopy was not considered necessary, and right thoracotomy was advised. This revealed congenital absence of the fissures between the right upper lobe and the right middle lobe and superior segment of the right lower lobe (RB6). A mass was present near the apex of the upper lobe. Right upper lobectomy was performed with the use of multiple rows of staples to separate the upper lobe from the middle lobe and RB6 (Fig. 3).

On pathologic examination of the upper lobe, there was a cavitary tumor, 2.5 cm in diameter, in the periphery of the apical segment (RB1). The tumor extended to within 3 mm of the pleural surface. Approximately half of the tumor was scar tissue; the remainder was bronchiolo-alveolar adenocarcinoma (Fig. 4). Peribronchial and hilar lymph nodes were negative.

Fig. 3. Sketch of right lung shows location of mass and stapled line of pulmonary resection.

Fig. 4. A, Low-power microscopic view of tumor shows adenocarcinoma of bronchiolo-alveolar type. **B,** Magnified microscopic view of tumor.

After recovery from surgery, the patient was followed by chest x-rays and sputum cytology tests every 4 months. The initial follow-up studies were satisfactory (Fig. 5).

The patient continued his recheck examinations. He remained asymptomatic and without evidence of tumor recurrence or metastasis for another full year.

A chest x-ray taken 20 months after surgery was considered stable. However, in retrospect, there was a small area of increased density, not present earlier, located behind the medial aspect of the right clavicle (Fig. 6).

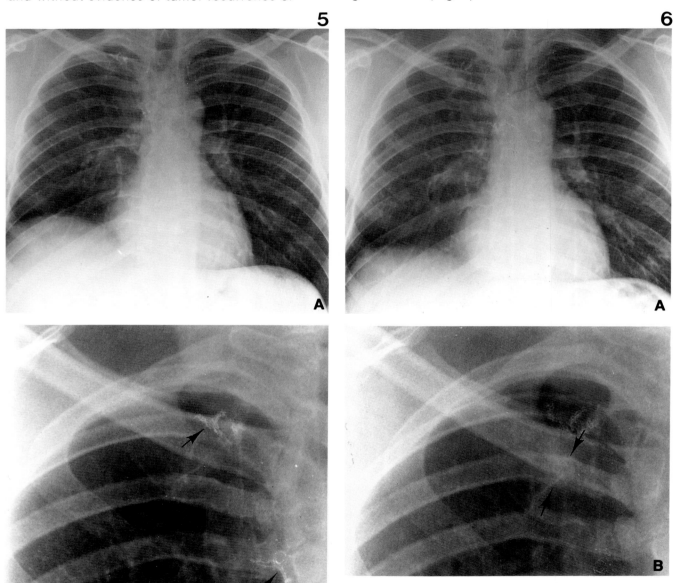

Fig. 5. A, Chest x-ray 4 months after surgery. There are postoperative elevation of right diaphragm and blunting of right costophrenic angle. **B,** Localized view of right upper lung field shows surgical staples (**arrows**) above right hilum and at apex of right hemithorax.

Fig. 6. A, Chest x-ray 20 months postoperatively, interpreted as stable. **B,** Enlarged view of right upper lung field. There is an area of increased density behind medial aspect of right clavicle and immediately below collection of staples in apical region (**arrows**).

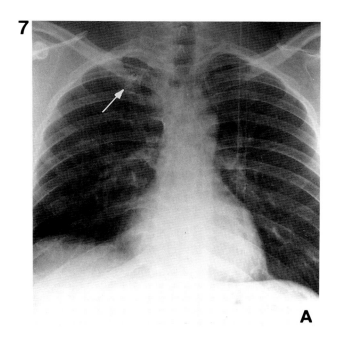

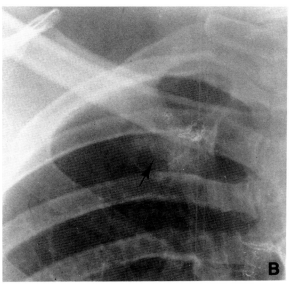

Fig. 7. A, Chest x-ray 2 years after surgery. Localized density is now obvious below medial end of right clavicle (**arrow**). **B,** Enlarged view of right upper lung field. Lobulated density extends below medial portion of right clavicle (**arrow**). **C,** Tomogram of right upper lung. Density is inferior to, but partially engulfs, apical collection of staples.

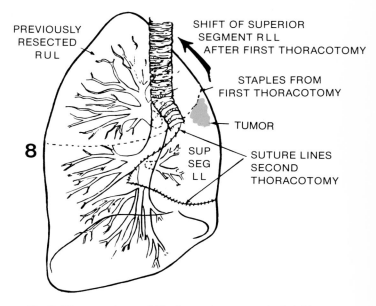

Fig. 8. Diagram shows shift of superior segment of right lower lobe (RB6) after upper lobectomy (**arrow**) and location of mass in RB6 at time of second thoracotomy.

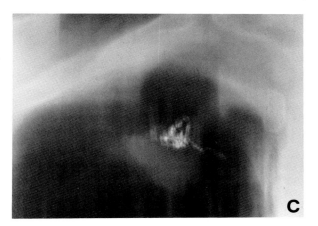

Four months after this, and 2 years after surgery, the chest x-ray was definitely abnormal. An area of increased density was now visible below the clavicle (Fig. 7).

The patient was asymptomatic. The remainder of his examination, including the sputum cytology test, was negative.

Again right thoracotomy was performed. A 2-cm mass was encountered in the superior segment of the right lower lobe (RB6), which now occupied the uppermost portion of the right hemithorax as a result of the previous upper lobectomy (Fig. 8). Superior segmentectomy was carried out.

9

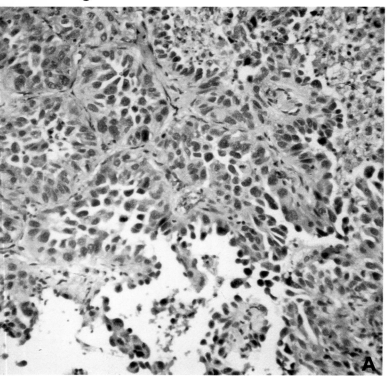

Fig. 9. A, Low-power view of microscopic section of second tumor shows bronchiolo-alveolar adenocarcinoma.

Pathologic examination of the resected mass revealed another adenocarcinoma of the bronchiolo-alveolar type (Fig. 9). The line of the bronchial transection, the pleura, and the hilar lymph nodes were free of tumor.

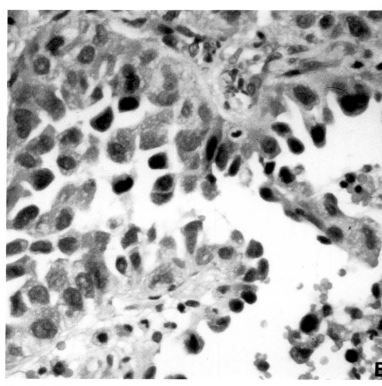

Fig. 9. B, Higher magnification of microscopic section of tumor.

Comment

1. In this case the tumor was discovered during a routine medical examination. The bronchiolo-alveolar type of adenocarcinoma actually bears little relationship to cigarette smoking.

2. The case illustrates the importance of careful comparison of sequential chest x-rays obtained at frequent intervals. It also demonstrates that, despite such comparisons, the earliest radiographic changes of an evolving tumor may be extremely subtle and as a consequence can be overlooked.

3. The first tumor was half scar tissue, whereas the second tumor was associated with a collection of surgical staples adjacent to the site of the previous pulmonary resection. Localized bronchiolo-alveolar adenocarcinoma has been associated with scar tissue often enough to have been termed "scar cancer."

4. Bronchiolo-alveolar adenocarcinomas have a well-documented tendency to be multicentric, and the second tumor doubtless represents a nonsynchronous primary cancer. The value of close postoperative follow-up of patients with bronchiolo-alveolar cancers is well demonstrated.

CASE 14

A 56-year-old welding inspector had smoked an average of 36 cigarettes a day for 32 years. He consulted his physician because of hearing loss that proved to be secondary to occupational noise trauma. For many years he had experienced a chronic productive cough. Two of his four brothers were victims of lung cancer.

On auscultation of his chest, there were bilateral rhonchi and distinct expiratory wheezes. A chest x-ray and a sputum cytology test were negative (Fig. 1). A diagnosis of chronic bronchitis due to excess smoking was recorded.

During the subsequent 2 years, lung cancer screening by chest radiography and sputum cytology was pursued. Both tests were repeated every 4 months and were consistently negative (Fig. 2). He continued to smoke.

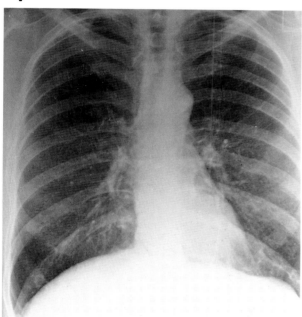

1

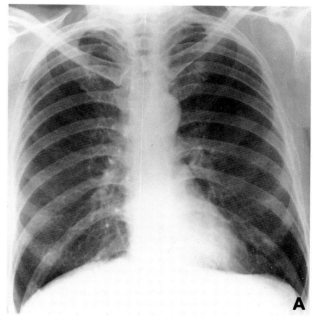

2

A

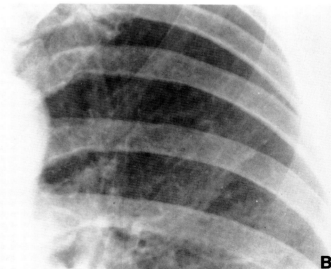

B

Fig. 1. Chest x-ray, reported as negative.

Fig. 2. A, Negative chest x-ray 2 years after previous film. **B,** Localized view of left upper lung field.

Four months later, a chest x-ray revealed an ill-defined new density, about 1.5 cm in diameter, in the periphery of the left upper lung (Fig. 3).

Tomography revealed no calcification within the lesion. The sputum remained negative for cancer cells.

Because of the strong possibility of cancer, the patient was hospitalized for evaluation and in anticipation of surgical resection. At the time, he was smoking 40 cigarettes a day and had a cough productive of thick, whitish sputum. Pulmonary function studies were consistent with moderately severe obstructive pulmonary disease.

Another sputum cytologic examination revealed no cancer cells. Bronchoscopy was not considered necessary.

Two days after admission to the hospital, a left thoracotomy was performed. The lung was described as very heavy, deeply pigmented, and somewhat stiff. A mass, approximately 2 cm in diameter, was palpated within the left upper lobe. This lobe was resected.

On gross pathologic inspection, the tumor measured 1.7 cm in diameter. It was located in the apical-posterior segment of the left upper lobe (LB1&2), 6 mm beneath the pleural surface. The subpleural pulmonary parenchyma exhibited pronounced dilatation of air spaces consistent with emphysema. There were several small peribronchial lymph nodes removed along with the tumor. Grossly, these appeared normal, but microscopically one node contained a small focus of metastatic cancer (Fig. 4).

Microscopically, the tumor proved to be a large cell undifferentiated type of bronchogenic carcinoma (Fig. 5).

3

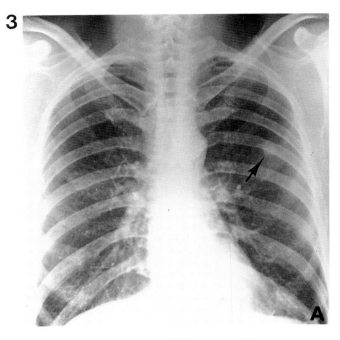

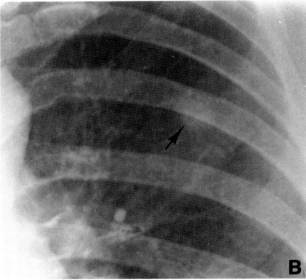

Fig. 3. A, Chest x-ray shows small circumscribed density in left upper lung (**arrow**). **B,** Enlarged view of left upper lung. Margin of lesion (**arrow**) is indistinct — a characteristic of peripheral lung cancer.

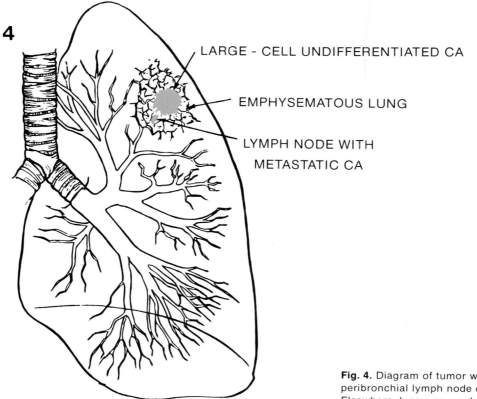

4

LARGE - CELL UNDIFFERENTIATED CA

EMPHYSEMATOUS LUNG

LYMPH NODE WITH
METASTATIC CA

Fig. 4. Diagram of tumor within left upper lobe. One peribronchial lymph node contained metastatic cancer. Elsewhere, lung was emphysematous.

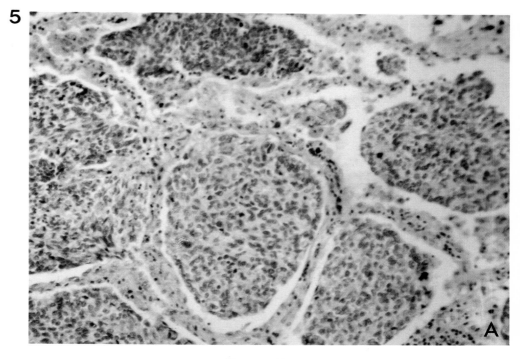

5

A

Fig. 5. A, Microscopic section of large cell undifferentiated cancer.

5

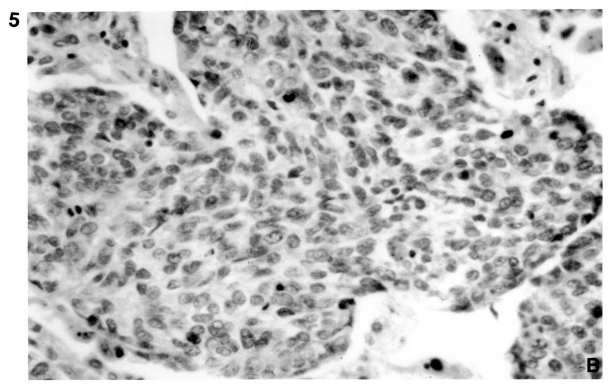

Fig. 5. B, Enlarged view of microscopic section.

The postoperative course was a stormy one, complicated by excessive bronchial secretions, pneumonia, and respiratory failure. At first the patient required tracheal intubation and ventilatory assistance, but eventually, 6 days after surgery, tracheostomy was necessary. Thereafter, the patient's condition improved. He was able to leave the hospital 18 days later.

Comment

1. This case demonstrates some of the features shared by large cell undifferentiated cancer of the lung and by the bronchogenic type of adenocarcinoma. Both of these tumors tend to arise peripherally. Both tend to become visible radiographically before they can be detected cytologically. Patients with both types of cancer have similar survival rates.

2. The tumor in this case was undemonstrable radiographically 127 days before it presented as a 1.5-cm density. Early radiographic detection of lung cancer requires that chest x-rays be repeated frequently and that they be carefully compared with any previous films that may be available.

3. Finally, this case serves as a reminder that chronic heavy cigarette smoking is usually accompanied by chronic bronchitis and increased bronchial secretion. Vigorous preoperative treatment of the bronchitis is important, in order to minimize postoperative complications of retention of secretions and infection. Discontinuance of smoking is essential.

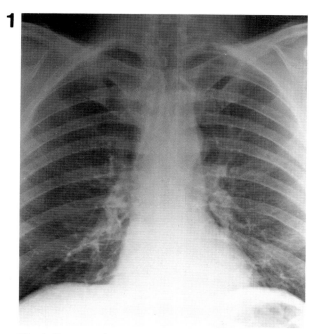

Fig. 1. Preoperative chest x-ray shows scattered fibrosis, especially in left base.

CASE 15

A 52-year-old food-plant supervisor had a history of cigarette smoking of 150 pack-years. His presenting medical problem was chronic dysphagia, which proved to be due to achalasia of the esophagus. Treatment consisted of esophagomyotomy. The initial results of surgery were excellent. Preoperatively, a chest x-ray showed scattered pulmonary fibrosis but was otherwise unremarkable (Fig. 1).

Four months later, he submitted a sputum specimen and a chest x-ray as screening tests for lung cancer. The sputum specimen was negative, and the chest x-ray showed the usual post-thoracotomy changes on the left, including periosteal reaction at the rib-spreader site between the left sixth and seventh ribs posteriorly (Fig. 2).

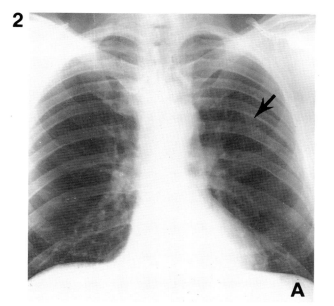

Fig. 2. A, Chest x-ray 4 months after thoracotomy. Periosteal reaction is evident between left sixth and seventh ribs posteriorly (**arrow**).

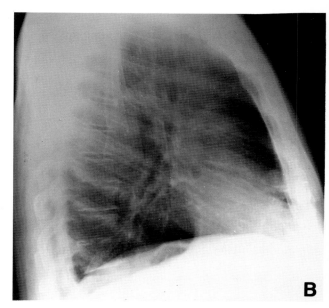

Fig. 2. B, Lateral chest x-ray taken at same time.

Screening chest x-rays and sputum cytology studies remained unchanged during the next year (Fig. 3).

Four months later, the sputum cytology test was again negative. The chest x-ray was interpreted as showing no change, and this interpretation is probably correct. However, in retrospect there may have been slight prominence of the right hilar density (Fig. 4).

During the next 4 months, the patient began

3

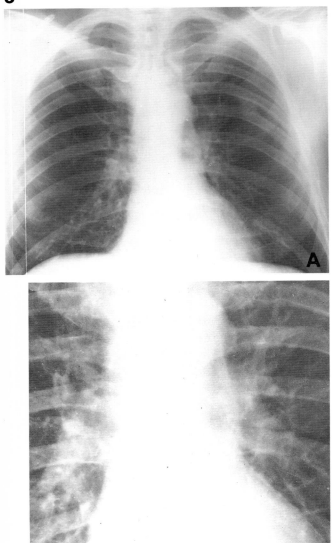

Fig. 3. A, Chest x-ray 16 months after esophagomyotomy. No change is noted. **B**, Enlarged view of heart and both hilar regions.

4

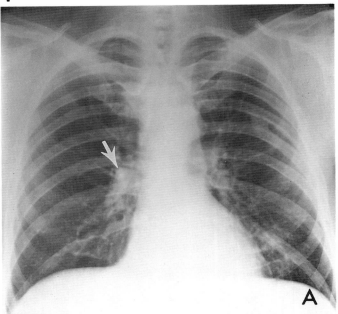

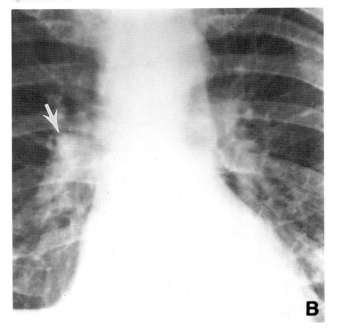

Fig. 4. A, Chest x-ray 4 months after film shown in Figure 3. There is questionable increase in size of right hilar density (**arrow**). **B**, Enlarged view of heart and hilar areas shows questionable right hilar enlargement (**arrow**).

to experience exertional dyspnea and pain in the back and neck. The sputum cytology test remained negative, but now the chest x-ray was obviously abnormal, with lobulated enlargement of the right hilar density (Fig. 5).

Tomograms of the right hilar region were obtained. These showed pronounced hilar lymphadenopathy and concentric tapering of the lobar bronchi characteristic of the small cell type of bronchogenic carcinoma (Fig. 6).

5

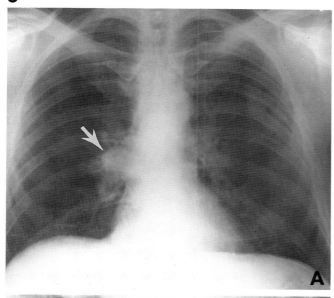

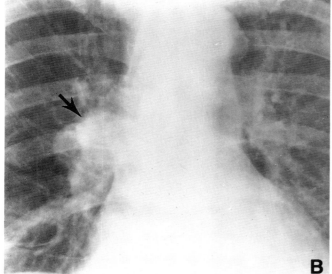

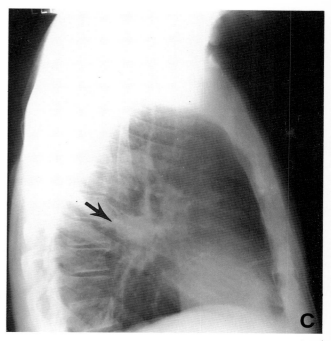

Fig. 5. A, Chest x-ray 4 months after that illustrated in Figure 4 and 2 years after esophagomyotomy. Note pronounced increase in size of right hilar density (**arrow**). **B**, Localized view of heart and hilar areas of both lungs. Increased right hilar density (**arrow**) has lobulated configuration. **C**, Lateral view of chest also demonstrates lobulated hilar enlargement (**arrow**).

6

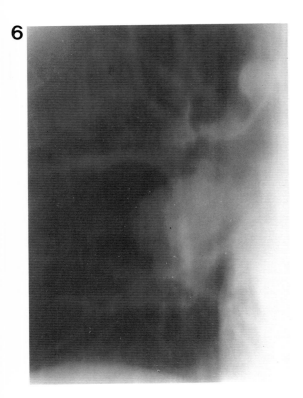

Fig. 6. Tomogram of right hilar area. Lobular densities presumably represent markedly enlarged lymph nodes involved by tumor.

7

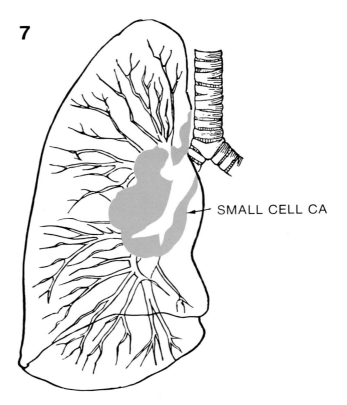

SMALL CELL CA

Fig. 7. Diagram of right lung shows pronounced hilar enlargement and tapering of lobar bronchi.

8

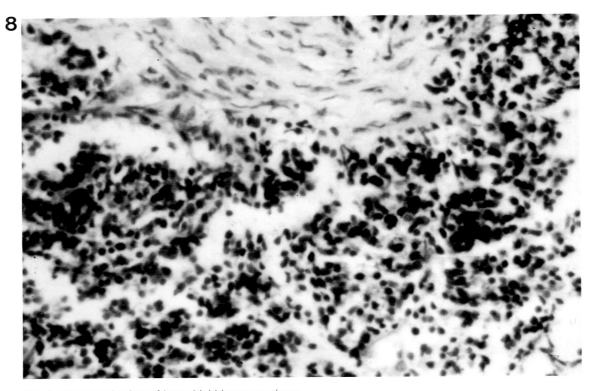

Fig. 8. Microscopic view of bronchial biopsy specimen shows small cell carcinoma.

In view of the recent onset of symptoms and the rapid and considerable enlargement of the right hilar density, this diagnosis seemed likely (Fig. 7).

The patient was hospitalized for further investigation. Examination revealed no obvious cervical or axillary adenopathy, but the liver was enlarged. In addition, the upper abdomen was tender to palpation.

Repeated sputum cytology tests were negative. Bronchoscopy was performed, and biopsy specimens from the right upper lobe bronchus disclosed small cell carcinoma (Fig. 8). Cytologic examination of bronchial secretion was positive for cancer cells of the small cell type.

Scintigraphic examination of the liver after injection of ^{99m}Tc-labeled sulfur colloid substantiated hepatic enlargement. There were also numerous large areas of decreased concentration of the isotope, suggesting metastatic tumor. Liver biopsy confirmed this (Fig. 9 and 10).

Fig. 9. Scintigram of liver shows multiple areas of decreased concentration of isotope (**arrows**) which strongly suggest metastatic disease.

With proof of metastatic small cell bronchogenic carcinoma, chemotherapy was begun. Unfortunately, there was no response, and the medications were discontinued. The patient returned home, where he died within a week.

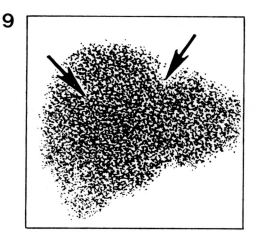

Fig. 10. Needle biopsy specimen from liver shows undifferentiated cancer cells of small cell type.

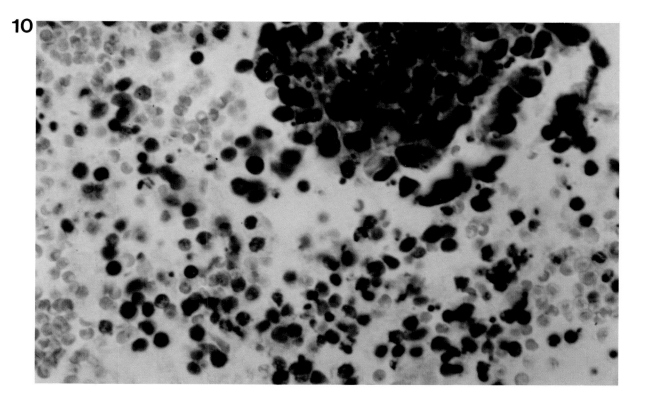

Comment

1. This is a typical case of small (oat) cell carcinoma of the lung, and it vividly illustrates the numerous frustrations that the disease creates.

2. Even in retrospect, the tumor was detected about as early as current screening procedures will permit. Yet symptoms severe enough to require medical attention actually began during the interval between regular 4-monthly chest x-rays and sputum cytology tests. It is possible that the x-ray preceding the onset of symptoms may have been abnormal. If so, the abnormality was certainly not a striking one.

3. By the time the disease was detected, metastasis had already occurred. Liver biopsy confirmed this. Treatment commenced as soon as possible, but 10 days later the patient was dead.

4. Some small cell lung cancers begin as **localized** peripheral (or perihilar) tumors. These localized tumors are uncommon manifestations of small cell cancer, yet they are not so rare as was once thought; they account for perhaps 20% of all bronchogenic carcinomas of this cell type. On the other hand, the present case represents the **typical** hilar type of small cell cancer, and it demonstrates graphically why this tumor is not generally considered a surgical disease.

5. Because small cell cancer tends to spread submucosally and rapidly, the chest x-ray will usually become positive before the sputum cytology test. However, since the tumor tends to grow so rapidly, the interval during which the tumor is demonstrable by x-ray but undetectable cytologically is probably short and of doubtful significance clinically.

CASE 16

A 55-year-old painter with a cigarette-smoking history of 80 pack-years consulted his physician because of episodic chest discomfort and shortness of breath associated with rapid heart rate.

Physical examination of the heart and lungs was normal, as was an electrocardiogram.

A chest x-ray showed some calcified areas and fibrosis in the right costophrenic angle, the residuals of an old infection (Fig. 1). A sputum specimen was negative for cancer cells.

Screening chest x-rays and sputum cytology tests at 4-monthly intervals were repeatedly negative during the ensuing 16 months. Four months after this they were also reported as negative, but in retrospect the chest x-ray may have shown a small, ovoid density just below the right hilus (Fig. 2).

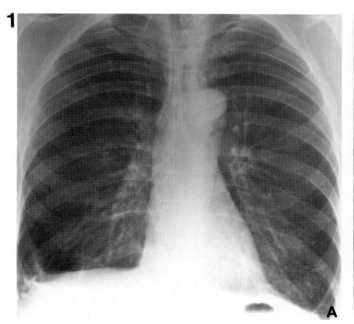 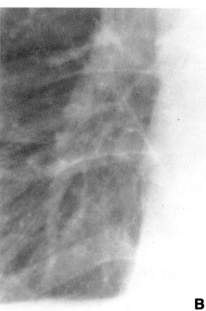

Fig. 1. **A**, Chest x-ray shows old stable calcification and fibrosis in right costophrenic angle. **B**, Enlarged view of right lower hilus and lower medial lung. No abnormality is visible.

Four months later (2 years after initiation of screening), the patient's sputum cytology test was still negative. However, the chest x-ray now showed a conspicuous rounded density below the right hilus (Fig. 3).

At first the patient was reluctant to accept a presumptive diagnosis of bronchogenic carcinoma. However, after a delay of 2 months, he entered a hospital near his home. There, chest x-rays confirmed the presence of a new and enlarging lesion. Three sputum cytologic examinations were negative.

2

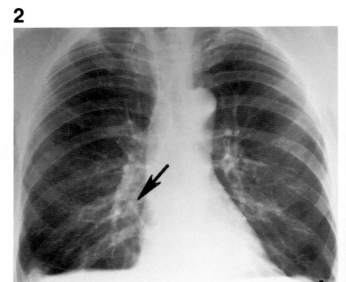

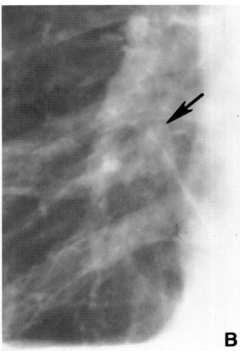

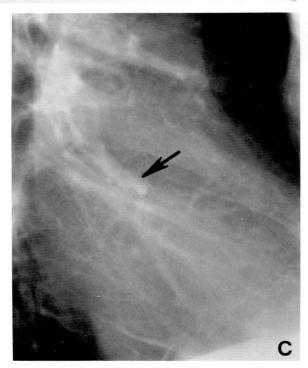

Fig. 2. A, Chest x-ray 20 months after initial film. Small, ill-defined ovoid density is present below right hilus (**arrow**). **B**, Enlarged view of right lower hilus and lower medial lung. Ovoid density appears more obvious (**arrow**). **C**, Localized view of lateral chest x-ray. It is difficult to separate ovoid density from surrounding vascular shadows (**arrow**).

Flexible fiberoptic bronchoscopy was performed. The orifice of the right middle lobe bronchus and especially its medial segmental bronchus (RB5) appeared partially obstructed, with mucosal thickening and friability suggesting carcinoma. Yet brushings, biopsy specimens, and secretions from this site were all negative.

Surgical exploration of the right chest was recommended and agreed on. At thoracotomy, a mass was palpated in the middle lobe near the hilus. There was no significant hilar lymphadenopathy, and a right middle lobectomy was performed with

3

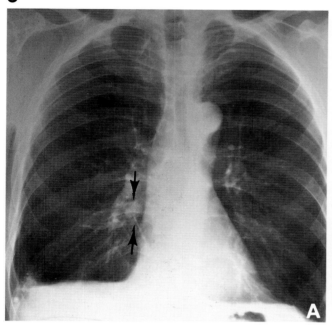

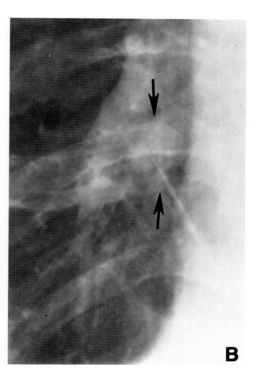

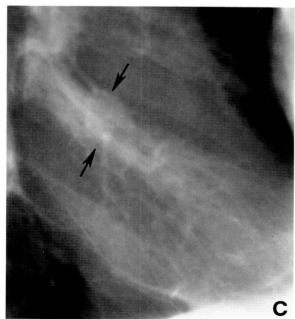

Fig. 3. A, Chest x-ray shows rounded density, 2 cm in diameter, below right hilus (**arrows**). **B,** Enlarged view of lesion (**arrows**). **C,** Lateral view, which now clearly shows lesion (**arrows**).

relative ease. Surprisingly, frozen section study of the mass revealed small (oat) cell bronchogenic carcinoma (Fig. 4).

Grossly, the tumor measured 18 mm in greatest dimension and arose from the bronchial mucosa 6 mm from the line of bronchial transection. The tumor dissected proximally beneath the bronchial cartilages to within 2 mm of the margin of resection. Lymph node involvement could not be demonstrated.

Microscopic examination confirmed that the tumor was indeed a localized perihilar small

cell carcinoma. As might have been predicted, the tumor was more extensive microscopically than was apparent grossly. Longitudinal sections through the margin of the resected bronchus showed several large cartilages completely surrounded by cancer cells. Yet so far as could be determined histologically, all of the tumor had been resected (Fig. 5).

The patient was given postsurgical adjuvant chemotherapy. He was alive without evidence of recurrence or metastasis 3 years later.

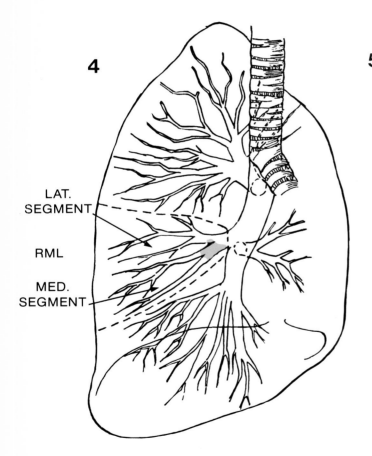

Fig. 4. Diagram of location of small (oat) cell bronchogenic cancer. It was situated near right middle lobe bronchial orifice and involved this bronchus and its medial subdivision (RB5). Fibrocalcific tissue was present in posterior and lateral pleural reflections.

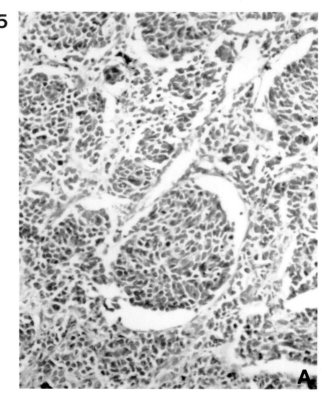

Fig. 5. A, Low-power view of histologic section of small cell cancer, right middle lobe.

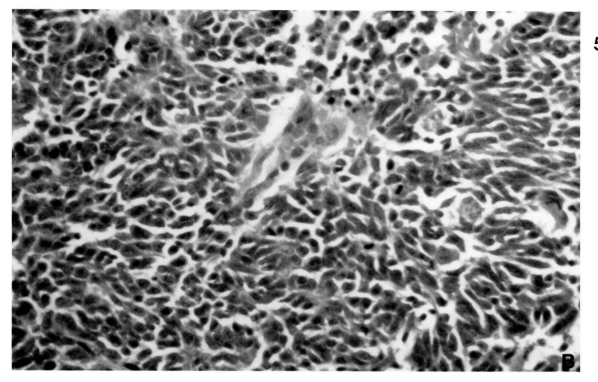

5

Fig. 5. B, High-power view of section of tumor.

Comment

1. It is commonly accepted that small (oat) cell lung cancer is not amenable to surgical treatment because the disease has almost always spread beyond the confines of the thorax by the time the diagnosis has been established.

2. There may be some exceptions to this generalization. Theoretically, at least, there must be some stage in the development of a small cell cancer when resection is possible.

3. The problem has been one of detecting the disease early enough. At present, the chances of doing so are bleak, even with frequent screening examinations.

4. Currently, the main reason for operating on any patient with small cell cancer is the inability to confirm the diagnosis by simpler procedures, as in the present case, or doubt concerning the preoperative impression.

5. The small cell cancer in the present case appeared to be localized, although detailed microscopic study disclosed tumor dissecting beneath and around bronchial cartilages, almost to the level of bronchial transection.

6. Obviously the prognosis in this case remains guarded. Any patient with small cell cancer of the lung, no matter how small or "localized," should receive aggressive surgical adjuvant radiotherapy or chemotherapy or both.

7. At present it would seem reasonable at least to consider resection of "localized" small cell cancers, such as the present one, provided that operative treatment is combined with vigorous adjuvant therapy. Success may be rare, but the effort seems justifiable until better therapy becomes available. However, surgical resection as the only therapeutic modality has no place in the management of small cell lung cancer today.